DRUGS

Contemporary Issues

Series Editors: Robert M. Baird
                Stuart E. Rosenbaum

Other titles in this series:

DRUGS

SHOULD WE LEGALIZE,

DECRIMINALIZE

OR DEREGULATE?

EDITED BY

Jeffrey A. Schaler

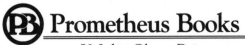 Prometheus Books

59 John Glenn Drive
Amherst, New York 14228-2197

Published 1998 by Prometheus Books

02 01 00 99 98   5 4 3 2 1

Library of Congress Cataloging-in-Publication Data

Drugs : should we legalize, decriminalize or deregulate? / edited by Jeffrey A. Schaler.
     p.   cm. — (Contemporary issues)
   Includes bibliographical references.
   ISBN 1–57392–196–3 (alk. paper)
   1. Drug legalization—United States. 2. Narcotics, Control of—United States.
3. Narcotic laws—United States. I. Schaler, Jeffrey A. II. Series: Contemporary issues (Buffalo, N.Y.)
HV5825.D88   1998
364.1′77′0973—dc21   97–48988
                                                    CIP

Printed in the United States of America on acid-free paper

Contents

5

PART EIGHT: STATE-SUPPORTED AND COURT-ORDERED
           TREATMENT FOR ADDICTION
           IS UNCONSTITUTIONAL
           (AND COUNTERPRODUCTIVE)

Introduction

The Drug *Policy* Problem

Jeffrey A. Schaler

Policies are based on values and on explanations for events. To evaluate the efficacy of our federal drug policy in a comprehensive and responsible way, we must examine the values and explanations that are associated with various possible courses of action. To that end, we must ask and honestly answer a question that challenges the status quo: What values and beliefs about illegal drugs and drug addiction are embraced and acted on by the leading drug policymakers, and what are the alternatives?

The reasoning behind current drug policies is often unstated for moral, political, economic, and even existential reasons. The reticence of policymakers on this subject is remarkable, given that the current institutional forms of the "war on drugs" are justified by the claim that drugs are destroying the "moral fabric of American society."

Americans tend to take at face value the unproved theories about drugs that are the foundation of current drug policy. For example, many Americans accept as fact the theories that drugs cause addiction, that they cause crime, and that addiction is a treatable disease. Most people are not aware of the existence of conflicting theories based on the results of empirical research. Yet abundant and convincing evidence exists to support the view that illegal drug use has more to do with choice, values, and expectations than with addiction, compulsion, or disease. With each new class of students at American University, Johns Hopkins University, Montgomery College, and Chestnut Hill College, I am asked, "Why weren't we told about this before?"

Drug policy is always based on explanations for drug use. Because there are diverse explanations for drug use as an event and these explanations differ *radically* from one another, drug policy can be implemented in ways radically different from current practice. But the average American citizen, like my numerous college students, has not been exposed to a range of views on drugs and addiction. The less people know about the range of theories, the more likely they are to be influenced by the status of the individuals who present a

9

particular message (scientists, doctors, public health officials, law enforcement professionals, politicians, and so on) rather than by the rationality or irrationality of the message itself. In order to exert democratic control in the drug policy debate—based on what is being said, not on who is saying it—Americans need to know the facts about drugs and addiction. Without complete information they cannot comprehend the meaning and implications of various proposed policies. Therefore, they will continue to assume that all qualified professionals in the field hold essentially the same views.

The prevailing policies can be faulted not only for their disregard of research but also for fundamental logical errors. The contradictory reasoning of drug policymakers needs to be subjected to public scrutiny. For example, many policymakers attribute abstinence from drugs both to the exercise of free will and to circumstances imposed from outside the individual, such as drug prohibition. They overlook the fact that, by definition, self-control cannot be the result of formal institutional controls backed by the threat of legal punishment. The same individuals typically assert that drug addiction is situational—that it is caused by the addict's physiological disposition or by the drug itself; thus they further contradict their avowed belief in free will.

When confronted with inconsistencies in their views, people often produce further theories or beliefs, perhaps to reduce the sense of dissonance and discomfort, or else they simply minimize the importance of a contradictory belief or policy. This simply creates more problems.

To understand the values and beliefs behind our federal drug policy, it is necessary to ask some unpopular questions:

- Do illegal drugs cause crime? Given that drugs are inanimate objects, are they capable of causing a human action? Can drugs "act" in the way that people can?
- Does drug use in the form of "addiction" encourage people to commit crimes other than the purchase and use of the drug itself? And if so, do the crimes stem from the addiction or from circumstances involved in the trade in illegal drugs, such as competition between dealers?
- Should drug policies that are based on the relationship between drug use and crime be consistent with legal precedents? Should drug policies reflect court opinions regarding the nature of addiction and criminal responsibility, and vice versa?

For the most part, U.S. drug policies are based on the assumption that drugs cause addiction. But many leading researchers and thinkers question the very existence of addiction as an empirical entity in the sociological "positivist" sense, viewing it rather as a social construct.

Does addiction exist? Do drugs cause addiction? The answers to these questions depend on what we mean by "addiction." If by addiction we are referring to *what drugs do to the physical body,* then the answer to both questions is yes. We know for a fact that drugs create changes in the body, a physiological dependency often characterized by tolerance, withdrawal symptoms, and death. However, if by addiction we are referring to *how drugs get into the body,* the answer is less clear. Research has produced no empirical evidence for the belief that drugs can cause drug users to lose control of their behavior. Furthermore, from a logical point of view, behavior is by definition a matter of choice. Do the bodily changes effected by drugs *cause* people to ingest more drugs in the same way that epilepsy causes people to have seizures? Most people would say no. The two cases are categorically different.

It is important to be clear about the meanings of words. When applied to human action, the term "behavior" refers to a mode of conduct or deportment. Human behavior *is* moral agency and as such can never be caused. *Things* are caused; *people* make choices. This difference is what makes us human. To speak of human behavior as caused makes no more sense than to speak of things as capable of choosing. Such confusion of language is inaccurate and irrational. The English philosopher Gilbert Ryle called this kind of mistake a "category error."

Shall we then create and implement policy on the assumption that addiction is simply a metaphor—that drug use is a moral issue ruled by choice? In that case, how much policymaking is called for? If we agree that drug use is a choice—one that harms no one but the user—should the government make any effort to control it?

Philosophical as these questions are, they should not be confined to the ivory tower as some politicians and academicians may prefer. If the advocates of a particular drug policy invoke science to justify their actions, they should be required by a discerning public to examine all available evidence, not just that which supports their political, economic, or moral interests. If they invoke moral principles, they should be challenged to defend those principles in a clear and rational manner.

Any meaningful discussion of the values expressed in drug policies raises large philosophical questions. We might begin by asking which is more important, health or liberty? Is it better to be sick and free from coercion in a society where medicine and state are separate, or to be healthy under the control of a therapeutic state? Can we trust our medical guardians to refrain from the paternalism and the persecution of "undesirables" exercised by theocracies throughout history? Who will guard us from the guardians?

The issue might be rephrased this way: Does the constitutional right to life, liberty, and the pursuit of happiness include the right to harm oneself? We accept the need for government to protect us from one another, and we agree that the exercise of liberty at the expense of another's freedom constitutes crime. But should the values of the majority dictate the personal behaviors of a minority when such actions harm no one else? Is it constitutionally proper for the government to protect us from ourselves?

Finally, can institutional methods of social control such as those advanced by our current federal drug policies increase responsibility and decrease liberty simultaneously? Or are these outcomes logically incompatible? If they are incompatible, what is actually going on in the field of drug control," and *cui bono* (who benefits)? Could it be that any drug policy short of total repeal of prohibition is simply a problem masquerading as a solution? These are questions we rarely hear discussed in a public forum.

The principal contenders in the current national debate represent three perspectives on drug policy in a free society: the prohibitionist or "drug warrior" perspective, the public health perspective, and the classical liberal or "libertarian" perspective.

The "drug warrior" perspective is the foundation of our present drug control policies. The drug warrior values a paternalistic state, which plays the role of protective parent in relation to vulnerable citizen-children. His focus is on strict enforcement of prohibition and on the regulation of currently legal drugs (for example, prescription drugs). Many drug warriors also advocate the expansion of sanctions to include tobacco and alcohol. General Barry McCaffrey and William J. Bennett—current and past "drug czars" respectively—former director of the National Institute on Drug Abuse, Robert J. Dupont, and Congressman Charles B. Rangel are drug warriors sharing this point of view here. They typically believe that drugs cause addiction and crime. In their view, public policies should aim to limit supply and punish users and dealers. Thus we have the "war on drugs." Illegal drugs such as heroin, cocaine, crack, LSD, "speed," and marijuana, and the people who profit by selling them, are the enemy.

Here are some questions we need to ask in evaluating the "drug warrior" perspective: Do drugs cause crime and addiction? Does prohibition itself create lawlessness? Is it proper for government to regulate behavior if that behavior harms no one but the user? Do people have a right to own and use drugs as personal property? Is drug supply the best predictor of use? Are social, economic, and psychological problems related to drug use ignored and thereby perpetuated when policy focuses on eliminating supply and punishing drug users and dealers? Is the war on drugs a scapegoating device to distract citizens from other social problems which they may feel helpless to solve? Does prohibition serve the economic interests of prison builders, policymakers, and drug dealers? Can drugs ever be controlled? If drug prohibition can work outside a total police state, why is the drug trade flourishing in prisons, the most totalitarian institutions of our society?

The public health perspective on drug policy is represented by people who advocate the legalization and medicalization of drug use. They regard addiction as a disease and criminal sanctions as inhumane and wasteful of tax money. Hence they advocate treatment rather than punishment for drug use. As Mayor Kurt Schmoke of Baltimore put it years ago, "The war on drugs should be led by the Surgeon General, not the Attorney General." Today the slogan of medicalization is "harm reduction." The advocates of medicalization generally also support "medical marijuana" laws such as those passed recently in California and Arizona. Ironically, prohibitionists and legalizers both embrace the medical model of addiction: they believe that drug addiction exists, that it is a disease, and thus that it is "treatable" as a disease.

In examining the public health perspective, we need to raise questions like the following: Does medical treatment of addiction work? Can it ever work, or is it based on a logical mistake? Will medical control (e.g., through prescription drugs) create the same problems of lawlessness that are associated with prohibition? Jerome P. Kassirer, George J. Annas, and Thomas S. Szasz address these important issues here. Does court-ordered and state-supported treatment violate the drug user's First Amendment rights? The late American Civil Liberties Union attorney Ellen M. Luff addresses that issue here. In an important case that received national attention in 1988 (*Maryland* v. *Norfolk*), Luff successfully argued that court-ordered attendance in Alcoholics Anonymous constitutes state entanglement with religion. Similar cases have emerged since then (e.g., *Griffin* v. *Coughlin,* 88 N.Y. 2d 674, New York Court of Appeals, decided 11 June 1996; *Kerr* v. *Farrey,* 95 F.3d 472, 7th Cir. 1996; *Warner* v. *Orange County Dept. of Probation,* No. 95-7055, 1997 WL 321553, 2nd Cir., 9 September 1996, amended 14 May 1997). Should public funds be spent on moral indoctrination in the name of public health? Again, should the government control behavior that harms no one but the individual involved?

In the classical liberal, or libertarian, perspective (represented in somewhat different ways by psychiatrist Thomas Szasz and economist Milton Friedman), drug use is regarded not as a disease but as a behavior based on personal values. It is regarded as an ethical rather than a medical issue. Classical liberals cite the scientific evidence that drug use is a function more of mindset and environment than of chemistry or physiology. They challenge the notion of "loss of control" that is integral to the prohibitionist and public health perspectives, basing their claims on studies of drug users who controlled their habits when motivated to do so. They do not believe that drugs or addiction can cause crime. In their view drugs are property and as such are protected by the Constitution; drug users need not be treated as "barbarians at the gate" requiring exceptions to the constitutional rule of law. The classical liberals believe that a free-market approach to the trade of currently illegal drugs would reduce the crime and lawlessness associated with them under prohibition. Valuing liberty over health, they criticize medicalization as paternalistic and statist. In their view, informal social controls, either relational or self-imposed, are the appropriate focus of drug policy.

In judging the classical liberal perspective, we need to ask questions like the following: If drug prohibition is repealed, will there be a substantial increase in drug use? If there is, will the problems associated with increased drug use pose a greater threat to freedom than drug prohibition has? Will an American free market in currently illegal drugs create international problems in trade with prohibitionist countries?

The purpose of this anthology is to improve the reader's legal and policy-oriented thinking about drug control in a free society. The articles were selected to promote greater comprehension of the ideological, economic, and political investments integral to various perspectives on drug policy. They challenge both the prohibitionist and the public health perspectives. They can help students to develop skill in debating important policy issues.

The anthology begins with an historical overview of attitudes toward drugs in America by noted medical historian David F. Musto. It is followed by the U.S. government's official drug policy position supporting continued prohibition. The federal position is supported with several articles by leading American intellectuals and politicians. Perspectives on the "medical marijuana" issue follows with important position statements and analysis appearing in the *New England Journal of Medicine*—and criticism of the movement by one of the first and most consistent defenders of drug prohibition repeal, psychiatrist Thomas S. Szasz.

The repeal position is presented next: Here we have anthropological, libertarian, and rights-based perspectives on the "war on drugs." The arguments presented here are supported with important research on heroin led by epidemiologist Lee N. Robins, research on cocaine and morphine led by psychologists Alexander and Erickson—and summaries of similar studies on alcohol. This is an example of the evidence supporting the idea that addiction has more to do with mind and environment than chemistry and physiology. New definitions of addiction, i.e., definitions consistent with these findings, are offered by Alexander and myself.

Further research led by Erickson on cocaine use, and philosopher Herbert Fingarette's classic article on addiction and criminal responsibility, complement the preceding articles. They present important arguments against the idea that crime stems from drug use, and that addiction and criminal activity are involuntary.

Since calls for state-supported treatment are echoed by prohibitionists and legalizers alike, I've enclosed Luff's article on First Amendment rights violations too. An important point here is that whether treatment for addiction is voluntary or involuntary, state involvement in any capacity—e.g., court-ordered attendance, state licensure of treatment facilities, or state subsidies for treatment programs—violates the invisible wall separating church and state. This is because all treatment for addiction is essentially a religious activity. The state has no business inside a person's head. The volume concludes by summarizing and introducing new ways of thinking about addiction—ways of thinking consistent with empirical findings on addiction and inconsistent with mainstream ideas about drugs and the policies based on them.

I've used these writings with my students for many years, and they say they've never been the same since we read and discussed them together.

This material provides no easy answers to the difficult questions posed earlier. It's purpose is simply to stimulate clear thinking. It is important that we as a nation choose the right course in drug policy, based on fact, not fiction—and even more important that we once again be free to choose.

Part One

Those Who Cannot Remember the Past . . .

1

Opium, Cocaine, and Marijuana in American History

David F. Musto

Dramatic shifts in attitude have characterized America's relation to drugs. During the nineteenth century, certain mood altering substances, such as opiates and cocaine, were often regarded as compounds helpful in everyday life. Gradually this perception of drugs changed. By the early 1900s, and until the 1940s, the country viewed these and some other psychoactive drugs as dangerous, addictive compounds that needed to be severely controlled. Today, after a resurgence of a tolerant attitude toward drugs during the 1960s and 1970s, we find ourselves, again, in a period of drug intolerance.

America's recurrent enthusiasm for recreational drugs and subsequent campaigns for abstinence present a problem to policymakers and to the public. Since the peaks of these episodes are about a lifetime apart, citizens rarely have an accurate or even a vivid recollection of the last wave of cocaine or opiate use.

Phases of intolerance have been fueled by such fear and anger that the record of times favorable toward drug taking has been either erased from public memory or so distorted that it becomes useless as a point of reference for policy formation. During each attack on drug taking, total denigration of the preceding, contrary mood has seemed necessary for public welfare. Although such vigorous rejection may have value in further reducing demand, the long term effect is to destroy a realistic perception of the past and of the conflicting attitudes toward mood-altering substances that have characterized our national history.

The absence of knowledge concerning our earlier and formative encounters with drugs unnecessarily impedes the already difficult task of establishing a workable and sustainable drug policy. An examination of the period of drug use that peaked around 1900 and the decline that followed it may enable us to approach the current drug problem with more confidence and reduce the likelihood that we will repeat past errors.

Until the nineteenth century, drugs had been used for millennia in their natural form. Cocaine and morphine, for example, were available only in coca leaves or poppy plants that were chewed, dissolved in alcoholic beverages, or taken in some way that diluted the impact of the active agent. The advent of organic chemistry in the 1800s changed the available forms of these drugs. Morphine was isolated in the first decade and cocaine by 1860; in 1874 diacetylmorphine was synthesized from morphine (although it became better known as heroin when the Bayer Company introduced it in 1898).

By mid-century the hypodermic syringe was perfected, and by 1870 it had become a familiar instrument to American physicians and patients.[1] At the same time, the astounding growth of the pharmaceutical industry intensified the ramifications of these accomplishments. As the century wore on, manufacturers grew increasingly adept at exploiting a marketable innovation and moving it into mass production, as well as advertising and distributing it throughout the world.

During this time, because of a peculiarity of the U.S. Constitution, the powerful new forms of opium and cocaine were more readily available in America than in most nations. Under the Constitution, individual states assumed responsibility for health issues, such as regulation of medical practice and the availability of pharmacological products. In fact, America had as many laws regarding health professions as it had states. For much of the nineteenth century, many states chose to have no controls at all; their legislatures reacted to the claims of contradictory health-care philosophies by allowing free enterprise for all practitioners. The federal government limited its concern to communicable diseases and the provision of health care to the merchant marine and to government dependents.

Nations with a less restricted central government, such as Britain and Prussia, had a single, preeminent pharmacy law that controlled availability of dangerous drugs. In those countries, physicians had their right to practice similarly granted by a central authority. Therefore, when we consider consumption of opium, opiates, coca, and cocaine in nineteenth-century America, we are looking at an era of wide availability and unrestrained advertising. The initial enthusiasm for the purified substances was only slightly affected by any substantial doubts or fear about safety, long-term health injuries, or psychological dependence.

History encouraged such attitudes. Crude opium, alone or dissolved in some liquid such as alcohol, was brought by European explorers and settlers to North America. Colonists regarded opium as a familiar resource for pain relief. Benjamin Franklin regularly took laudanum—opium in alcohol extract—to alleviate the pain of kidney stones during the last few years of his life. The poet Samuel Taylor Coleridge, while a student at Cambridge in 1791, began using laudanum for pain and developed a lifelong addiction to the drug. Opium use in those early decades constituted an "experiment in nature" that has been largely forgotten, even repressed, as a result of the extremely negative reaction that followed.

Americans had recognized, however, the potential danger of continually using opium long before the availability of morphine and the hypodermic's popularity. The American Dispensatory of 1818 noted that the habitual use of opium could lead to "tremors, paralysis, stupidity and general emaciation." Balancing this danger, the text proclaimed the extraordinary value of opium in a multitude of ailments ranging from cholera to asthma. (Considering the treatments then in vogue—blistering, vomiting, and bleeding—we can understand why opium was as cherished by patients as by their physicians.)

Opium's rise and fall can be tracked through U.S. import-consumption statistics compiled while importation of the drug and its derivative, morphine, was unrestricted and carried moderate tariffs. The per capita consumption of crude opium rose gradually during the 1800s, reaching a peak in the last decade of the century. It then declined, but after 1915 the data no longer reflect trends in drug use, because that year new federal laws severely restricted legal imports. In contrast, per capita consumption of smoking opium rose until a 1909 act outlawed its importation.

Americans had quickly associated smoking opium with Chinese immigrants who arrived after the Civil War to work on railroad construction. This association was one of the earliest examples of a powerful theme in the American perception of drugs: linkage between a drug and a feared or rejected group within society. Cocaine would be similarly linked with blacks and marijuana with Mexicans in the first third of the twentieth century. The association of a drug with a racial group or a political cause, however, is not unique to America. In the nineteenth century, for instance, the Chinese came to regard opium as a tool and symbol of Western domination. That perception helped to fuel a vigorous antiopium campaign in China early in the twentieth century.

During the 1800s, increasing numbers of people fell under the influence of opiates—substances that demanded regular consumption or the penalty of withdrawal, a painful but rarely life-threatening experience. Whatever the cause—overprescribing by physicians, over-the-counter medicines, self-indulgence, or "weak will"—opium addiction brought shame. As consumption increased, so did the frequency of addiction.

At first, neither physicians nor their patients thought that the introduction of the hypodermic syringe or pure morphine contributed to the danger of addiction. On the contrary, because pain could be controlled with less morphine when injected, the presumption was made that the procedure was less likely to foster addiction.

Figure 1.1

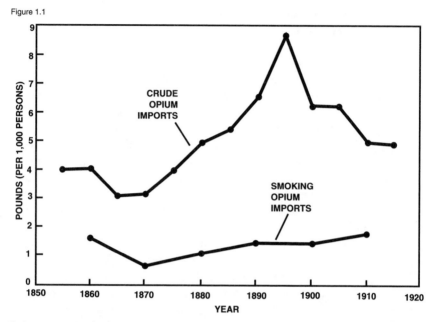

Opiate consumption was documented by the Treasury and the Commerce Departments, starting in the mid-nineteenth century. The importation of smoking opium became illegal in 1909, and crude opium and its derivatives were severely restricted in 1915. After 1915, the data reflected medicinal use.

Late in the century some states and localities enacted laws limiting morphine to a physician's prescription, and some laws even forbade refilling these prescriptions. But the absence of any federal control over interstate commerce in habit-forming drugs, of uniformity among the state laws, and of effective enforcement meant that the rising tide of legislation directed at opiates—and later cocaine—was more a reflection of changing public attitude toward these drugs than an effective reduction of supplies to users. Indeed, the decline noted after the mid-1890s was probably related mostly to the public's growing fear of addiction and of the casual social use of habit-forming substances rather than to any successful campaign to reduce supplies.

At the same time, health professionals were developing more specific treatments for painful diseases, finding less dangerous analgesics (such as aspirin) and beginning to appreciate the addictive power of the hypodermic syringe. By now the public had learned to fear the careless, and possibly addicted, physician. In *A Long Day's Journey into Night,* Eugene O'Neill dramatized the painful and shameful impact of his mother's physician-induced addiction.

In a spirit not unlike that of our times, Americans in the last decade of the nineteenth century grew increasingly concerned about the environment, adulterated foods, destruction of the forests, and the widespread use of mood-altering drugs. The concern embraced alcohol as well. The Anti-Saloon League, founded in 1893, led a temperance movement toward prohibition, which later was achieved in 1919 and became law in January 1920.

After overcoming years of resistance by over-the-counter, or patent, medicine manufacturers, the federal government enacted the Pure Food and Drug Act in 1906. This act did not prevent sales of addictive drugs like opiates and cocaine, but it did require accurate labeling of contents for all patent remedies sold in interstate commerce. Still, no national restriction existed on the availability of opiates or cocaine. The solution to this problem would emerge from growing concern, legal ingenuity, and the unexpected involvement of the federal government with the international trade in narcotics.

Responsibility for the Philippines in 1898 added an international dimension to the growing domestic alarm about drug abuse. It also revealed that Congress, if given the opportunity, would prohibit nonmedicinal uses of opium among its new dependents. Civil Governor William Howard Taft proposed reinstituting an opium monopoly—through which the previous Spanish colonial government had obtained revenue from sales to opium merchants—and using those profits to help pay for a massive public education campaign. President Theodore Roosevelt vetoed this plan, and in 1905 Congress mandated an absolute prohibition of opium for any purpose other than medicinal use.

To deal efficiently with the antidrug policy established for the Philippines, a committee from the Islands visited various territories in the area to see how others dealt with the opium problem. The benefit of controlling narcotics internationally became apparent.

In early 1906 China had instituted a campaign against opium, especially smoking opium, in an attempt to modernize and to make the empire better able to cope with continued Western encroachments on its sovereignty. At about the same time, Chinese anger at maltreatment of their nationals in the United States seethed into a voluntary boycott of American goods. Partly to appease the Chinese by aiding their antiopium efforts and partly to deal with uncontrollable smuggling within the Philippine Archipelago, the United States convened a meeting of regional powers. In this way, the United States launched a campaign for worldwide narcotics traffic control that would extend through the years in an unbroken diplomatic sequence from the League of Nations to the present efforts of the United Nations.

The International Opium Commission, a gathering of thirteen nations, met in Shanghai in February 1909. The Protestant Episcopal bishop of the Philippines, Charles Henry Brent, who had been instrumental in organizing the meeting, was chosen to preside. Resolutions noting problems with opium and opiates were adopted, but they did not constitute a treaty, and no decisions bound the nations attending the commission. In diplomatic parlance, what was needed now was a conference not a commission. The United States began to pursue this goal with determination.

The antinarcotics campaign in America had several motivations. Appeasement of China was certainly one factor for officials of the State Department. The department's opium commissioner, Hamilton Wright, thought the whole matter could be "used as oil to smooth the troubled water of our aggressive commercial policy there." Another reason was the belief, strongly held by the federal government today, that controlling crops and traffic in producing countries could most efficiently stop U.S. nonmedical consumption of drugs.

To restrict opium and coca production required worldwide agreement and, thus, an international conference. After intense diplomatic activity, one was convened in the Hague in December 1911. Brent again presided, and on January 23, 1912, the twelve nations represented signed a convention. Provision was made for the other countries to comply before the treaty was brought into force. After all, no producing or manufacturing nation wanted to leave the market open to nonratifying nations.

The convention required each country to enact domestic legislation controlling narcotics trade. The goal was a world in which narcotics were restricted to medicinal use. Both the producing and consuming nations would have control over their boundaries.

After his return from Shanghai, Wright labored to craft a federal antinarcotics law. In his path loomed the problem of states' rights. The health professions were considered a major cause of patient addiction. Yet how could federal law interfere with the prescribing practices of physicians or require that pharmacists keep records? Wright settled on the federal government's power to tax; the result, after prolonged bargaining with pharmaceutical, import, export, and medical interests, was the Harrison Act of December 1914.

Representative Francis Burton Harrison's association with the act was an accidental one, the consequence of his introduction of the administration's bill. If the chief proponent and negotiator were to be given eponymic credit, it should have been called the Wright Act. It could even have been called a second Mann Act, after Representative James Mann, who saw the bill through to passage in the House of Representatives, for by that time Harrison had become governor-general of the Philippines.

The act required a strict accounting of opium and coca and their derivatives from entry into the United States to dispensing to a patient. To accomplish this control, a small tax had to be paid at each transfer, and permits had to be obtained by applying to the Treasury Department. Only the patient paid no tax, needed no permit, and, in fact, was not allowed to obtain one.

Initially Wright and the Department of Justice argued that the Harrison Act forbade indefinite maintenance of addiction unless there was a specific medical reason such as cancer or tuberculosis. This interpretation was rejected in 1916 by the Supreme Court—even though the Justice Department argued that the Harrison Act was the domestic implementation of the Hague

Opium Convention and therefore took precedence over states' rights. Maintenance was to be allowed.

That decision was short-lived. in 1919 the Supreme Court, led by Oliver Wendell Holmes and Louis Brandeis, changed its mind by a 5-4 vote. The court declared that indefinite maintenance for "mere addiction" was outside legitimate medical practice and that, consequently, prohibiting it did not constitute interference with a state's right to regulate physicians. Second, because the person receiving the drugs for maintenance was not a bona fide patient but just a recipient of drugs, the transfer of narcotics defrauded the government of taxes required under the Harrison Act.

During the 1920s and 1930s, the opiate problem, chiefly morphine and heroin, declined in the United States, until much of the problem was confined to the periphery of society and the outcasts of urban areas. There were exceptions: some health professionals and a few others of middle class or higher status continued to take opiates.

America's international efforts continued. After World War I, the British and U.S. governments proposed adding the Hague Convention to the Versailles Treaty. As a result, ratifying the peace treaty meant ratifying the Hague Convention and enacting a domestic law controlling narcotics. This incorporation led to the British Dangerous Drugs Act of 1920, an act often misattributed to a raging heroin epidemic in Britain. In the 1940s some Americans argued that the British system provided heroin to addicts and, by not relying on law enforcement, had almost eradicated the opiate problem. In fact, Britain had no problem to begin with. This argument serves as an interesting example of how the desperate need to solve the drug problem in the United States tends to create misperceptions of a foreign drug situation.

The story of cocaine use in America is somewhat shorter than that of opium, but it follows a similar plot. In 1884 purified cocaine became commercially available in the United States. At first the wholesale cost was very high— $5 to $10 a gram—but it soon fell to 25 cents a gram and remained there until the price inflation of World War I. Problems with cocaine were evident almost from the beginning, but popular opinion and the voices of leading medical experts depicted cocaine as a remarkable, harmless stimulant.

William A. Hammond, one of America's most prominent neurologists, extolled cocaine in print and lectures. By 1887 Hammond was assuring audiences that cocaine was no more habit-forming than coffee or tea. He also told them of the "cocaine wine" he had perfected with the help of a New York druggist: two grains of cocaine to a pint of wine. Hammond claimed that this tonic was far more effective than the popular French coca wine, probably a reference to Vin Mariani, which he complained had only half a grain of cocaine to the pint.

Coca-Cola was also introduced in 1886 as a drink offering the advantages of coca but lacking the danger of alcohol. It amounted to a temperance coca beverage. The cocaine was removed in 1900, a year before the city of Atlanta, Georgia, passed an ordinance (and a state statute the following year) prohibiting provision of any cocaine to a consumer without a prescription.

Cocaine is one of the most powerful of the central nervous system euphoriants. This fact underlay cocaine's quickly growing consumption and the ineffectiveness of the early warnings. How could anything that made users so confident and happy be bad? Within a year of cocaine's introduction, the Parke-Davis Company provided coca and cocaine in fifteen forms, including coca cigarettes, cocaine for injection, and cocaine for sniffing. Parke-Davis and at least one other company also offered consumers a handy cocaine kit. (The Parke-Davis kit contained a hypodermic syringe.) The firm proudly supplied a drug that, it announced, "can supply the place of food, make the coward brave, the silent eloquent and . . . render the sufferer insensitive to pain."

Cocaine spread rapidly throughout the nation. In September 1886 a physician in Puyallup, Washington Territory, reported an adverse reaction to cocaine during an operation. Eventually reports of overdoses and idiosyncratic reactions shifted to accounts of the social and behavioral effects of long-term cocaine use. The ease with which experimenters became regular users and the increasing instances of cocaine being linked with violence and paranoia gradually took hold in popular and medical thought.

In 1907 an attempt was made in New York State to shift the responsibility for cocaine's availability from the open market to medical control. Assemblyman Alfred E. Smith, later the governor of New York and in 1928 the Democratic party's presidential candidate, sponsored such a bill. The cost of cocaine on New York City streets, as revealed by newspaper and police accounts after the law's enactment, was typically 25 cents a packet, or "deck."

Although 25 cents may seem cheap, it was actually slightly higher than the average industrial wage at that time, which was about 20 cents an hour. Packets, commonly glycine envelopes, usually contained one to two grains (65 to 130 milligrams), or about a tenth of a gram. The going rate was roughly ten times that of the wholesale price, a ratio not unlike recent cocaine street prices, although in the past few years the street price has actually been lower in real value than what it was in 1910.

Several similar reports from the years before the Harrison Act of 1914 suggest that both the profit margin and the street price of cocaine were unaffected by the legal availability of cocaine from a physician. Perhaps the formality of medical consultation and the growing antagonism among physicians and the public toward cocaine helped to sustain the illicit market.

In 1910 William Howard Taft, then president of the United States, sent to Congress a report that cocaine posed the most serious drug problem America had ever faced. Four years later President Woodrow Wilson signed into law the Harrison Act, which, in addition to its opiate provisions, permitted the sale of cocaine only through prescriptions. It also forbade any trace of cocaine in patent remedies, the most severe restriction on any habit-forming drug to that date. (Opiates, including heroin, could still be present in small amounts in nonprescription remedies, such as cough medicines.)

Although the press continued to reveal Hollywood scandals and underworld cocaine practices during the 1920s, cocaine use gradually declined as a societal problem. The laws probably hastened the trend, and certainly the tremendous public fear reduced demand. By 1930 the New York City Mayor's Committee on Drug Addiction was reporting that "during the last 20 years cocaine as an addiction has ceased to be a problem."

Unlike opiates and cocaine, marijuana was introduced during a period of drug intolerance. Consequently, it was not until the 1960s, forty years after marijuana cigarettes had arrived in America, that it was widely used. The practice of smoking cannabis leaves came to the United States with Mexican immigrants, who had come north during the 1920s to work in agriculture, and it soon extended to white and black jazz musicians.

As the Great Depression of the 1930s settled over America, the immigrants became an unwelcome minority linked with violence and with growing and smoking marijuana. Western states pressured the federal government to control marijuana use. The first official response was to urge adoption of a uniform state antinarcotics law. Then a new approach became feasible in 1937, when the Supreme Court upheld the National Firearms Act. This act prohibited the transfer of machine guns between private citizens without purchase of a transfer tax stamp—and the government would not issue the necessary stamp. Prohibition was implemented through the taxing power of the federal government.

Within a month of the Supreme Court's decision, the Treasury Department testified before Congress for a bill to establish a marijuana transfer tax. The bill became law, and until the Comprehensive Drug Abuse Act of 1970, marijuana was legally controlled through a transfer tax for which no stamps or licenses were available to private citizens. Certainly some people were smoking marijuana in the 1930s, but not until the 1960s was its use widespread.

Around the time of the Marihuana Tax Act of 1937, the federal government released dramatic and exaggerated portrayals of marijuana's effects. Scientific publications during the 1930s also fearfully described marijuana's dangers. Even Walter Bromberg, who thought that marijuana made only a small contribution to major crimes, nevertheless reported the drug was "a primary stimulus to the impulsive life with direct expression in the motor field."

Marijuana's image shifted during the 1960s, when it was said that its use at the gigantic Woodstock gathering kept peace—as opposed to what might have happened if alcohol had been the drug of choice. In the shift to drug toleration in the late 1960s and early 1970s, investigators found it difficult to associate health problems with marijuana use. The 1930s and 1940s had marked the nadir of drug toleration in the United States, and possibly the mood of both times affected professional perception of this controversial plant.

After the Harrison Act, the severity of federal laws concerning the sale and possession of opiates and cocaine gradually rose. As drug use declined, penalties increased until 1956, when the death penalty was introduced as an option by the federal government for anyone older than eighteen providing heroin to anyone younger than eighteen (apparently no one was ever executed under this statute). At the same time, mandatory minimum prison sentences were extended to ten years.

After the youthful counterculture discovered marijuana in the 1960s, demand for the substance grew until about 1978, when the favorable attitude toward it reached a peak. In 1972 the Presidential Commission on Marihuana and Drug Abuse recommended "decriminalization" of marijuana, that is, legal possession of a small amount for personal use. In 1977 the Carter administration formally advocated legalizing marijuana in amounts up to an ounce.

The Gallup Poll on relaxation of laws against marijuana is instructive. In 1980, 53 percent of Americans favored legalization of small amounts of marijuana; by 1986 only 27 percent supported that view. At the same time, those favoring penalties for marijuana use rose from 43 to 67 percent. This reversal parallels the changes in attitude among high school students revealed by the Institute of Social Research at the University of Michigan.

The decline in favorable attitudes toward marijuana that began in the late 1970s continues. In the past few years we have seen penalties rise again against users and dealers. The recriminalization of marijuana possession by popular vote in Alaska in 1990 is one example of such a striking reversal.

In addition to stricter penalties, two other strategies, silence and exaggeration, were implemented in the 1930s to keep drug use low and prevent a occurrence of the decades-long, frustrating, and fearful antidrug battle of the late nineteenth and early twentieth centuries. Primary and secondary schools instituted educational programs against drugs. Then policies shifted amid fears that talking about cocaine or heroin to young people, who now had less exposure to drugs, would arouse their curiosity. This concern led to a decline in drug-related information given during school instruction as well as to the censorship of motion pictures.

The Motion Picture Association of America, under strong public and religious pressure, decided in 1934 to refuse a seal of approval for any film that showed narcotics. This prohibition was enforced with one exception—*To the Ends of the Earth,* a 1948 film that lauded the Federal Bureau of Narcotics— until *Man with a Golden Arm* was successfully exhibited in 1956 without a seal.

Associated with a decline in drug information was a second, apparently paradoxical strategy: exaggerating the effects of drugs. The middle ground was abandoned. In 1924 Richmond P. Hobson, a nationally prominent campaigner against drugs, declared that one ounce of heroin could addict two thousand persons. In 1936 an article in the *American Journal of Nursing* warned that a marijuana user "will suddenly turn with murderous violence upon whomever [*sic*] is nearest to him. He will run amuck with knife, axe, gun, or anything else that is close at hand, and will kill or maim without any reason."

A goal of this well-meaning exaggeration was to describe drugs so repulsively that anyone reading or hearing of them would not be tempted to experiment with the substances. One contributing factor to such a publicity campaign, especially regarding marijuana, was that the Depression permitted little money for any other course of action.

Severe penalties, silence, and, if silence was not possible, exaggeration became the basic strategies against drugs after the decline of their first wave of use. But the effect of these tactics was to create ignorance and false images that would present no real obstacle to a renewed enthusiasm for drugs in the 1960s. At the time, enforcing draconian and mandatory penalties would have filled to overflowing all jails and prisons with the users of marijuana alone.

Exaggeration fell in the face of the realities of drug use and led to a loss of credibility regarding any government pronouncement on drugs. The lack of information erased any awareness of the first epidemic, including the gradually obtained and hard-won public insight into the hazards of cocaine and opiates. Public memory, which would have provided some context for the antidrug laws, was a casualty of the antidrug strategies.

The earlier and present waves of drug use have much in common, but there is at least one major difference. During the first wave of drug use, antidrug laws were not enacted until the public demanded them. In contrast, today's most severe antidrug laws were on the books from the outset; this gap between law and public opinion made the controls appear ridiculous and bizarre. Our current frustration over the laws' ineffectiveness has been greater and more lengthy than before because we have lived through many years in which antidrug laws lacked substantial public support. Those laws appeared powerless to curb the rise in drug use during the 1960s and 1970s.

The first wave of drug use involved primarily opiates and cocaine. The nation's full experience with marijuana is now under way (marijuana's tax regulation in 1937 was not the result of any lengthy or broad experience with the plant). The popularity and growth in demand for opiates and cocaine in mainstream society derived from a simple factor: the effect on most people's physiology and emotions was enjoyable. Moreover, Americans have recurrently hoped that the technology of drugs would maximize their personal potential. That opiates could relax and cocaine energize seemed wonderful opportunities for fine-tuning such efforts.

Two other factors allowed a long and substantial rise in consumption during the 1800s. First, casualties accumulate gradually; not everyone taking cocaine or opiates becomes hooked on the drug. In the case of opiates, some users have become addicted for a lifetime and have still been productive.

Yet casualties have mounted as those who could not handle occasional use have succumbed to domination by drugs and by drug-seeking behavior.

These addicts become not only miserable themselves but also frightening to their families and friends. Such cases are legion today in our larger cities, but the percentage of those who try a substance and acquire a dependence or get into serious legal trouble is not 100 percent. For cocaine, the estimate varies from 3 to 20 percent, or even higher, and so it is a matter of time before cocaine is recognized as a likely danger.

Early in the cycle, when social tolerance prevails, the explanation for casualties is that those who succumb to addiction are seen as having a physiological idiosyncrasy or "foolish trait." Personal disaster is thus viewed as an exception to the rule. Another factor minimizing the sense of risk is our belief in our own invulnerability—that general warnings do not include us. Such faith reigns in the years of greatest exposure to drug use, ages fifteen to twenty-five. Resistance to a drug that makes a user feel confident and exuberant takes many years to permeate a society as large and complex as the United States.

The interesting question is not why people take drugs, but rather why they stop taking them. We perceive risk differently as we begin to reject drugs. One can perceive a hypothetical 3 percent risk from taking cocaine as an assurance of 97 percent safety, or one can react as if told that 3 percent of New York/Washington shuttle flights crash. Our exposure to drug problems at work, in our neighborhood, and within our families shifts our perception, gradually shaking our sense of invulnerability.

Cocaine has caused the most dramatic change in estimating risk. From a grand image as the ideal tonic, cocaine's reputation degenerated into that of the most dangerous of drugs, linked in our minds with stereotypes of mad, violent behavior. Opiates have never fallen so far in esteem, nor were they repressed to the extent cocaine had been between 1930 and 1970.

Today we are experiencing the reverse of recent decades, when the technology of drug use promised an extension of our natural potential. Increasingly we see drug consumption as reducing what we could achieve on our own with healthy food and exercise. Our change of attitude about drugs is connected to our concern over air pollution, food adulteration, and fears for the stability of the environment.

Ours is an era not unlike that early in this century, when Americans made similar efforts at self-improvement accompanied by an assault on habit-forming drugs. Americans seem to be the least likely of any people to accept the inevitability of historical cycles. Yet if we do not appreciate our history, we may again become captive to the powerful emotions that led to draconian penalties, exaggeration, or silence.

NOTE

1. See Norman Howard-Jones, "The Origins of Hypodermic Medication," *Scientific American,* January 1971.

Part Two

A "War on Drugs" or a War on People?: The Federal Government's Position

2

The National Drug-Control Strategy

Office of National Drug-Control Policy

I. THE PURPOSES OF THIS STRATEGY

The National Drug Control Strategy organizes a collective American effort to achieve a common purpose. The Strategy provides general guidance and specific direction to the efforts of the more than fifty federal agencies involved in the struggle against illegal drugs and substance abuse. Further, this Strategy offers a common framework to state and local government agencies, to educators and health care professionals, to law enforcement officials and community groups, and to religious organizations, mass media, and American business to build a unified American counterdrug effort. The common purpose of that collective effort is to reduce illegal drug use and its consequences in America.

II. WHY WE MUST RESPOND TO THE DRUG PROBLEM IN AMERICA TODAY

Drugs affect the lives of millions of Americans. According to a recent Gallup Poll, almost one-half (45 percent) of Americans report that either they, someone in their family, or a close friend has used illegal drugs. Of these, 28 percent characterized the drug use as moderate, while 29 percent described it as a serious addiction. More than half of those who reported knowing someone with a moderate or serious drug problem were living in households with incomes of $35,000 or more, and most were white. Clearly,

The National Drug Control Strategy: 1996. Reprinted by permission of the Diane Publishing Corporation.

drugs are not a problem just for inner city residents, or the poor, or members of some minority group—they affect all Americans from every social, ethnic, racial, and economic background.

Americans are especially concerned about the increased use of drugs by youth. In 1991, after several years of decline, the number of people trying marijuana for the first time showed a marked increase. The majority of these "initiates" to drug use were young people. Several recent surveys confirm that the rate of drug use among youth has continued to climb. Past-month use of all drugs among youth aged twelve to seventeen increased by the rate of 50 percent between 1992 and 1994. With the exception of alcohol, drugs of all kinds are being used increasingly by youth. However, it is marijuana that is used most often. Among youth aged twelve to seventeen, the use of marijuana almost doubled between 1992 and 1994.

Americans are also troubled by hardcore drug use and its devastating consequences to society. Fewer individuals are using drugs on an occasional or nonaddicted basis. In fact, this number has declined dramatically from its peak seventeen years ago. However, the insidious nature of addiction has been realized as many of these formerly occasional users have progressed to chronic, hardcore drug use. Families and neighborhoods are being torn apart by the crime and health consequences that so often accompany addiction. While only one in four drug users is a hardcore drug abuser, this minority consumes the majority of the illegal drugs and commits a disproportionate number of drug-related crimes. About two-thirds of these hardcore users come in contact with the criminal justice system each year. We can and must reduce the number of hardcore drug users.

The numbers underscore the unacceptable costs of illegal drug use to our society:

America has suffered 100,000 drug-related deaths in the 1990s alone—over 20,000 of our citizens die every year because of illicit drugs.

- In 1993, the year from which the most recent data is available, Americans spent an estimated $49 billion on illegal drugs: $31 billion on cocaine, $7 billion on heroin, $9 billion on marijuana, and $2 billion on other illegal drugs.
- Federal, state, and local governments collectively spend about $30 billion a year to reduce illegal drug use and trafficking and deal with their consequences.
- The annual social cost of illicit drug use is $67 billion, mostly from the consequences of drug-related crime.
- Drug-related hospital emergency department visits continue to be at record levels—over one-half million annually—owing in large part to the consequences of drug addiction.
- Drug use contributes significantly to property and violent crimes. Of nearly

712,000 prison inmates interviewed in June 1991, 62 percent reported they had used drugs regularly at some time in their lives, 50 percent reported drug use in the month before committing the offense that had sent them to prison, 31 percent said they were under the influence of drugs when they committed their crime, and 17 percent said they were trying to get money for drugs when they committed the crime. Of more than 20,000 adult, male arrestees tested in 1994 under the Drug Use Forecasting program, 66 percent were positive for use of at least one drug at the time of arrest.

• Each year over one million persons are arrested on drug-related charges.

Other drugs are now beginning to emerge that further threaten all Americans. Heroin presents a particularly grave threat to the American people. The surveys that track heroin-use patterns are discouraging. In 1993, the rate of heroin-related emergency room episodes was 64 per 100,000 population among persons ages 35 to 44, almost double of what it was in 1988 for this age group. The users of heroin are also initiating use of the drug at a younger age (the Monitoring the Future [MTF] study reports increased heroin use by tenth and twelfth graders) and they are beginning to rely on routes of administration such as smoking and snorting, rather than injecting. This may make heroin use more accessible to a wider range of users, particularly those users of other drugs that were unwilling to inject drugs.

The continued rise in popularity of methamphetamine (also know as speed, crystal, crank, and ice) is also of increasing concern. For many years, methamphetamine use has been confined to certain areas of the country (the West and Southwest) and to certain distinct groups of users (motorcycle gangs and older polydrug users). The drug is now becoming more attractive to young users, and its use is expanding into other areas of the country such as Denver, Des Moines, Dallas, Atlanta, Philadelphia, and Minneapolis/St. Paul. Methamphetamine, used for its stimulant effect, is often combined in use with alcohol, heroin, and cocaine. An estimated 4 million persons in the United States have used methamphetamine at least once in their lives. . . .

The National Office of Drug Control Policy (ONDCP) is also monitoring two additional emerging drugs: LSD and PCP. The distribution pattern for LSD, which is now available in nearly every state, is unique within the drug culture. A proliferation of mail order sales has created a marketplace where the LSD sellers are generally unknown to the buyers, providing the highest-level traffickers with considerable insulation from drug law enforcement operations. The vast majority of users are white, middle-class high school and college students attracted by low prices, who perceive the drug as harmless.

PCP production appears to be centered in the greater Los Angeles, California, metropolitan area. PCP use peaked in the early to mid-1980s and was supplanted by the use of crack-cocaine. However, there are recent indications that PCP use has increased somewhat in a limited number of cities.

And finally, due to the serious problems posed by the increased use of marijuana, it must logically be included in any discussion of emerging drugs. While marijuana has been a problem in the United States for many years, the recent increases in use among young people and its rise in potency also warrant our concern as an emerging drug of abuse.

The drug trade is a growing threat to America's interests abroad. Drug-related corruption, intimidation, and dirty money undermine democratic governments and free-market economies around the world. This jeopardizes important political and commercial relationships the United States has with many countries.

III. THERE IS CAUSE FOR GUARDED OPTIMISM

Despite the recent upturn in casual drug use by our youth, we have made real progress in the past decade as a result of a principled, long-term effort. Thanks to the bipartisan efforts of the Congress and three successive administrations, along with the broad-based efforts of citizens and communities throughout the United States, we have made substantial progress since the 1970s when drug use was at its peak. We have moved from widespread social tolerance of drug abuse to a current environment in which the vast majority of Americans strongly disapprove of substance abuse and do not use illegal drugs. Consider how far we have progressed:

- While 72 million Americans have experimented with illegal drugs, the overwhelming majority quit of their own accord and oppose the use of illicit drugs.
- As a result of aggressive prevention efforts, the number of illegal drug users has fallen by half since 1985, from 22.3 million to 12.2 million "past-month" users.
- The number of new cocaine users plummeted from a million and a half in 1980 to about half a million in 1992. Overall, cocaine use has fallen 30 percent in the last three years alone.
- Between 1975 and the early 1990s, the number of new heroin users dropped by 25 percent.
- Homicides have decreased by 5 percent, and those that are judged to be drug-related are down approximately 25 percent.
- Workplaces are safer and more productive: drug use among U.S. workers decreased from 19 percent in 1979 to 8.1 percent in 1993, and three out of four companies with more than 250 employees have formal antidrug programs and policies in place.
- Since the late 1980s, U.S. government seizures of drug trafficker assets have been about $700 million a year.

- Drug treatment programs have improved dramatically and are better linked with offender management and drug court programs, creating a mutually supporting dynamic between law enforcement and rehabilitation. Progress is being made in helping those who want help.
- Internationally, we moved from a standing start to a web of increasingly effective alliances, partnerships, and cooperative agreements:

   —We essentially blocked the free flow of cocaine through the western Caribbean into Florida and the Southeast.

   —Our interdiction efforts in South America have disrupted the trafficking patterns of cocaine traffickers in Peru, causing them to change flight routes and modes of transportation.

   —Six of the seven ringleaders of the Cali Cartel were arrested in 1995, and one recently was killed by the Colombian police while resisting arrest. Continued pressure on Colombian drug lords has resulted in a recent flurry of surrenders and arrests of "next generation" traffickers, causing further disruption of cartel operations.

   —A third of the cocaine produced in South America is intercepted before it hits our streets or those of other countries.

   —Due to increased enforcement activity and greater international focus and cooperation, money laundering has become tougher for traffickers and their front businesses.

   —Key Asian countries have begun to arrest kingpins involved in heroin trafficking and to extradite them to the United States. Such efforts to attack these drug trafficking organizations are being intensified.

IV. RECENT DRUG CONTROL INITIATIVES

Recent drug-control initiatives by the U.S. Government have helped to maintain the overall progress of the last decade. Highlights of current efforts to address the problems of illicit drug use and trafficking include:

- **A Reaffirmation of Anti-Legalization Sentiments.** ONDCP helped to reaffirm the sentiment of millions of Americans who oppose the legalization of drugs. In May 1995, the Office, in coordination with other federal agencies, co-sponsored the 1995 "American Cities against Drugs" conference in Atlanta, Georgia. Officials representing dozens of American cities, large and small, signed a declaration of resolute opposition to the legalization of illicit drugs.
- **A Comprehensive Marijuana Strategy Targeting Youth.** The Marijuana Strategy is targeted primarily at the nation's youth. It coordinates efforts at the federal, state, and local level and includes both supply and demand reduction components. A 1995 highlight of the Marijuana Strategy was the Department of Health and Human Services National Conference on Mari-

juana Use Prevention, Treatment and Research. Also in 1995, the U.S. Department of Health and Human Services launched a national anti-marijuana information campaign.

- **A Methamphetamine Strategy.** To more effectively address the emerging methamphetamine problem, a comprehensive law enforcement, prevention, and treatment strategy coordinating the efforts at the federal, state, and local levels has been developed. This project, begun at the request of the president, brings ONDCP, the Department of Justice, the Department of Health and Human Services, and other concerned federal agencies together to lay the ground work for a response to the serious threat posed by methamphetamine use and trafficking. In conjunction with this effort, the Substance Abuse Mental Health Administration's Center for Substance Abuse Prevention and the National Institute on Drug Abuse will be developing a methamphetamine information awareness and prevention initiative.
- **Regulations to Reduce Children's Use of Tobacco Products.** In August 1995, the Food and Drug Administration (FDA) proposed (i) restricting youth access to tobacco products, (ii) reducing the advertising and promotional activities that make these products appealing to young persons, and (iii) an educational campaign, funded by the tobacco industry, aimed at teaching children the real health risks of tobacco products. Also, the Substance Abuse and Mental Health Services Administration (SAMHSA) recently published regulations to implement the Public Health Services Act, requiring as a condition of receiving federal substance abuse block grant funds, that each state enact and enforce laws banning the sale and distribution of tobacco products to people under eighteen. Further, each state is required to perform annual, random, unannounced inspections of outlets that sell and distribute tobacco products, with the outcome of these inspections to be used as a measure of state success in enforcing their laws.
- **Progress against the Illegal Use of Alcohol by Underage Users.** President Clinton signed into law the "National Highway System Designation Act of 1995," which requires states to adopt a Zero Tolerance standard for drivers under the age of twenty-one. This law makes it illegal for young people who have been drinking to drive an automobile. Alcohol-related crashes involving teenage drivers are down as much as 20 percent in those states which have Zero Tolerance laws on the books.
- **A National Media Literacy Campaign for Parents, Youth, and Communities.** ONDCP has initiated a national effort to empower youth, parents, and communities with critical cognitive skills needed to challenge and resist the powerful media messages that glamorize or condone the use of alcohol, tobacco, and other illegal substances. The Media Literacy campaign is part of an overall increased emphasis on empowering youth to recognize the true risks associated with the use of illegal substances.
- **Public-Private Prevention Partnership with Pharmaceutical Compa-**

nies. Fourteen major pharmaceutical companies have agreed to participate in a federal-private sector prevention partnership. The goal will be the development and dissemination of prevention information to physicians throughout the nation for distribution to their patients.

- **A Presidential Initiative to Improve Community Oriented Policing Services (COPS).** The Department of Justice has provided resources to state, local, and Indian tribal governments to put an additional 34,000 police officers on the streets to keep Americans safe from drugs and crime. Employing community policing strategies, these new officers will work in partnership with communities to tackle drug trafficking, drug use, and related crime.

- **High-Intensity Drug Trafficking Areas (HIDTA).** The HIDTA program takes a strategic approach to drug trafficking in those areas of the country most impacted by drugs. It focuses on the major retailers and wholesalers of illicit drugs through efforts to coordinate better the drug enforcement efforts of federal, state, and local law enforcement agencies. In addition, the HIDTA Executive Committee works to facilitate the flow of intelligence information among member agencies. In each HIDTA, the Executive Committee, upon the release of this new Strategy, is required to update its threat assessment and strategy annually, select cochairpersons who serve, and select a full time Director, approved by the Director, ONDCP. Section IV provides detailed information on the HIDTA program.

- **DEA's Mobile Enforcement Team (MET) Initiative.** This project has been successful in reducing drug-related crime and violence in over fifty locations where such teams have been deployed. After approving a request from a chief or sheriff who is facing escalating drug-related violence, federal agents work with state and local officers to target local drug organizations and their leaders. These federal, state, and local law enforcement teams reduce the influence of drug gangs and restore public confidence in the government; this is crucial in order to find witnesses who will come forward and cooperate to ensure that proper convictions are obtained, making streets and neighborhoods safe from those who would continue to perpetrate violent, drug-related crimes.

- **Safe Streets Violent Crimes Initiative.** The Federal Bureau of Investigation has established the Safe Streets Violent Crimes Initiative, designed to allow the special agent in charge of each FBI field office to address the problems of street, gang, and drug-related violence. Through Safe Streets Task Forces (SSTFs)—FBI-sponsored long-term task forces manned by federal, state, and local law enforcement officers and prosecutors—the FBI is able to better focus enforcement and investigative efforts on violent gangs, crimes of violence, and the apprehension of violent fugitives. As of January 30, 1996, 138 SSTFs have been established in 53 field offices. SSTFs involve the coordinated efforts of 708 FBI special agents, 1,033 state and local officers, and 183 federal law enforcement officers from other agencies. Currently there are 32 Fugitive Task Forces, 64 Violent Crimes Task Forces, 33 Violent Crimes/Fugitive Task Forces, and 9 Major Offenders (property crime/car jacking) Task Forces in operation under this initiative.

- **Drug Testing Accountability for Federal Arrestees.** The Department of Justice is developing a systematic multi-year approach to end drug abuse among offenders who cycle through the federal, state, and local criminal justice systems, called: *Operation Drug TEST (Testing, Effective Sanctions, and Treatment).* Under this initiative, defendants are tested for drugs as soon as possible after their arrest; judges use the test results in making pretrial detention determinations and in setting conditions of continued testing, sanctions, and treatment for defendants released into the community; and appropriate treatment and other drug abuse deterrence programs are made available to defendants, using the levers of criminal justice supervision to break the cycle of drug abuse and crime. The first steps of Operation Drug TEST include establishing a program providing for universal pretrial drug testing throughout the federal system and implementing related prosecutorial guidelines. Simultaneously, linkages will be established between the testing program, sanctions, and treatment, both in correctional institutions and the community. Operation Drug TEST also calls for implementation of a coordinated program of federal assistance to state and local jurisdictions to help them develop their own parallel systematic accountability programs of testing, effective sanctions, and treatment.
- **Investigation, Apprehension, and Removal of Criminal Aliens Involved in Narcotics Violations.** During fiscal year 1995, efforts by the Immigration and Naturalization Service (INS), in cooperation with other federal, state, and local law enforcement agencies, have resulted in the joint investigation, apprehension, and removal from the United States of 17,555 illegal aliens who either possessed, imported, transported, or manufactured controlled substances.
- **Research Breakthrough in the Treatment of Cocaine Addiction.** Researchers from the National Institute on Drug Abuse and Columbia University, bolstered by ONDCP support, have made progress in the "Cocaine Treatment Discovery Program." They have discovered compounds that show promise in blocking the effects of cocaine without interfering with the normal mood modulating effects of dopamine, one of the brain's essential neurotransmitters. This finding removes a major obstacle in the development of medications to address cocaine addiction.
- **Increased Border Security against Smuggling.** U.S. Customs "Operation Hard Line" has reduced instances of port running along the Southwest border by 42 percent. Since Operation Hard Line was instituted, smuggling has shifted away from passenger vehicles into commercial cargo. The success against smuggling has continued with a 125 percent increase in narcotics seizures in commercial cargo along the Southwest border in fiscal year 1995.

- **Presidential Directive against International Organized Crime.** The president in October 1995 used, for the first time ever, the authority provided him in the International Emergency Economic Powers Act for counternarcotics purposes. The president signed Executive Order Number 12978, directing the secretary of the treasury, in consultation with the secretary of state and the attorney general, to identify the leaders, cohorts, and front companies of the Cali organizations and to block their assets in the United States. The Executive Order also bars individuals and companies in the United States from trading with those identified individuals and their front companies.

- **An International Cocaine Strategy.** Drug trafficking organizations continue to target the U.S. drug market effectively, despite the unprecedented international and U.S. domestic law enforcement pressure that they face. Latin American producers are the sole suppliers of cocaine to the United States. They remain intent on meeting the demands of their most profitable market. The Cocaine Strategy focuses on the growing and processing areas of the source countries. This strategy reflects the need to target the available resources on areas where they can have the greatest effect. This approach responds to evidence that patterns of drug production and flow are changing and that a comprehensive regional approach is essential. From a tactical standpoint, antidrug efforts in the source countries should provide us with the best opportunities to eradicate production, arrest drug kingpins and destroy their organizations, and interdict drug flow. This Cocaine Strategy has already led to substantial success:

—Disruption in the cocaine production and distribution network. A regional air interdiction program has disrupted the major air route for smugglers between Peru and Colombia. The cooperative effort between the United States, Peru, and other governments in the region has disrupted the coca markets on the ground, making coca cultivation financially less attractive to the farmers who initiate the cocaine production process.

—Arrests of Colombian Drug Cartel leadership. Colombian law enforcement authorities, with U.S. assistance, arrested six of the seven Cali Drug Cartel leaders in 1995. One suspect subsequently escaped and was killed by Colombian National Police while resisting arrest.

—Arrest of a major Mexican drug trafficker. In January 1996, the leader of one of Mexico's four major cocaine smuggling organizations was arrested in Mexico and expelled to face U.S. charges.

—Largest maritime cocaine seizure in U.S. history. A multi-agency operation, comprised of elements of both the U.S. Coast Guard and Navy, seized more than twelve tons of cocaine from the *Nataly I,* a 112-foot Panamanian fishing vessel boarded in the Pacific Ocean 180 miles west of Peru. This action exemplifies interagency cooperation and the importance of maintaining a strong transit zone presence and flexible interdiction capability.

- **An International Heroin Strategy.** The president recently developed a new international heroin strategy to blunt the impact of the growing potential heroin problem. It reflects the need for a significantly different approach than that prescribed for cocaine. The heroin industry is more decentralized, more diversified, and more resistant to law enforcement operations. International criminal groups, attracted by huge profits, are moving larger quantities of heroin to the United States. With the increased availability of heroin and a drastic increase in the purity of heroin on the street, consumption is increasing, even among adolescents. If left unchecked, these factors could lead to an epidemic of heroin use.
- **Disruption of Money Laundering Operations.** The Departments of the Treasury, Justice, and State have been actively engaged in carrying out anti-money laundering efforts, both nationally and internationally. At the Summit of the Americas hosted by the president in 1994, the leaders of thirty-four nations in the Western Hemisphere agreed to a set of principles that included a commitment to fight drug trafficking and money laundering. The U.S. subsequently coordinated the development of a Communique on Money Laundering which was adopted by the international community in 1995 and which laid out a series of steps for countries to take to implement an effective anti-money laundering program.
- **Aggressive Use of the Annual Certification Process.** Certification involves evaluating the counternarcotics performance of countries that have been defined as major drug-producing or drug-transit countries. That performance is judged on the basis of their meeting the antidrug objectives enunciated in the 1988 United Nations Convention against Illicit Traffic in Narcotic Drugs and Psychotropic Substances. For countries that are not certified, the United States cuts off most forms of assistance and votes against loans by six multilateral development banks.
- **Successful Attacks on Major Drug Traffickers.** Efforts of one component of the Miami HIDTA; principally U.S. Customs, the DEA and FBI, and the U.S. Attorney, resulted in the Operation Cornerstone indictments of 252 major drug traffickers. The Miami HIDTA task forces include all major federal, state, and local law enforcement agencies.

V. STRATEGIC GOALS AND OBJECTIVES OF THE 1996 NATIONAL DRUG CONTROL STRATEGY

These goals:

- Facilitate objective measurement of the nation's progress toward reducing illicit drug use and its consequences;
- Are in accordance with Section 1005 of Public Law 100-690, as amended,

which states that the National Drug Control Strategy must include "comprehensive, research-based, long-range goals for reducing drug abuse"; and
- Represent a strategic approach to solving the current major aspects of the drug problem.

Despite past strides in addressing drug use and trafficking, tough challenges must be faced. An upsurge in drug use by teens reflects the need to refocus and reinvigorate prevention efforts. We have yet to substantially influence either the availability or the purity of cocaine and heroin within the United States. Nor have we yet been able to reduce the number of hardcore drug users who sustain the criminal infrastructure of drug traffickers and fuel drug-related violence. International criminal organizations are building momentum along the Southwest border with Mexico and in the eastern Caribbean and Puerto Rico. Finally, emerging drugs threaten to spur new drug "epidemics" and accompanying waves of crime and violence.

The five goals and their supporting objectives underscore our central purpose and mission—reducing illicit drug use and its consequences. They acknowledge that antidrug efforts do not occur in isolation and must be long-term in focus. Our efforts must also be linked with efforts to curb the use of alcohol and tobacco by those who are underage and the illicit use of other controlled substances. We must also recognize the need for prevention programs to deter first-time drug use among adolescents and other high-risk populations and to reduce the progression from casual use to addiction. We must uphold the belief that those who have started using drugs may need a hand in stopping. We also reaffirm that those who seek to profit from the drug trade must face the certainty of punishment. The smaller number of strategic goals does not imply a rejection of past goals or existing programs. Rather, the smaller number ensures that our message is unambiguous and that our commitment is clear. All Americans must understand our central purposes if this strategy is to be a worthwhile guide for action.

This strategy is founded in a firm belief that America can no longer tolerate the negative effects of drug use on the lives of our citizens—the personal tragedies of millions of Americans whose children have been seduced by the glamour and availability of dangerous and illicit drugs and substances; the members of our families who have been killed, wounded, or assaulted by drug users and traffickers; and our schools, neighborhoods, and workplaces that have been ravaged by drugs. We cannot be satisfied with managing the drug problem so that its consequences are acceptable to the majority. Our task must be to break the cycle of addiction so that we can significantly reduce both illicit drug use and its consequences.

Figure 2.1
Adolescent Drug Use

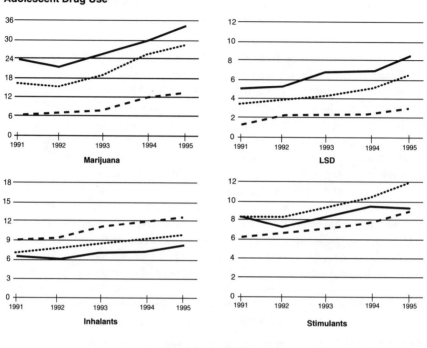

Source: Monitoring the Future

Strategic Goals and Objectives of the 1996 National Drug Control Strategy

Goal 1: Motivate America's youth to reject illegal drugs and substance abuse.

Objective 1: Increase the number of state governments and community organizations participating in the development of national prevention standards and a national prevention infrastructure.

Objective 2: Increase the number of schools with comprehensive drug prevention and early intervention strategies with a focus on family involvement.

Objective 3: Increase the number of community drug coalitions through a focus on the need for public support of local drug prevention empowerment efforts.

Objective 4: Increase, through public education, the public's awareness of the consequences of illicit drug use and the use of alcohol and tobacco by underage populations.

Figure 2.2
Annual U.S. Consumption of Cocaine by Type of User, 1972-92

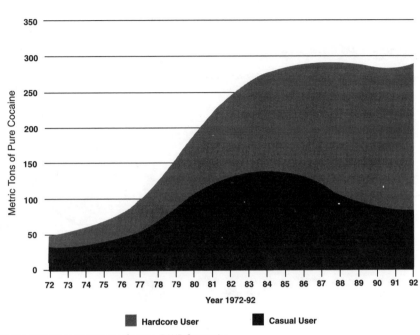

Source: *Modeling the Demand for Cocaine, RAND Corporation*

Objective 5: Reverse the upward trend in marijuana use among young people and raise the average age of initial users of all illicit drugs.

Goal 2: Increase the safety of America's citizens by substantially reducing drug-related crime and violence.

Objective 1: Increase the effectiveness of local police through the implementation of community and problem-oriented policing with a focus on youth and gang violence, drug-related homicides, and domestic violence.

Objective 2: Break the cycle of drug abuse and crime by integrating drug testing, court-authorized graduated sanctions, treatment, offender tracking and rehabilitation, and aftercare through drug courts and other offender management programs, prison rehabilitation and education, and supervised transition to the community.

Objective 3: Increase the effectiveness of federal, state, and local law enforcement task forces that target all levels of trafficking to reduce the flow of drugs to neighborhoods and make our streets safe for the public.

Figure 2.3
Health Consequences

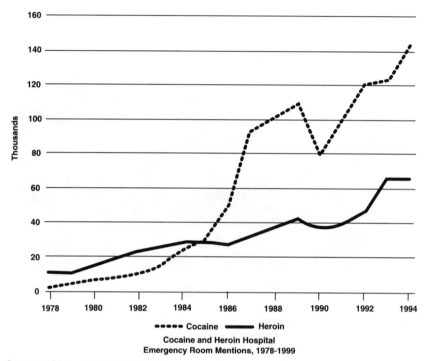

Cocaine and Heroin Hospital
Emergency Room Mentions, 1978-1999

Source: HHS Drug Abuse Warning Network

Objective 4: Improve the efficiency of Federal drug law enforcement investigative and intelligence programs to apprehend drug traffickers, seize their drugs, and forfeit their assets.

Objective 5: Increase the number of schools that are free of drugs and violence.

Goal 3: Reduce health, welfare, and crime costs resulting from illegal drug use.

Objective 1: Increase treatment efficiency and effectiveness.

Objective 2: Use effective outreach, referral, and case management efforts to facilitate early access to treatment.

Objective 3: Reduce the spread of infectious diseases and other illnesses related to drug use.

Objective 4: Expand and enhance drug education and prevention strategies in the workplace.

Figure 2.4
Cocaine Seizures Versus Production

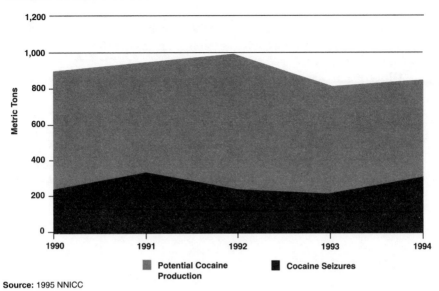

Source: 1995 NNICC

Goal 4: Shield America's air, land, and sea frontiers from the drug threat.

Objective 1: Identify and implement options, including science and technology options, to improve the effectiveness of law enforcement to stop the flow of drugs into the United States, especially along the Southwest Border.

Objective 2: Lead efforts to develop stronger bilateral and multilateral intelligence sharing to thwart the use of international commercial air, maritime, and land cargo shipments for smuggling.

Objective 3: Conduct flexible interdiction in the transit zone to ensure effective use of maritime and aerial interdiction capabilities.

Goal 5: Break foreign and domestic drug sources of supply.

Objective 1: Destroy major trafficking organizations by arresting, convicting, and incarcerating their leaders and top associates, and seizing their drugs and assets.

Objective 2: Reduce the foreign availability of drugs through eradication and other programs that reduce drug crop cultivation and through enforcement efforts to attack chemical, money laundering, and transportation networks that support trafficking organizations.

Objective 3: Reduce all domestic drug production and availability and continue to target for investigation and prosecution those who illegally divert pharmaceuticals and listed chemicals.

Objective 4: Increase the political will of countries to cooperate with the United States on drug control efforts through aggressive diplomacy, certification, and carefully targeted foreign assistance.

Objective 5: Strengthen host nation institutions so that they can conduct more effective drug-control efforts on their own and withstand the threat that narcotics trafficking poses to sovereignty, democracy, and free-market economies. In the source countries, aggressively support the full range of host nation interdiction efforts by providing training and operational support.

Objective 6: Make greater use of multilateral organizations to share the burdens and costs of international narcotics control to complement the efforts of the United States and to institute programs where the United States has limited or no access. . . .

Part Three

Just Say No to Drug Legalization

3

Against the Legalization of Drugs

James Q. Wilson

In 1972, the president appointed me chairman of the National Advisory Council for Drug Abuse Prevention. Created by Congress, the Council was charged with providing guidance on how best to coordinate the national war on drugs. (Yes, we called it a war then, too.) In those days, the drug we were chiefly concerned with was heroin. When I took office, heroin use had been increasing dramatically. Everybody was worried that this increase would continue. Such phrases as "heroin epidemic" were commonplace.

That same year, the eminent economist Milton Friedman published an essay in *Newsweek* in which he called for legalizing heroin. His argument was on two grounds: As a matter of ethics, the government has no right to tell people not to use heroin (or to drink or to commit suicide); as a matter of economics, the prohibition of drug use imposes costs on society that far exceed the benefits. Others, such as the psychoanalyst Thomas Szasz, made the same argument.*

We did not take Friedman's advice. (Government commissions rarely do.) I do not recall that we even discussed legalizing heroin, though we did discuss (but did not take action on) legalizing a drug, cocaine, that many people then argued was benign. Our marching orders were to figure out how to win the war on heroin, not to run up the white flag of surrender.

That was 1972. Today, we have the same number of heroin addicts that we had then—half a million, give or take a few thousand. Having that many heroin addicts is no trivial matter; these people deserve our attention. But not having had an increase in that number for over fifteen years is also something

Reprinted from *Commentary,* February 1990, by permission; all rights reserved.

*See Szasz, "Medics in the War on Drugs" and "Drugs as Property: The Right We Rejected," chapters 16 and 19, respectively, in this volume.

that deserves our attention. What happened to the "heroin epidemic" that many people once thought would overwhelm us?

The facts are clear: A more or less stable pool of heroin addicts has been getting older, with relatively few new recruits. In 1976 the average age of heroin users who appeared in hospital emergency rooms was about twenty-seven; ten years later it was thirty-two. More than two-thirds of all heroin users appearing in emergency rooms are now over the age of thirty. Back in the early 1970s, when heroin got onto the national political agenda, the typical heroin addict was much younger, often a teenager. Household surveys show the same thing—the rate of opiate use (which includes heroin) has been flat for the better part of two decades. More fine-grained studies of inner-city neighborhoods confirm this. John Boyle and Ann Brunswick found that the percentage of young blacks in Harlem who used heroin fell from 8 percent in 1970–71 to about 3 percent in 1975–76.

Why did heroin lose its appeal for young people? When the young blacks in Harlem were asked why they stopped, more than half mentioned "trouble with the law" or "high cost" (and high cost is, of course, directly the result of law enforcement). Two-thirds said that heroin hurt their health; nearly all said they had had a bad experience with it. We need not rely, however, simply on what they said. In New York City in 1973–75, the street price of heroin rose dramatically and its purity sharply declined, probably as a result of the heroin shortage caused by the success of the Turkish government in reducing the supply of opium base and of the French government in closing down heroin-processing laboratories located in and around Marseilles. These were short-lived gains for, just as Friedman predicted, alternative sources of supply—mostly in Mexico—quickly emerged. But the three-year heroin shortage interrupted the easy recruitment of new users.

Health and related problems were no doubt part of the reason for the reduced flow of recruits. Over the preceding years, Harlem youth had watched as more and more heroin users died of overdoses, were poisoned by adulterated doses, or acquired hepatitis from dirty needles. The word got around: heroin can kill you. By 1974 new hepatitis cases and drug-overdose deaths had dropped to a fraction of what they had been in 1970.

Alas, treatment did not seem to explain much of the cessation in drug use. Treatment programs can and do help heroin addicts, but treatment did not explain the drop in the number of *new* users (who by definition had never been in treatment) nor even much of the reduction in the number of experienced users.

No one knows how much of the decline to attribute to personal observation as opposed to high prices or reduced supply. But other evidence suggests strongly that price and supply played a large role. In 1972 the National Advisory Council was especially worried by the prospect that U.S. servicemen returning to this country from Vietnam would bring their heroin habits with them. Fortunately, a brilliant study by Lee Robins of Washington University in St. Louis put that fear to rest. She measured drug use of Vietnam veterans shortly after they had returned home. Though many had used heroin regularly while in Southeast Asia, most gave up the habit when back in the United States. The reason: Here, heroin was less available and sanctions on its use were more pronounced. Of course, if a veteran had been willing to pay enough—which might have meant traveling to another city and would certainly have meant making an illegal contact with a disreputable dealer in a threatening neighborhood in order to acquire a (possibly) dangerous dose— he could have sustained his drug habit. Most veterans were unwilling to pay this price, and so their drug use declined or disappeared.

RELIVING THE PAST

Suppose we had taken Friedman's advice in 1972. What would have happened? We cannot be entirely certain, but at a minimum we would have placed the young heroin addicts (and, above all, the prospective addicts) in a very different position from the one in which they actually found themselves. Heroin would have been legal. Its price would have been reduced by 95 percent (minus whatever we chose to recover in taxes). Now that it could be sold by the same people who make aspirin, its quality would have been assured—no poisons, no adulterants. Sterile hypodermic needles would have been readily available at the neighborhood drugstore, probably at the same counter where the heroin was sold. No need to travel to big cities or unfamiliar neighborhoods—heroin could have been purchased anywhere, perhaps by mail order.

There would no longer have been any financial or medical reason to avoid heroin use. Anybody could have afforded it. We might have tried to prevent children from buying it, but as we have learned from our efforts to prevent minors from buying alcohol and tobacco, young people have a way of penetrating markets theoretically reserved for adults. Returning Vietnam veterans would have discovered that Omaha and Raleigh had been converted into the pharmaceutical equivalent of Saigon.

Under these circumstances, can we doubt for a moment that heroin use would have grown exponentially? Or that a vastly larger supply of new users would have been recruited? Professor Friedman is a Nobel Prize-winning economist whose understanding of market forces is profound. What did he think would happen to consumption under his legalized regime? Here are his words: "Legalizing drugs might increase the number of addicts but it is not clear that it would. Forbidden fruit is attractive, particularly to the young."

Really? I suppose that we should expect no increase in Porsche sales if we cut the price by 95 percent, no increase in whiskey sales if we cut the price by a comparable amount—because young people only want fast cars and strong liquor when they are "forbidden." Perhaps Friedman's uncharacteristic lapse from the obvious implications of price theory can be explained by a misunderstanding of how drug users are recruited. In his 1972 essay he said that "drug addicts are deliberately made by pushers, who give likely prospects their first few doses free." If drugs were legal it would not pay anybody to produce addicts, because everybody would buy from the cheapest source. But as every drug expert knows, pushers do not produce addicts. Friends or acquaintances do. In fact, pushers are usually reluctant to deal with nonusers because a nonuser could be an undercover cop. Drug use spreads in the same way any fad or fashion spreads: Somebody who is already a user urges his friends to try, or simply shows already eager friends how to do it.

But we need not rely on speculation, however plausible, that lowered prices and more abundant supplies would have increased heroin usage. Great Britain once followed such a policy and with almost exactly those results. Until the mid-1960s, British physicians were allowed to prescribe heroin to certain classes of addicts. (Possessing these drugs without a doctor's prescription remained a criminal offense.) For many years this policy worked well enough because the addict patients were typically middle-class people who had become dependent on opiate painkillers while undergoing hospital treatment. There was no drug culture. The British system worked for many years, not because it prevented drug abuse, but because there was no problem of drug abuse that would test the system.

All that changed in the 1960s. A few unscrupulous doctors began passing out heroin in wholesale amounts. One doctor prescribed almost 600,000 heroin tablets—that is, over thirteen pounds—in just one year. A youthful drug culture emerged with a demand for drugs far different from that of the older addicts. As a result, the British government required doctors to refer users to government-run clinics to receive their heroin.

But the shift to clinics did not curtail the growth in heroin use. Throughout the 1960s the number of addicts increased—the late John Kaplan of Stanford estimated by fivefold—in part as a result of the diversion of heroin from clinic patients to new users on the streets. An addict would bargain with the clinic doctor over how big a dose he would receive. The patient wanted as much as he could get, the doctor wanted to give as little as was needed. The patient had an advantage in this conflict because the doctor could not be certain how much was really needed. Many patients would use some of their "maintenance" dose and sell the remaining part to friends, thereby recruiting new addicts. As the clinics learned of this, they began to shift their treatment away from heroin and toward methadone, an addictive drug that, when taken orally, does not produce a "high" but will block the withdrawal pains associated with heroin abstinence.

Whether what happened in England in the 1960s was a mini-epidemic or an epidemic depends on whether one looks at numbers or at rates of change. Compared to the United States, the numbers were small. In 1960 there were sixty-eight heroin addicts known to the British government; by 1968 there were two thousand in treatment and many more who refused treatment. (They would refuse in part because they did not want to get methadone at a clinic if they could get heroin on the street.) Richard Hartnoll estimates that the actual number of addicts in England is five times the number officially registered. At a minimum, the number of British addicts increased by thirty-fold in ten years; the actual increase may have been much larger.

In the early 1980s the numbers began to rise again, and this time nobody doubted that a real epidemic was at hand. The increase was estimated to be 40 percent a year. By 1982 there were thought to be 20,000 heroin users in London alone. Geoffrey Pearson reports that many cities—Glasgow, Liverpool, Manchester, and Sheffield among them—were now experiencing a drug problem that once had been largely confined to London. The problem, again, was supply. The country was being flooded with cheap, high-quality heroin, first from Iran and then from Southeast Asia.

The United States began the 1960s with a much larger number of heroin addicts and probably a bigger at-risk population than was the case in Great Britain. Even though it would be foolhardy to suppose that the British system, if installed here, would have worked the same way or with the same results, it would be equally foolhardy to suppose that a combination of heroin available from leaky clinics and from street dealers who faced only minimal law-enforcement risks would not have produced a much greater increase in heroin use than we actually experienced. My guess is that if we had allowed either doctors or clinics to prescribe heroin, we would have had far worse results than were produced in Britain, if for no other reason than the vastly larger number of addicts with which we began. We would have had to find some way to police thousands (not scores) of physicians and hundreds (not dozens) of clinics. If the British civil service found it difficult to keep heroin in the hands of addicts and out of the hands of recruits when it was dealing with a few hundred people, how well would the American civil service have accomplished the same tasks when dealing with tens of thousands of people?

BACK TO THE FUTURE

Now cocaine, especially in its potent form, crack, is the focus of attention. Now as in 1972 the government is trying to reduce its use. Now as then some people are advocating legalization. Is there any more reason to yield to those arguments today than there was almost two decades ago?[1]

I think not. If we had yielded in 1972 we almost certainly would have had today a permanent population of several million, not several hundred thousand, heroin addicts. If we yield now we will have a far more serious problem with cocaine.

Crack is worse than heroin by almost any measure. Heroin produces a pleasant drowsiness and, if hygienically administered, has only the physical side effects of constipation and sexual impotence. Regular heroin use incapacitates many users, especially poor ones, for any productive work or social responsibility. They will sit nodding on a street corner, helpless but at least harmless. By contrast, regular cocaine use leaves the user neither helpless nor harmless. When smoked (as with crack) or injected, cocaine produces instant, intense, and short-lived euphoria. The experience generates a powerful desire to repeat it. If the drug is readily available, repeat use will occur. Those people who progress to "binging" on cocaine become devoted to the drug and its effects to the exclusion of almost all other considerations—job, family, children, sleep, food, even sex. Dr. Frank Gawin at Yale and Dr. Everett Ellinwood at Duke report that a substantial percentage of all high-dose, binge users become uninhibited, impulsive, hypersexual, compulsive, irritable, and hyperactive. Their moods vacillate dramatically, leading at times to violence and homicide.

Women are much more likely to use crack than heroin, and if they are pregnant, the effects on their babies are tragic. Douglas Besharov, who has been following the effects of drugs on infants for twenty years, writes that nothing he learned about heroin prepared him for the devastation of cocaine. Cocaine harms the fetus and can lead to physical deformities or neurological damage. Some crack babies have for all practical purposes suffered a disabling stroke while still in the womb. The long-term consequences of this brain damage are lowered cognitive ability and the onset of mood disorders. Besharov estimates that about 30,000 to 50,000 such babies are born every year, about 7,000 in New York City alone. There may be ways to treat such infants, but from everything we now know the treatment will be long, difficult, and expensive. Worse, the mothers who are most likely to produce crack babies are precisely the ones who, because of poverty or temperament, are least able and willing to obtain such treatment. In fact, anecdotal evidence suggests that crack mothers are likely to abuse their infants.

The notion that abusing drugs such as cocaine is a "victimless crime" is not only absurd but dangerous. Even ignoring the fetal drug syndrome, crack-dependent people are, like heroin addicts, individuals who regularly victimize their children by neglect, their spouses by improvidence, their employers by lethargy, and their coworkers by carelessness. Society is not and could never be a collection of autonomous individuals. We all have a stake in ensuring that each of us displays a minimal level of dignity, responsibility, and empathy. We cannot, of course, coerce people into goodness, but we can and should insist that some standards must be met if society itself—on which the very existence of the human personality depends—is to persist. Drawing the line that defines those standards is difficult and contentious, but if crack and heroin use do not fall below it, what does?

The advocates of legalization will respond by suggesting that my picture is overdrawn. Ethan Nadelmann of Princeton argues that the risk of legalization is less than most people suppose. Over 20 million Americans between the ages of eighteen and twenty-five have tried cocaine (according to a government survey), but only a quarter million use it daily. From this Nadelmann concludes that at most 3 percent of all young people who try cocaine develop a problem with it. The implication is clear: Make the drug legal and we only have to worry about 3 percent of our youth.

The implication rests on a logical fallacy and a factual error. The fallacy is this: The percentage of occasional cocaine users who become binge users *when the drug is illegal* (and thus expensive and hard to find) tells us nothing about the percentage who will become dependent when the drug is legal (and thus cheap and abundant). Drs. Gawin and Ellinwood report, in common with several other researchers, that controlled or occasional use of cocaine changes to compulsive and frequent use "when access to the drug increases" or when the user switches from snorting to smoking. More cocaine more potently administered alters, perhaps sharply, the proportion of "controlled" users who become heavy users.

The factual error is this: The federal survey Nadelmann quotes was done in 1985, before crack had become common. Thus the probability of becoming dependent on cocaine was derived from the responses of users who snorted the drug. The speed and potency of cocaine's action increases dramatically when it is smoked. We do not yet know how greatly the advent of crack increases the risk of dependency, but all the clinical evidence suggests that the increase is likely to be large.

It is possible that some people will not become heavy users even when the drug is readily available in its most potent form. So far there are no scientific grounds for predicting who will and who will not become dependent. Neither socioeconomic background nor personality traits differentiate between casual and intensive users. Thus, the only way to settle the question of who is correct about the effect of easy availability on drug use, Nadelmann or Gawin and Ellinwood, is to try it and see. But that social experiment is so risky as to be no experiment at all, for if cocaine is legalized and if the rate of its abusive use increases dramatically, there is no way to put the genie back in the bottle, and it is not a kindly genie.

HAVE WE LOST?

Many people who agree that there are risks in legalizing cocaine or heroin still favor it because, they think, we have lost the war on drugs. "Nothing we have done has worked" and the current federal policy is just "more of the same." Whatever the costs of greater drug use, surely they would be less than the costs of our present, failed efforts.

That is exactly what I was told in 1972—and heroin is not quite as bad a drug as cocaine. We did not surrender and we did not lose. We did not win, either. What the nation accomplished then was what most efforts to save people from themselves accomplish: The problem was contained and the number of victims minimized, all at a considerable cost in law enforcement and increased crime. Was the cost worth it? I think so, but others may disagree. What are the lives of would-be addicts worth? I recall some people saying to me then, "Let them kill themselves." I was appalled. Happily, such views did not prevail.

Have we lost today? Not at all. High-rate cocaine use is not commonplace. The National Institute of Drug Abuse (NIDA) reports that less than 5 percent of high school seniors used cocaine within the last thirty days. Of course this survey misses young people who have dropped out of school and miscounts those who lie on the questionnaire, but even if we inflate the NIDA estimate by some plausible percentage, it is still not much above 5 percent. Medical examiners reported in 1987 that about 1,500 died from cocaine use; hospital emergency rooms reported about 30,000 admissions related to cocaine abuse.

These are not small numbers, but neither are they evidence of a nationwide plague that threatens to engulf us all. Moreover, cities vary greatly in the proportion of people who are involved with cocaine. To get city-level data we need to turn to drug tests carried out on arrested persons, who obviously are more likely to be drug users than the average citizen. The National Institute of Justice, through its Drug Use Forecasting (DUF) project, collects urinalysis data on arrestees in twenty-two cities. As we have already seen, opiate (chiefly heroin) use has been net or declining in most of these cities over the last decade. Cocaine use has gone up sharply, but with great variation among cities. New York, Philadelphia, and Washington, D.C., all report that two-thirds or more of their arrestees tested positive for cocaine, but in Portland, San Antonio, and Indianapolis the percentage was one-third or less.

In some neighborhoods, of course, matters have reached crisis proportions. Gangs control the streets, shootings terrorize residents, and drug dealing occurs in plain view. The police seem barely able to contain matters. But in these neighborhoods—unlike at Palo Alto cocktail parties— the people are not calling for legalization, they are calling for help. And often not much help has come. Many cities are willing to do almost anything about the drug problem except spend more money on it. The federal government cannot change that; only local voters and politicians can. It is not clear that they will.

It took about ten years to contain heroin. We have had experience with crack for only about three or four years. Each year we spend perhaps $11 billion on law enforcement (and some of that goes to deal with marijuana) and perhaps $2 billion on treatment. Large sums, but not sums that should lead anyone to say, "We just can't afford this any more."

The illegality of drugs increases crime, partly because some users turn to crime to pay for their habits, partly because some users are stimulated by certain drugs (such as crack or PCP) to act more violently or ruthlessly than they otherwise would, and partly because criminal organizations seeking to control drug supplies use force to manage their markets. These also are serious costs, but no one knows how much they would be reduced if drugs were legalized. Addicts would no longer steal to pay black-market prices for drugs, a real gain. But some, perhaps a great deal, of that gain would be offset by the great increase in the number of addicts. These people, nodding on heroin or living in the delusion-ridden high of cocaine, would hardly be ideal employees. Many would steal simply to support themselves, since snatch-and-grab, opportunistic crime can be managed even by people unable to hold a regular job or plan an elaborate crime.Those British addicts who get their supplies from government clinics are not models of law-abiding decency. Most are in crime, and though their per capita rate of criminality may be lower thanks to the cheapness of their drugs, the total volume of crime they produce may be quite large. Of course, society could decide to support all unemployable addicts on welfare, but that would mean that gains from lowered rates of crime would have to be offset by large increases in welfare budgets.

Proponents of legalization claim that the costs of having more addicts around would be largely if not entirely offset by having more money available with which to treat and care for them. The money would come from taxes levied on the sale of heroin and cocaine.

To obtain this fiscal dividend, however, legalization's supporters must first solve an economic dilemma. If they want to raise a lot of money to pay for welfare and treatment, the tax rate on the drugs will have to be quite high. Even if they themselves do not want a high rate, the politicians' love of "sin taxes" would probably guarantee that it would be high anyway. But the higher the tax, the higher the price of the drug, and the higher the price the greater the likelihood that addicts will turn to crime to find the money for it and that criminal organizations will be formed to sell tax-free drugs at below-market rates. If we managed to keep taxes (and thus prices) low, we would get that much less money to pay for welfare and treatment and more people could afford to become addicts. There may be an optimal tax rate for drugs that maximizes revenue while minimizing crime, bootlegging, and the recruitment of new addicts, but our experience with alcohol does not suggest that we know how to find it.

THE BENEFITS OF ILLEGALITY

The advocates of legalization find nothing to be said in favor of the current system except, possibly, that it keeps the number of addicts smaller than it would otherwise be. In fact, the benefits are more substantial than that.

First, treatment. All the talk about providing "treatment on demand," implies that there is a demand for treatment. That is not quite right. There are some drug-dependent people who genuinely want treatment and will remain in it if offered; they should receive it. But there are far more who want only short-term help after a bad crash; once stabilized and bathed, they are back on the street again, hustling. And even many of the addicts who enroll in a program honestly wanting help drop out after a short while when they discover that help takes time and commitment. Drug-dependent people have very short time horizons and a weak capacity for commitment. These two groups—those looking for a quick fix and those unable to stick with a long-term fix—are not easily helped. Even if we increase the number of treatment slots—as we should—we would have to do something to make treatment more effective.

One thing that can often make it more effective is compulsion. Douglas Anglin of UCLA, in common with many other researchers, has found that the longer one stays in a treatment program, the better the chances of a reduction in drug dependency. But he, again like most other researchers, has found that drop-out rates are high. He has also found, however, that patients who enter treatment under legal compulsion stay in the program longer than those not subject to such pressure. His research on the California civil commitment program, for example, found that heroin users involved with its required drug-testing program had over the long term a lower rate of heroin use than similar addicts who were free of such constraints. If for many addicts compulsion is a useful component of treatment, it is not clear how compulsion could be achieved in a society in which purchasing, possessing, and using the drug were legal. It could be managed, I suppose, but I would not want to have to answer the challenge from the American Civil Liberties Union that it is wrong to compel a person to undergo treatment for consuming a legal commodity.

Next, education. We are now investing substantially in drug-education programs in the schools. Though we do not yet know for certain what will work, there are some promising leads. But I wonder how credible such programs would be if they were aimed at dissuading children from doing something perfectly legal. We could, of course, treat drug education like smoking education: Inhaling crack and inhaling tobacco are both legal, but you should not do it because it is bad for you. That tobacco is bad for you is easily shown; the Surgeon General has seen to that. But what do we say about crack? It is pleasurable, but devoting yourself to so much pleasure is not a good idea (though perfectly legal)? Unlike tobacco, cocaine will not give you cancer or emphysema, but it will lead you to neglect your duties to family, job, and neighborhood? Everybody is doing cocaine, but you should not?

Again, it might be possible under a legalized regime to have effective drug-prevention programs, but their effectiveness would depend heavily, I think, on first having decided that cocaine use, like tobacco use, is purely a matter of practical consequences; no fundamental moral significance attaches to either. But if we believe—as I do—that dependency on certain mind-altering drugs is a moral issue and that their illegality rests in part on their immorality, then legalizing them undercuts, if it does not eliminate altogether, the moral message.

That message is at the root of the distinction we now make between nicotine and cocaine. Both are highly addictive; both have harmful physical effects. But we treat the two drugs differently, not simply because nicotine is so widely used as to be beyond the reach of effective prohibition, but because its use does not destroy the user's essential humanity. Tobacco shortens one's life, cocaine debases it. Nicotine alters one's habits, cocaine alters one's soul. The heavy use of crack, unlike the heavy use of tobacco, corrodes those natural sentiments of sympathy and duty that constitute our human nature and make possible our social life. To say, as does Nadelmann, that distinguishing morally between tobacco and cocaine is "little more than a transient prejudice" is close to saying that morality itself is but a prejudice.

THE ALCOHOL PROBLEM

Now we have arrived where many arguments about legalizing drugs begin: Is there any reason to treat heroin and cocaine differently from the way we treat alcohol?

There is no easy answer to that question because, as with so many human problems, one cannot decide simply on the basis either of moral principles or of individual consequences; one has to temper any policy by a commonsense judgment of what is possible. Alcohol, like heroin, cocaine, PCP, and marijuana, is a drug—that is, a mood-altering substance—and consumed to excess it certainly has harmful consequences: auto accidents, barroom fights, bedroom shootings. It is also, for some people, addictive. We cannot confidently compare the addictive powers of these drugs, but the best evidence suggests that crack and heroin are much more addictive than alcohol.

Many people, Nadelmann included, argue that since the health and financial costs of alcohol abuse are so much higher than those of cocaine or heroin abuse, it is hypocritical folly to devote our efforts to preventing cocaine or drug use. But as Mark Kleiman of Harvard has pointed out, this comparison is quite misleading. What Nadelmann is doing is showing that a *legalized* drug (alcohol) produces greater social harm than *illegal* ones (cocaine and heroin). But of course. Suppose that in the 1920s we had made heroin and cocaine legal and alcohol illegal. Can anyone doubt that Nadelmann would now be writing that it is folly to continue our ban on alcohol because cocaine and heroin are so much more harmful?

And let there be no doubt about it—widespread heroin and cocaine use are associated with all manner of ills. Thomas Bewley found that the mortality rate of British heroin addicts in 1968 was 28 times as high as the death rate of the same age group of nonaddicts, even though in England at the time an addict could obtain free or low-cost heroin and clean needles from British clinics. Perform the following mental experiment: Suppose we legalized heroin and cocaine in this country. In what proportion of auto fatalities would the state police report that the driver was nodding off on heroin or recklessly driving on a coke high? In what proportion of spouse-assault and child-abuse cases would the local police report that crack was involved? In what proportion of industrial accidents would safety investigators report that the forklift or drill-press operator was in a drug-induced stupor or frenzy? We do not know exactly what the proportion would be, but anyone who asserts that it would not be much higher than it is now would have to believe that these drugs have little appeal except when they are illegal. And that is nonsense.

An advocate of legalization might concede that social harm—perhaps harm equivalent to that already produced by alcohol—would follow from making cocaine and heroin generally available. But at least, he might add, we would have the problem "out in the open" where it could be treated as a matter of "public health." That is well and good, *if* we knew how to treat—that is, cure—heroin and cocaine abuse. But we do not know how to do it for all the people who would need such help. We are having only limited success in coping with chronic alcoholics. Addictive behavior is immensely difficult to change, and the best methods for changing it—living in drug-free therapeutic communities, becoming faithful members of Alcoholics Anonymous or Narcotics Anonymous—require great personal commitment, a quality that is, alas, in short supply among the very persons—young people, disadvantaged people—who are often most at risk for addiction.

Suppose that today we had, not 15 million alcohol abusers, but half a million. Suppose that we already knew what we have learned from our long experience with the widespread use of alcohol. Would we make whiskey legal? I do not know, but I suspect there would be a lively debate. The Surgeon General would remind us of the risks alcohol poses to pregnant women. The National Highway Traffic Safety Administration would point to the likelihood of more highway fatalities caused by drunk drivers. The Food and Drug Administration might find that there is a nontrivial increase in cancer associated with alcohol consumption. At the same time the police would report great difficulty in keeping illegal whiskey out of our cities, officers being corrupted by bootleggers, and alcohol addicts often resorting to crime to feed their habit. Libertarians, for their part, would argue that every citizen has a right to drink anything he wishes and that drinking is, in any event, a "victimless crime."

However the debate might turn out, the central fact would be that the problem was still, at that point, a small one. The government cannot legislate away the addictive tendencies in all of us, nor can it remove completely even the most dangerous addictive substances. But it can cope with harms when the harms are still manageable.

SCIENCE AND ADDICTION

One advantage of containing a problem while it is still containable is that it buys time for science to learn more about it and perhaps to discover a cure. Almost unnoticed in the current debate over legalizing drugs is that basic science has made rapid strides in identifying the underlying neurological processes involved in some forms of addiction. Stimulants such as cocaine and amphetamines alter the way certain brain cells communicate with one another. That alteration is complex and not entirely understood, but in simplified form it involves modifying the way in which a neurotransmitter called dopamine sends signals from one cell to another.

When dopamine crosses the synapse between two cells, it is in effect carrying a message from the first cell to activate the second one. In certain parts of the brain that message is experienced as pleasure. After the message is delivered, the dopamine returns to the first cell. Cocaine apparently blocks this return, or "reuptake," so that the excited cell and others nearby continue to send pleasure messages. When the exaggerated high produced by cocaine-influenced dopamine finally ends, the brain cells may (in ways that are still a matter of dispute) suffer from an extreme lack of dopamine, thereby making the individual unable to experience any pleasure at all. This would explain why cocaine users often feel so depressed after enjoying the drug. Stimulants may also affect the way in which other neurotransmitters, such as serotonin and noradrenaline, operate.

Whatever the exact mechanism may be, once it is identified it becomes possible to use drugs to block either the effect of cocaine or its tendency to produce dependency. There have already been experiments using desipramine, imipramine, bromocriptine, carbamazepine, and other chemicals. There are some promising results.

Tragically, we spend very little on such research, and the agencies funding it have not in the past occupied very influential or visible posts in the federal bureaucracy. If there is one aspect of the "war on drugs" metaphor that I dislike, it is its tendency to focus attention almost exclusively on the troops in the trenches, whether engaged in enforcement or treatment, and away from the research-and-development efforts back on the home front where the war may ultimately be decided.

I believe that the prospects of scientists in controlling addiction will be strongly influenced by the size and character of the problem they face. If the problem is a few hundred thousand chronic high-dose users of an illegal product, the chances of making a difference at a reasonable cost will be much greater than if the problem is a few million chronic users of legal substances. Once a drug is legal, not only will its use increase but many of those who then use it will prefer the drug to the treatment: They will want the pleasure, whatever the cost to themselves or their families, and they will resist—probably successfully—any effort to wean them away from experiencing the high that comes from inhaling a legal substance.

IF I AM WRONG . . .

No one can know what our society would be like if we changed the law to make access to cocaine, heroin, and PCP easier. I believe, for reasons given, that the result would be a sharp increase in use, a more widespread degradation of the human personality, and a greater rate of accidents and violence.

I may be wrong. If I am, then we will needlessly have incurred heavy costs in law enforcement and some forms of criminality. But if I am right, and the legalizers prevail anyway, then we will have consigned millions of people, hundreds of thousands of infants, and hundreds of neighborhoods to a life of oblivion and disease. To the lives and families destroyed by alcohol we will have added countless more destroyed by cocaine, heroin, PCP, and whatever else a basement scientist can invent.

Human character is formed by society; indeed, human character is inconceivable without society, and good character is less likely in a bad society. Will we, in the name of an abstract doctrine of radical individualism, and with the false comfort of suspect predictions, decide to take the chance that somehow individual decency can survive amid a more general level of degradation?

I think not. The American people are too wise for that, whatever the academic essayists and cocktail-party pundits may say. But if Americans today are less wise than I suppose, then Americans at some future time will look back on us now and wonder, what kind of people were they that they could have done such a thing?

NOTE

1. I do not here take up the question of marijuana. For a variety of reasons—its widespread use and its lesser tendency to addict—it presents a different problem from cocaine or heroin. For a penetrating analysis, see Mark Kleiman, *Marijuana: Costs of Abuse, Costs of Control* (Westport, Conn.: Greenwood Press, 1989).

4

Should Drugs Be Legalized?

William Bennett

Since I took command of the war on drugs, I have learned from former Secretary of State George Shultz that our concept of fighting drugs is "flawed." The only thing to do, he says, is to "make it possible for addicts to buy drugs at some regulated place." Conservative commentator William F. Buckley Jr. suggests I should be "fatalistic" about the flood of cocaine from South America and simply "let it in." Syndicated columnist Mike Royko contends it would be easier to sweep junkies out of the gutters "than to fight a hopeless war against the narcotics that send them there. Labeling our efforts "bankrupt," federal judge Robert W. Sweet opts for legalization, saying, "If our society can learn to stop using butter, it should be able to cut down on cocaine."

Flawed, fatalistic, hopeless, bankrupt! I never realized surrender was so fashionable until I assumed this post.

Though most Americans are overwhelmingly determined to go toe-to-toe with the foreign drug lords and neighborhood pushers; a small minority believe that enforcing drug laws impose greater costs on society than do drugs themselves. Like addicts seeking immediate euphoria, the legalizers want peace at any price, even though it means the inevitable proliferation of a practice that degrades, impoverishes, and kills.

I am acutely aware of the burdens drug enforcement places upon us. It consumes economic resources we would like to use elsewhere. It is sometimes frustrating, thankless, and often dangerous. But the consequences of *not* enforcing drug laws would be far more costly. Those consequences involve the intrinsically destructive nature of drugs and the toll they exact

William Bennett, "Should Drugs Be Legalized?" *Reader's Digest,* March 1990. Reprinted with permission from the March 1990 *Reader's Digest.* Copyright © 1990 by the Reader's Digest Association, Inc.

from our society in hundreds of thousands of lost and broken lives . . . human potential never realized . . . time stolen from families and jobs . . . precious spiritual and economic resources squandered.

That is precisely why virtually every civilized society has found it necessary to exert some form of control over mind-altering substances and why this war is to important. Americans feel up to their hips in drugs now. They would be up to their necks under legalization.

Even limited experiments in drug legalization have shown that when drugs are more widely available, addiction skyrockets. In 1975 Italy liberalized its drug law and now has one of the highest heroin-related death rates in Western Europe. In Alaska, where marijuana was decriminalized in 1975, the easy atmosphere has increased usage of the drug, particularly among children. Nor does it stop there. Some Alaskan schoolchildren now tout "coca puffs," marijuana cigarettes laced with cocaine.

Many legalizers concede that drug legalization might increase use, but they shrug off the matter. "It may well be that there would be more addicts, and I would regret that result," says Nobel laureate economist Milton Friedman. The late Harvard Medical School psychiatry professor Norman Zinberg, a long-time proponent of "responsible" drug use, admitted that "use of now illicit drugs would certainly increase. Also, casualties probably would increase."

In fact, Dr. Herbert D. Kleber of Yale University, my deputy in charge of demand reduction, predicts legalization might cause "a five-to-sixfold increase" in cocaine use. But legalizers regard this as a necessary price for the "benefits" of legalization. What benefits?

1. *Legalization will take the profit out of drugs.* The result supposedly will be the end of criminal drug pushers and the big foreign drug wholesalers, who will turn to other enterprises because nobody will need to make furtive and dangerous trips to his local pusher.

But what, exactly, would the brave new world of legalized drugs look like? Buckley stresses that "adults get to buy the stuff at carefully regulated stores." (Would you want one in *your* neighborhood?) Others, like Friedman, suggest we sell the drugs at "ordinary retail outlets."

Former City University of New York sociologist Georgette Bennett assures us that "brand-name competition will be prohibited" and that strict quality control and proper labeling will be overseen by the Food and Drug Administration. In a touching egalitarian note, she adds that "free drugs will be provided at government clinics" for addicts too poor to buy them.

Almost all the legalizers point out that the price of drugs will fall, even though the drugs will be heavily taxed. Buckley, for example, argues that somehow federal drugstores will keep the price "low enough to discourage a black market but high enough to accumulate a surplus to be used for drug education."

Supposedly, drug sales will generate huge amounts of revenue, which will then be used to tell the public not to use drugs and to treat those who don't listen.

In reality, this tax would only allow government to *share* the drug profits now garnered by criminals. Legalizers would have to tax drugs heavily in order to pay for drug education and treatment programs. Criminals could undercut the official price and still make huge profits. What alternative would the government have? Cut the price until it was within the lunch-money budget of the average sixth-grade student?

2. *Legalization will eliminate the black market.* Wrong. And not just because the regulated prices could be undercut. Many legalizers admit that drugs such as crack or PCP are simply too dangerous to allow the shelter of the law. Thus criminals will provide what the government will not. "As long as drugs that people very much want remain illegal, a black market will exist," says legalization advocate David Boaz of the libertarian Cato Institute.

Look at crack. In powdered form, cocaine was an expensive indulgence. But street chemists found that a better and far less expensive—and far more dangerous—high could be achieved by mixing cocaine with baking soda and heating it. Crack was born, and "cheap" coke invaded low-income communities with furious speed.

An ounce of powdered cocaine might sell on the street for $1200. That same ounce can produce 370 vials of crack at $10 each. Ten bucks seems like a cheap hit, but crack's intense ten- to fifteen-minute high is followed by an unbearable depression. The user wants more crack, thus starting a rapid and costly descent into addiction.

If government drugstores do not stock crack, addicts will find it in the clandestine market or simply bake it themselves from their legally purchased cocaine.

Currently, crack is being laced with insecticides and animal tranquilizers to heighten its effect. Emergency rooms are now warned to expect victims of "sandwiches" and "moon rocks," life-threatening smokable mixtures of heroin and crack. Unless the government is prepared to sell these deadly variations of dangerous drugs, it will perpetuate a criminal black market by default.

And what about children and teenagers? They would obviously be barred from drug purchases, just as they are prohibited from buying beer and liquor. But pushers will continue to cater to these young customers with the old, favorite come-ons—a couple of free fixes to get them hooked, and what good will anti-drug education be when these youngsters observe their older brothers and sisters, parents and friends lighting up and shooting up with government permission?

Legalization will give us the worst of both worlds: millions of *new* drug users *and* a thriving criminal black market.

3. *Legalization will dramatically reduce crime.* "It is the high price of drugs that leads addicts to robbery, murder, and other crimes," says Ira Glasser, executive director of the American Civil Liberties Union. A study by the Cato Institute concludes: "Most, if not all, 'drug-related murders' are the result of drug prohibition."

But researchers tell us that many drug-related felonies are committed by people involved in crime *before* they started taking drugs. The drugs, so routinely available in criminal circles, make the criminals more violent and unpredictable.

Certainly there are some kill-for-a-fix crimes, but does any rational person believe that a cut-rate price for drugs at a government outlet will stop such psychopathic behavior? The fact is that under the influence of drugs, normal people do not act normally, and abnormal people behave in chilling and horrible ways. DEA agents told me about a teenage addict in Manhattan who was smoking crack when he sexually abused and caused permanent internal injuries to his one-month-old daughter.

Children are among the most frequent victims of violent, drug-related crimes that have nothing to do with the cost of acquiring the drugs. In Philadelphia in 1987 more than half the child-abuse fatalities involved at least one parent who was a heavy drug user. Seventy-three percent of the child-abuse deaths in New York City in 1987 involved parental drug use.

In my travels to the ramparts of the drug war, I have seen nothing to support the legalizers' argument that lower drug prices would reduce crime. Virtually everywhere I have gone, police and DEA agents have told me that crime rates are highest where crack is cheapest.

4. *Drug use should be legal since users only harm themselves.* Those who believe this should stand beside the medical examiner as he counts the thirty-six bullet wounds in the shattered corpse of a three-year-old who happened to get in the way of his mother's drug-crazed boyfriend. They should visit the babies abandoned by cocaine-addicted mothers—infants who already carry the ravages of addiction in their own tiny bodies. They should console the devastated relatives of the nun who worked in a homeless shelter and was stabbed to death by a crack addict enraged that she would not stake him to a fix.

Do drug addicts only harm themselves? Here is a former cocaine addict describing the compulsion that quickly draws even the most "responsible" user into irresponsible behavior: "Everything is about getting high, and any means necessary to get there becomes rational. If it means stealing something from somebody close to you, lying to your family, borrowing money from people you know you can't pay back, writing checks you know you can't cover, you do all those things—things that are totally against everything you have ever believed in."

Society pays for this behavior, and not just in bigger insurance premiums, losses from accidents, and poor job performance. We pay in the loss of a priceless social currency as families are destroyed, trust between friends is betrayed, and promising careers are never fulfilled. I cannot imagine sanctioning behavior that would increase that toll.

I find no merit in the legalizers' case. The simple fact is that drug use is wrong. And the moral argument, in the end, is the most compelling argument. A citizen in a drug-induced haze, whether on his backyard deck or on a mattress in a ghetto crack house, is not what the founding fathers meant by the "pursuit of happiness." Despite the legalizers' argument that drug use is a matter of "personal freedom," our nation's notion of liberty is rooted in the ideal of a self-reliant citizenry. Helpless wrecks in treatment centers, men chained by their noses to cocaine—these people are slaves.

Imagine if, in the darkest days of 1940, Winston Churchill had rallied the West by saying, "This war looks hopeless, and besides, it will cost too much. Hitler can't be *that* bad. Let's surrender and see what happens." That is essentially what we hear from the legalizers.

This war *can* be won. I am heartened by indications that education and public revulsion are having an effect on drug use. The, National Institute on Drug Abuse's latest survey of current users shows a 37 percent *decrease* in drug consumption since 1985. Cocaine is down 50 percent; marijuana use among young people is at its lowest rate since 1972. In my travels I've been encouraged by signs that Americans are fighting back.

I am under no illusion that such developments, however hopeful, mean the war is over. We need to involve more citizens in the fight, increase pressure on drug criminals and build on antidrug programs that have proved to work. This will not be easy. But the moral and social costs of surrender are simply too great to contemplate.

5

Drug Legalization:
Asking for Trouble

Robert L. DuPont and Ronald L. Goldfarb

The world's most reasonable-sounding but dumb idea is the one that advocates solving the country's drug problem by legalizing drugs.

Its fundamental flaw is the premise that the drug problem is not one of drug use but of drug prohibition. The reality is otherwise: Drug use is the core drug problem. Legalization cures the problem of prohibition at the cost of more drug use.

Legalization advocates emphasize the high cost of maintaining the prohibition of such drugs as marijuana, cocaine, PCP, and heroin. The costs of prohibition are high and rising. But the debates about legalization generally overlook the costs attributed to drug use itself—the lost potential and the lost lives. A few people die now in America because they cannot get drugs cheaply. Far more die and suffer because they can, despite prohibition. Fourteen million Americans now pay $100 billion a year for illicit drugs. How many more Americans would consume how much more if drug prices were cut by 90 percent or more as the legalization advocates propose?

The litmus test of any legalization plan is what to do with dangerous drugs such as crack and PCP. Crack, or smokable cocaine, is the only drug problem that is getting worse in the United States. Legalizing limited use of small quantities of marijuana or giving IV drug users sterile needles will not dent the crack problem.

Watch what happens when you ask advocates of legalization how their scheme would work: they turn silent, or they talk about how bad prohibition is. Which drugs would be legalized, in what forms, at what potencies and for

Originally published in the *Washington Post,* January 26, 1990. Reprinted by permission.

whom? Imagine your junior high school—or college-age—son or daughter, or your neighbor, dropping into the local, government-run package store. "A packet of crack, please, some PCP for my date, and a little heroin for the weekend."

"Yes, sir. Will that be cash or charge?"

Some legalizers have talked about doctors writing prescriptions for legalized cocaine, heroin, or other drugs. The idea is ridiculous. Doctors don't and shouldn't write prescriptions for chemical parties.

Drug abuse treatment, both public and private, is expensive and a growth industry because of the national drug epidemic, not because of drug prohibition. Using drugs such as methadone in the treatment of heroin addiction is a far cry from legalization, because methadone is only available in tightly controlled settings and only for therapeutic purposes. This fits with the long-standing U.S. approach, which allows dependence-producing substances to be used in medical practice to treat diseases but not outside medical settings and not for recreational purposes.

Advocates of legalization point to the "failure" of Prohibition. But during Prohibition—of manufacture, not use, of alcohol—consumption did decline drastically, and alcohol-related arrests dropped by half. Thus, laws do cut drug consumption, prevent new users, and decrease casualties. Correctly or not, society seems to have made a costly, special deal with recreational drinking.

The most recent National Institute on Drug Abuse survey of Americans over the age of twelve showed that in 1988 there were 106 million alcohol users, 57 million cigarette smokers, but only 12 million users of marijuana and 3 million users of cocaine. All four numbers were down from 1985 levels. Alcohol use dropped 6 percent, cigarette use dropped 5 percent, marijuana use dropped 33 percent, and cocaine use dropped 50 percent. It is not easy to look at these numbers and conclude that prohibition of illegal drugs is not working to reduce use or that we are losing the war on drugs.

The best way to cut the drug market is to decrease society's tolerance for illicit drug use. That means creating painful consequences for illicit drug use to help the nonuser stay clean. There need to be more and better programs to help the current drug users get clean. This country needs less debate on the legalization of drugs and more discussion about how best to deter drug users and provide drug treatment.

Law enforcement aimed at the supply of drugs is an important but small part of the solution. We do not believe that the drug problem will be solved by criminal sanction. No social problems are. We agree with the Harlem barbershop owner who said the idea that jails stop drugs is "like saying cemeteries stop death." Along with deterring use and punishing sales, we also must learn more about causes and prevention of drug use.

The battle to end the drug abuse epidemic is likely to be won or lost in families and neighborhoods, in workplaces and schools. Do we, individually and collectively, tolerate or do we reject illicit drug use? The debate about legalization simply delays the important commitment to reject the use of illicit drugs. It also demoralizes the people most committed to ending the drug problem by raising questions about national support for their vital efforts.

Debating legalization is a dangerous decision. Why now, when only a few months ago the federal government released new statistics that showed a 37 percent decline in the regular use of illicit drugs in America, a fall that included every region in the nation, all races, both sexes, and all social classes? With that sort of progress in the war on drugs, this is a particularly odd time to give up a battle.

The problem with drugs is drug use. Every proposed reform that makes drugs more available or acceptable is going to increase drug use. It would also increase the suffering and unhappiness that flows from drug use for both users and nonusers of drugs.

6

Legalizing Drugs Would Sidestep the Moral Issue

Rushworth M. Kidder

Should drugs be legalized?

In the wake of the State Department report earlier this month showing soaring levels of global drug production and abuse, the arguments for legalization seem seductive. Look what would happen, proponents say, if the price of a packet of white stuff fell from a few thousand dollars to a few cents. In one swoop, they claim, you would gut the gangsters' budgets, encourage addicts to seek help openly, and clean up street crime. Isn't that the answer?

No, says Boston University's Edwin Delattre. Legalization, says the quiet-spoken philosopher and former president of St. John's College in Annapolis, Maryland, is "not only implausible—it's downright foolish, it's dangerous, and I hasten to add, I think it's immoral."

Professor Delattre, who consults with the FBI and police departments when he's not teaching ethics, knows whereof he speaks. For years he's been riding with police officers on their inner-city beats. Out of that experience has come his latest book, *Character and Cops: Ethics in Policing.* Out of it, too, comes his conviction about the perils of legalization.

First, he notes, even proponents of legalization admit that "if you legalize, consumption and therefore addiction will rise substantially." That's been the case with alcohol, he observes, which now claims 23,000 lives on American highways each year. That's been the experience in Italy, where legalization of drugs has produced "an enormous addict population and a very high AIDS rate." And that's what happened in the United States when, from 1912 to 1925, heroin clinics were legalized. In those years, he notes,

Originally published in the *Christian Science Monitor,* March 12, 1990.

"levels of corruption were so high and the distribution of the drug [to new users] so great that it made the heroin problem worse, not better."

Second, there is no evidence that legalization destroys black markets or the crimes that go with those markets. Case in point: gambling. Since it was legalized in Atlantic City in 1977, says Delattre, every category of indexed crime [in that city] has increased by over 400 percent. Six of the last seven mayors have been indicted, and the public service agencies are among the most corrupt in the country."

Why should that be? Because, he reasons, legalization involves a tremendous regulatory network. And there are always profits to be made by breaking regulations. Drug dealers won't stop dealing. They'll simply shift gears—underselling the government, targeting people who can't legally buy, or offering more attractive conditions to addicts.

Third, the idea that legalization will sweep all current addicts into treatment clinics is naive. Many won't go. Some will go only sporadically. Others will find that the research has not yet produced the so-called maintenance drugs that can help them. After all, yesterday's somewhat treatable cocaine and heroin have already been joined by crack and ice, which are much more difficult to treat. "Given that the drug traffickers could introduce a new free-base drug into the marketplace every year," says Delattre, "how the research would keep up with them is beyond imagination."

What most concerns him, however, is the essential immorality of the quick-fix legalize-now mentality. Legalization, he says, would "undermine the efforts of parents, corporations, and schools, to show that drugs are not wrong because they are illegal—they are illegal because they are wrong."

That message, he feels, has recently been getting through. But "if you legalize stuff that's as lethal as this, what else will you legalize? It seems to me that you have declared there are no limits to the tolerable."

In the end, that's the point: that there *are* limits to the tolerable. A society in despair may wish to redefine its way out of its problems. Simply declaring that wrong is right, however, is no way to address the situation. Hats off to Delattre for bringing the clear insights of philosophy to bear on that point.

7

Legalizing Drugs:
A "Dangerous Idea"

Charles B. Rangel

On the surface, the call by Baltimore Mayor Kurt Schmoke [May 15, 1988] and others for a national debate on decriminalizing illicit narcotics seems reasonable. Schmoke is clearly right that more narcotics entering the United States are generating more addicts and more crime.

The answer, however, is not surrender before we have even fought the war. When we consider that the [Reagan] administration has no one in charge, full-time, of the No. 1 problem facing the nation, and that the person the president has placed in charge, Attorney General Edwin Meese, is obviously concerned with other personal as well as substantive issues, the lack of seriousness of the national effort to date is obvious. Top administration officials, including Office of Management and Budget Director James Miller and Secretary of Education William Bennett, have testified that drug use, drug-related crime, and school-based prevention are "state and local" problems, not national issues. To me, this is absurd, considering that practically not one ounce of cocaine or heroin is grown in any community in the United States. We clearly have a national and international crisis mandating a federal commitment.

To be given serious consideration, the advocates of a "debate" on legalization or decriminalization of drugs would have to bring some answers to the table. I would ask the following questions:

- Which narcotic and psychotropic drugs should be legalized? On what criteria should this decision be based?

Originally published in the *Washington Post*, June 11, 1988. Reprinted by permission of the author.

- Should narcotic and psychotropic drugs be made available to anyone who wishes to try them—or just to people already dependent on them?
- Would an unlimited supply of drugs be made available to habitual users or addicts? Or would they have to pay the market price, even for drugs for which an increasing tolerance would require the purchase of ever larger quantities? Could those who were heavily dependent or addicted work or even hold a job? Or would they resort to crime to support their legal habit and to provide livelihoods for themselves and their dependents?
- Who would provide drugs? Private companies? The government? Would they be provided at cost or for a profit—or be subject to a tax? If taxed, what would be a fair rate?
- Where would these drugs be made available? Pharmacies? Supermarkets? Special shops? Dispensaries? Clinics?
- Would use of legalized drugs by employees in certain occupations be prohibited? Since marijuana can remain in the body for weeks after use, would marijuana use by employees in jobs in which security and safety are at issue be forbidden even off duty? What about airline pilots, surgeons, police, firefighters, military personnel, railroad engineers, bus drivers, cross-country truckers, nuclear reactor operators— even Wall Street brokers and teachers?
- What rate of addiction and dependency would one project if drugs were legalized and thereby made cheaper and more readily available? Wouldn't cheap and readily available legal drugs result in more people using more drugs? What would one project the accidental drug-related death rate to be?
- What is the opinion of medical experts as to the potential effects of legalization? And of drug-treatment experts?
- Would legalization affect medical insurance rates and the overall cost of health care?
- Would we be adding to the spread of AIDS by having more addicts using more needles?

It just may be that when these questions are answered, the very dangerous idea of legalization of drugs will be put to rest once and for all. Then I hope we can get on with the battle with a true federal commitment to confronting our greatest crisis.

8

Just Say "No!" to
Proposal to Make Drug Use Legal

Joseph R. Biden Jr.

Recently, I have heard a number of intellectuals and radio and TV talk-show hosts advocating the legalization of drugs. I suspect they are voicing the frustration many Americans feel in trying to deal with this serious issue. But as the old adage goes: "To every difficult and complex problem there is a simple solution, and it is wrong."

The same holds true for drug legalization. Its simplicity is enticing, but it would create far more problems than it would solve.

Advocates of legalization raise a number of arguments. For instance, they say there will be fewer people selling drugs, because it will be regulated and profits will be cut. In addition, they claim with drug-dealing criminals out of the picture, crime and violence will drop.

These arguments depend on the price of drugs, such as heroin and cocaine, dropping so low that criminal organizations will have little incentive to sell in a black market. But if legal drugs are loaded up with taxes to raise enough money to pay for the treatment and education programs needed for drug addicts, drug dealers still would sell untaxed drugs for illegal profits. And it would be harder to stop this new black market than it is today, because it would be legal to possess and ship drugs.

Furthermore, drug buyers, not drug sellers, commit most drug-related crimes. It is addicts who have no jobs or whose jobs cannot support a drug habit who rob and mug people.

The hard-core users will not stop committing crimes because the price is lower. The cocaine and heroin addict's appetite for drugs is practically insa-

---

Originally published in the *Philadelphia Tribune,* April 3, 1990.

tiable. If prices drop, addicts will use more. If they have no jobs, they will steal to buy as much as they can afford.

Even if hard-core drug users could support their habits with less criminal activity, an increase in drug use itself would give rise to more violence in America. People who use drugs like crack and ice become paranoid, irritable, and prone to violence. They abuse their children; they assault other people— not just for money, but because violence itself is often a drug-induced behavior.

In addition, the majority of crack-cocaine users in this country are under the age of twenty-one. I am not aware of any legalization proponent who believes we should sell drugs to minors. So half of the existing crack market, and a large portion of the market for other drugs, would still be in the illegal domain.

Drug legalization advocates also base their arguments on the comparison between the prohibition of alcohol with the illegal status of drugs. They say prohibition of alcohol didn't work. But the truth is that between 1916 and 1922 alcohol consumption declined by 30 to 50 percent, alcohol-related deaths and disease declined, and arrests for drunkenness and disorderly conduct dropped 50 percent.

I am not proposing to reinstate the prohibition of alcohol, but when it is used as an argument for legalizing drugs, we should examine the facts. Knowing the harm alcohol abuse has caused our society, we would be extremely foolish to welcome a more addictive set of chemicals into our lives.

9

Mistakes of the Legalizers

Charles Krauthammer

Little was expected from the three-day global conference, completed Wednesday [April 11, 1990] in London, on the world drug trade. But there was one result that should be important to Americans: the 112 participating nations unanimously rejected legalization as a solution to the drug problem.

This is important for Americans because drug talk, like drug use, has its cycles, and we are now in the midst of the first real burst of legalization talk since 1979. The legalizers, who now include such establishment types as George Shultz, Baltimore Mayor Kurt Schmoke, and the [London] *Economist,* have a very simple theme: things cannot get worse. Prohibition, as they like to call it, leads to crime, corruption, and ruinous cost. We have to do something, they insist. Take the crime out of drugs, and the residue will be a mere public health problem.

Like all arguments born of desperation, this one has little appeal to reason. Just how desperate becomes clear whenever you ask a legalization advocate to spell out exactly what his brave new world would look like. Late last year, Judge Robert Sweet of New York became the latest establishment figure to earn his fifteen minutes of fame by advocating legalization. But at least Sweet, the first federal judge to go over to the legalization side, had the candor to offer a rather precise picture of the world after prohibition.

A charming picture indeed. You come in and browse at a government-run store that prices and sells the stuff. After checking out competing brands of hashish, heroin, crack, and PCP, you pay for what you want and take the lot home. But—this is my favorite touch—you are not permitted to buy a

Originally published in the *Washington Post,* April 13, 1990. © 1990, Washington Post Writers Group. Reprinted with permission.

lethal dose unless you have a doctor's prescription. Derangement on demand but death by prescription. Solomonic reasoning for an Aldous Huxley world.

What to do about all the new junkies? Here the legalizers split along party lines. Liberals want to pour the money saved from drug enforcement into treatment for all the addicts they have created—a brilliant Humphrey-Hawkins job creation program for ex-addicts and social workers. Conservatives, such as libertarian Milton Friedman, say that if someone wants to poison himself with drugs, that is his business, but it does not entitle him to any special sympathy or subsidy from the state.

Take your pick: the liberal dream of state-run coke stores subsidizing state-run coke clinics or the conservative vision of a new generation of ruggedly individual addicts turned loose on the street. Whichever you prefer, you must admit one thing: While the corner coke store would undoubtedly cut down habit-supporting crime, it would just as surely increase addiction. In order to undercut the black market, legalization must radically reduce the price of drugs. And the price of drugs is the surest predictor of use. Drugs are like any other commodity: the lower the price, the higher the consumption.

The cost to society of increased drug abuse would dwarf the $8 million now allocated to the "war on drugs." The cost in cocaine-addicted newborns and cocaine-ravaged families, in broken homes and abused children, in traffic death and absenteeism, in spontaneous violence and plain random street looniness would be immense. A recent report from the Bahamas studied what happened when the price of cocaine declined by 80 percent. Cocaine-related admissions at the one psychiatric hospital in Nassau went from zero to three hundred.

The historical record, too, is clear. Whatever else it was, the prohibition of alcohol was a public health success: The incidence of cirrhosis and alcoholic psychosis declined dramatically during Prohibition. In fact, it took until 1971 for alcohol consumption to resume pre-Prohibition levels.

In discussing the social costs of increased drug use, legalization advocates are rather disingenuous. Judge Sweet evinces concern for the abandoned and abused kids from crack-destroyed homes. This phenomenon, he argues, "demonstrates the failure of our present prohibition. . . . There is no present evidence that prohibition has, or will, break this vicious cycle of dependence and abandonment."

Of course it won't, and no one claims it will. The only claim is that prohibition at least *contains* this vicious cycle. Lifting prohibition can only make it worse. It is simply perverse to suggest that because criminalizing crack doesn't prevent abandoned children, the answer is to legalize crack, a sure prescription for more abandoned children.

To make their case come out right the legalizers are forced to resort to the most tortured logic. Take the likelihood that there will be some increasing crime caused directly by drug-induced violence. The chief guru of the legalization movement, Ethan Nadelmann, tries to diffuse that argument by pointing out that 54 percent of inmates convicted in the United States are already under the influence of alcohol at the time of the crime. An odd defense for legalizing yet another drug that can induce violent behavior.

And who would dispense the stuff? The *Economist,* another pro-legalization heavy, weighs in with the helpful suggestion that it should be distributed by the "glum state liquor stores of Sweden or New Hampshire" or "the post office, which has perfected the art of driving customers away." The *Economist* has a deserved reputation for wit. Wit is indeed the only defense left against the certainty that legal dope, even if dispensed in less than boutique surroundings, would bring a nightmarish increase in drug abuse.

The critics are right. The current drug situation is intolerable. But only America the comfortable could possibly imagine that things cannot get worse. They can get infinitely worse, and if drugs are legalized they will.

10

Some among Us Would Seek to Surrender

Daryl F. Gates

History teaches that no matter how violent and unprovoked the enemy's attack or how just and winnable the war, there will always be some among us who will work for our defeat or surrender. We call them fifth columnists.

Today, we have a fifth column in the war on drugs. "People of America, let us give in to our enemy," it urges. The enemy, the fifth column argues, is not all that bad; if approached in the right way, it could even be our friend. So why continue to waste valuable resources and national energy on an unwinnable war? Let's legalize drugs and get on with living the good life, the fifth column advises.

I suppose that calling pushers of drug legalization treasonous would be too extreme. But I'll continue to wonder why they choose to weaken our war effort just when we, as a nation, are beginning to take the offensive.

We *are* on the offensive. In Washington, there is a comprehensive, fully funded national strategy in place that includes use of armed forces and diplomatic initiatives to fight the drug war. The Colombian government has reestablished its authority over the Medellin cartel. Manuel Noriega is in jail, and Mexico has been pressured to further clamp down on traffickers and marijuana growers. At home, drug-infested neighborhoods in city after city are being liberated by a combination of good people and good policing. Six thousand police officers are in classrooms across the nation each day teaching millions of kids the DARE (Drug Abuse Resistance Education) curriculum. Teaching our children self-esteem, self-discipline, a reverence for the law, and our moral values is beginning to pay off. And Operation Cul de

Originally published in the *Los Angeles Times,* March 15, 1990. Reprinted by permission of the author.

Sac in South Central Los Angels has proved so successful that two hundred youngsters who were too afraid to leave their homes to attend Jefferson High School are now back in class.

Despite these and other examples of progress, the fifth columnists chant, "Legalize drugs, and crime will automatically go down." That would happen, they argue, because decriminalization would take the profit out of dealing. The fact is that the kind of crime that puts fear into the hearts of citizens was lowest during Prohibition. People were not burglarized, robbed, and killed by drinkers who needed money to buy a bottle of illegal whiskey.

In any event, the economic argument for legalization is perhaps the most interesting—and the most spurious. As James Q. Wilson wrote . . . in *Commentary*:*

> Addicts would no longer steal to pay black-market prices for drugs, a real gain. But some, perhaps a great deal, of that gain would be offset by the great increase in the number of addicts. These people, nodding on heroin or living in the delusion-ridden high of cocaine, would hardly be ideal employees. Many would steal simply to support themselves. . . . Society could decide to support all unemployable addicts on welfare, but that would mean that gains from lowered rates of crime would have to be offset by large increases in welfare budgets.

Advocates of drug legalization say that the money would come from a tax on drugs. But such a levy couldn't be too high, lest our druggies do their buying in a tax-free black market. Once again, we are being asked to accept what bulls excrete.

Dr. Herbert Kleber, the Bush administration official in charge of demand reduction, predicts that legalization might lead to a five- to sixfold increase in cocaine use. Why wouldn't the number of murders in Los Angeles increase by a similar factor of five or six? (Half of the 874 murders in Los Angeles last year were drug-related.) That translates to 2,400 homicides. A Los Angeles with that murder rate would be a very exciting and interesting place in which to be chief of police, but I would not want to live here.

Some sentimentalists (myself included) worry about babies who have been prenatally exposed to drugs. In 1988, 375,000 addicted babies were born in the United States. Researchers say these infants lack the enthusiasm of healthy newborns, that their facial expressions are flat and joyless. What kind of people would we be if we allowed such joyless faces to be born into our society in ever-increasing numbers? Probably people who should find a holiday to celebrate other than Mother's Day.

Addicted babies will require special treatment and assistance as they grow up, probably for the rest of their lives. Their drug-using mothers will certainly not provide the necessary help. Of course, society could use some

---

*Chapter 3 in this volume.

of the revenue generated by a drug tax to help offset this huge welfare cost—
if there is any money left after the increased number of addicts are taken care
of. If there is no money, the problem might be solved by sterilizing all
women of child-bearing age who play around with drugs. Clearly, either
alternative is incompatible with our values.

History repeatedly teaches us that advanced societies cannot survive if
their fundamental values are not continuously nourished. [Los Angeles]
Times columnist Jim Murray said it best when he wrote about proposals to
get government involved in legalized sports betting.

> The state has apparently succumbed to the argument that gambling is always
> going to be around, so why not get in on it? OK? But, why stop there? People
> are always going to rob banks. So why not get in on that? Let's license bank rob-
> bers for a percentage of the take. Humanity is always going to sell dope,
> embezzle funds, cheat widows and orphans, rig the stock market. Should gov-
> ernment get in on that, too? The government's notion seems to be, why should
> the crooks get all the money? We'll become the crooks.

Murray doesn't believe that is what the Founding Fathers had in mind
when they created our republic. Neither do I.

Come on, folks. We can, we will, we must win the war on drugs—not for
the "Gipper"* but for ourselves, our kids, and the future of our nation. If we
don't, we do not deserve to survive.

---

*A reference to former President Ronald Reagan. (Ed.)

11

Should We Legalize Drugs?
History Answers . . . No

David T. Courtwright

One thing that all parties in the American drug-policy debate agree on is that they want to eliminate the traffic in illicit drugs and the criminal syndicates that control it. There are two divergent strategies for achieving this end: the drug war and drug legalization, or, more precisely, controlled legalization, since few people want the government to simply abandon drug control and proclaim laissez faire.

The drug war was launched during the Reagan administration. It is actually the fourth such campaign, there having been sustained legislative and governmental efforts against drug abuse between 1909 and 1923, 1951 and 1956, and 1971 and 1973. What distinguishes the current war is that it is more concerned with stimulants like cocaine than with opiates, it is larger, and—no surprise in our age of many zeros—it is much more expensive.

The war against drugs has included the treatment of addicts and educational programs designed to discourage new users, but the emphasis has been on law enforcement, with interdiction, prosecution, imprisonment, and the seizure of assets at the heart of the campaign. The news from the front has been mixed. Price and purity levels, treatment and emergency-room admissions, urinalyses, and most other indices of drug availability showed a worsening of the problem during the 1980s, with some improvement in 1989 and 1990. The number of casual cocaine users has recently declined, but cocaine addiction remains widespread, affecting anywhere from about 650,000 to 2.4 million compulsive users, depending on whose definitions and estimates one chooses to accept. There has been some success in stopping marijuana im-

Originally published in *American Heritage* (February–March 1993). Reprinted by permission of *American Heritage* magazine, a division of Forbes, Inc. © Forbes, Inc., 1993.

ports—shipments of the drug are relatively bulky and thus easier to detect—but this has been offset by the increased domestic cultivation of high-quality marijuana, which has more than doubled since 1985. Heroin likewise has become both more available and more potent than it was in the late 1970s.

But cocaine has been the drug of greatest concern. Just how severe the crisis has become may be gauged by federal cocaine seizures. Fifty years ago the annual haul for the entire nation was one or two pounds, an amount that could easily be contained in the glove compartment of a car. As late as 1970 the total was under five hundred pounds, which would fit in the car's trunk. In fiscal year 1990 it was 235,000 pounds—about the weight of sixty mid-size cars. And this represented a fraction, no more than 10 percent, of what went into the nostrils and lungs and veins of the approximately seven million Americans who used cocaine during 1990. Worse may be in store. World-wide production of coca surged during 1989 to a level of 225,000 metric tons, despite U.S. efforts to eradicate cultivation. Global production of opium, marijuana, and hashish has likewise increased since President Reagan formally declared war on drugs in 1986.

The greatest obstacle to the supply-reduction strategy is the enormous amount of money generated by the illicit traffic. Drug profits have been used to buy off foreign and domestic officials and to secure protection for the most vulnerable stages of the drug-cultivation, -manufacturing, and -distribution process. These profits also hire various specialists, from assassins to money launderers to lawyers, needed to cope with interlopers; they pay for technological devices ranging from cellular phones to jet planes; and they ensure that should a trafficker die or land in jail, there will be no shortage of replacements.

It is hardly surprising that these stubborn economic realities, together with the drug war's uneven and often disappointing results, have led several commentators to question the wisdom of what they call the prohibition policy. What is unprecedented is that these disenchanted critics include mayors, prominent lawyers, federal judges, nationally syndicated columnists, a congressman, a Princeton professor, and a Nobel laureate in economics. They espouse variations of a position that is often called controlled legalization, meaning that the sale of narcotics should be permitted under conditions that restrict and limit consumption, such as no sales to minors, no advertising, and substantial taxation. They cite the numerous advantages of this approach: Several billion dollars per year would be realized from tax revenues and savings on law enforcement; crime would diminish because addicts would not have to hustle to keep themselves supplied with drugs; the murders associated with big-city drug trafficking would abate as lower-cost, legal drugs drive the traffickers out of business. Because these drugs would be of known quality and potency, and because they would not have to be injected with shared needles, the risk of overdose and infection would drop. The issue of foreign complicity in the drug traffic, which has complicated

American diplomatic relations with many countries, would disappear. Under a policy of controlled legalization, it would be no more criminal or controversial to import coca from Colombia than to import coffee.

The more candid of the legalization proponents concede that these advantages would be purchased at the cost of increased drug abuse. Widespread availability, lower prices, and the elimination of the criminal sanction would result in more users, some of whom would inevitably become addicts. But how many more? Herbert Kleber, a treatment specialist and former deputy director of the Office of National Drug Control Policy, has argued that there would be between twelve and fifty-five million addicted users if cocaine and heroin were legally available. While it is impossible to anticipate the exact magnitude of the increase, history does support Kleber's argument. In countries like Iran or Thailand, where narcotics have long been cheap, potent, and readily available, the prevalence of addiction has been and continues to be quite high. Large quantities of opium sold by British and American merchants created a social disaster in nineteenth-century China; that Chinese sailors and immigrants subsequently introduced opium smoking to Britain and America is a kind of ironic justice. Doctors, who constantly work with and around narcotics, have historically had a very serious addiction problem: Estimates of the extent of morphine addiction among American physicians at the turn of the century ran from 6 percent to an astonishing 23 percent. In a word, exposure matters.

Kleber has also attacked the crime-reduction rationale by pointing out that addicts will generally use much more of an illicit substance if the cost is low. They would spend most of their time using drugs and little of it working, thus continuing to resort to crime to acquire money. If the total number of addicts rose sharply as availability increased, total crime would also increase. There would be less crime committed by any single addict but more crime in the aggregate.

The debate over decriminalization is, in essence, an argument about a high-stakes gamble, and so far the opponents represent the majority view. At the close of the 1980s, four out of every five Americans were against the legalization of marijuana, let alone cocaine. But if the drug war produces another decade of indifferent results, growing disillusionment could conceivably prompt experiments in controlled legalization.

The controlled-legalization argument rests on the assumption that legal sales would largely eliminate the illicit traffic and its attendant evils. The history of drug use, regulation, and taxation in the United States suggests otherwise. The very phrase *controlled legalization* implies denying certain groups access to drugs. Minors are the most obvious example. No one advocates supplying narcotics to children, so presumably selling drugs to anyone under twenty-one would remain a criminal offense, since that is the cutoff point for sales of beverage alcohol. Unfortunately, illicit drug abuse in this century has become concentrated among the young—that is, among the very ones most likely to be made exceptions to the rule of legal sales.

Until about 1900 the most common pattern of drug dependence in the United States was opium or morphine addiction, brought about by the treatment of chronic diseases and painful symptoms. Addicts were mainly female, middle-class, and middle-aged or older; Eugene O'Neill's mother, fictionalized as Mary Tyrone in *Long Day's Journey into Night,* was one. Habitual users of morphine, laudanum, and other medicinal opiates in their adolescence were extremely rare, even in big cities like Chicago.

Another pattern of drug use was nonmedical and had its roots in marginal, deviant, and criminal subcultures. The "pleasure users," as they were sometimes called, smoked opium, sniffed cocaine, injected morphine and cocaine in combination, or, after 1910, sniffed or injected heroin. Nonmedical addicts began much younger than their medical counterparts. The average age of addiction (not first use, which would have been lower still) for urban heroin addicts studied in the 1910s was only nineteen or twenty years. They were also more likely to be male than those whose addiction was of medical origin, and more likely to have been involved in crime.

Initially the pleasure users were the smaller group, but during the first two decades of this century—the same period when the police approach to national drug control was formulated—the number of older, docile medical addicts steadily diminished. There were several reasons: doctors became better educated and more conservative in their use of narcotics; the population grew healthier; patent-medicine manufacturers were forced to reveal the contents of their products; and the numerous morphine addicts who had been created in the nineteenth century began to age and die off. Drug use and addiction became increasingly concentrated among young men in their teens and twenties, a pattern that continues to this day.

In 1980, 44 percent of drug arrests nationwide were of persons under the age of twenty-one. There were more arrests among teenagers than among the entire population over the age of twenty-five; eighteen-year-olds had the highest arrest rate of any age group. By 1987 the proportion of those arrested under twenty-one had declined to 25 percent. This was partly due to the aging of the population and to the effects of drug education on students. But when large numbers of "echo boomers"—the children of the baby boomers—become adolescents during the 1990s, the percentage of under-twenty-one drug arrests will likely increase.

So, depending on timing and demographic circumstances, at least a quarter and perhaps more than a third of all drug buyers would be underage, and there would be a great deal of money to be made by selling to them. The primary source of supply would likely be diversion—adults legally purchasing drugs and selling them to customers below the legal age. The sellers (or middlemen who collected and then resold the legal purchases) would make a profit through marking up or adulterating the drugs, and there might well be turf disputes and hence violence. Some of the dealers and their underage purchasers would be caught, prosecuted, and jailed, and the criminal-justice system would still be burdened with drug arrests. The black market would be altered and diminished, but it would scarcely disappear.

Potential for illegal sales and use extends far beyond minors. Pilots; police officers; firefighters; drivers of buses, trains, taxis, and ambulances; surgeons; active-duty military personnel; and others whose drug use would jeopardize public safety would be denied access to at least some drugs, and those of them who did take narcotics would be liable to criminal prosecution, as would their suppliers. Pregnant women would also pose a problem. Drugs transmitted to fetuses can cause irreversible and enormously costly harm. Federal and local governments may soon be spending billions of dollars a year just to prepare the impaired children of addicts for kindergarten. Society has the right and the obligation to stop this neurological carnage, both because it cruelly handicaps innocents and because it harms everyone else through higher taxes and health-insurance premiums. Paradoxically, the arguments for controlled legalization might lead to denying alcohol and tobacco to pregnant women along with narcotics. Alcohol and tobacco can also harm fetal development, and several legalization proponents have observed that it is both inconsistent and unwise to treat them as if they were not dangerous because they are legal. If cocaine is denied to pregnant women, why not alcohol too? The point here is simply that every time one makes an exception for good and compelling reasons—every time one accents the "controlled" as opposed to the "legalization"—one creates the likelihood of continued illicit sales and use.

The supposition that this illegal market would be fueled by diversion is well founded historically. There has always been an undercurrent of diversion, especially in the late 1910s and 1920s, when black-market operators like Legs Diamond got their supplies not so much by smuggling as by purchases from legitimate drug companies. One possible solution is to require of all legal purchasers that which is required of newly enrolled methadone patients: consumption of the drug on the premises. Unfortunately, unlike methadone, heroin and cocaine are short-acting, and compulsive users must administer them every few hours or less. The dayrooms of drug-treatment clinics set up in Britain after 1968 to provide heroin maintenance were often clogged with whining addicts. Frustrated and angry, the clinic staffs largely abandoned heroin during the 1970s, switching instead to methadone, which, having the advantages of oral administration and twenty-four-hour duration, is far more suitable for clinic-based distribution. Confining the use of heroin or cocaine or other street drugs to clinics would be a logistical nightmare. But the alternative, take-home supplies, invites illegal sales to excluded groups.

Another historical pattern of black-market activity has been the smuggling of drugs to prisoners. Contraband was one of the reasons the government built specialized narcotic hospitals in Lexington, Kentucky, and Fort

Worth, Texas, in the 1930s. Federal wardens wanted to get addicts out of their prisons because they were constantly conniving to obtain smuggled drugs. But when drug-related arrests multiplied after 1965 and the Lexington and Fort Worth facilities were closed, the prisons again filled with inmates eager to obtain drugs. Birch Bayh, chairing a Senate investigation of the matter in 1975, observed that in some institutions young offenders had a more plentiful supply of drugs than they did on the outside.

Since then more jails have been crammed with more prisoners, and these prisoners are more likely than ever to have had a history of drug use. In 1989, 60 to 80 percent of male arrestees in twelve large American cities tested positive for drugs. It is hard to imagine a controlled-legalization system that would permit sales to prisoners. Alcohol, although a legal drug, is not sold licitly in prisons, and for good reason, as more than 40 percent of prisoners were under its influence when they committed their crimes. If drugs are similarly denied to inmates, then the contraband problem will persist. If, moreover, we insist that our nearly three million parolees and probationers remain clean on the theory that drug use aggravates recidivism, the market for illegal sales would be so much the larger.

By now the problem should be clear. If drugs are legalized, but not for those under twenty-one, or for public-safety officers, or transport workers, or military personnel, or pregnant women, or prisoners, or probationers, or parolees, or psychotics, or any of several other special groups one could plausibly name, then just exactly who is going to buy them? Noncriminal adults, whose drug use is comparatively low to begin with? Controlled legalization entails a dilemma. To the extent that its controls are enforced, some form of black-market activity will persist. If, on the other hand, its controls are not enforced and drugs are easily diverted to those who are underage or otherwise ineligible, then it is a disguised form of wholesale legalization and as such morally, politically, and economically unacceptable.

One of the selling points of controlled legalization was also one of the decisive arguments for the repeal of Prohibition: taxation. Instead of spending billions to suppress the illicit traffic, the government would reap billions by imposing duties on legitimate imports and taxes on domestically manufactured drugs. Not only could these revenues be earmarked for drug treatment and education programs, but they would also increase the prices paid by the consumer, thus discouraging consumption, especially among adolescents.

The United States government has had extensive historical experience with the taxation of legal narcotics. In the nineteenth and early twentieth centuries, opium was imported and subject to customs duties. The imports were assigned to one of three categories. The first was crude opium, used mainly for medicinal purposes and for the domestic manufacture of morphine. Foreign-manufactured morphine, codeine, and heroin made up the second class of imports, while the third was smoking opium, most of it prepared in Hong Kong and shipped to San Francisco.

The imposts on these imported drugs fluctuated over the years, but they were generally quite stiff. From 1866 to 1914 the average ad valorem duty on crude opium was 33 percent; for morphine or its salts, 48 percent. From 1866 to 1908 the average duty on smoking opium was an extraordinarily high 97 percent. This last was in the nature of a sin tax; congressmen identified opium smoking with Chinese coolies, gamblers, pimps, and prostitutes and wished to discourage its importation and use.

These customs duties produced revenue; they also produced widespread smuggling, much of it organized by violent criminal societies like the Chinese tongs. The smugglers were as ingenious as their latter-day Mafia counterparts. They hid their shipments in everything from hollowed-out lumber to snake cages. Avoiding the customs collectors, they saved as much as three dollars a pound on crude opium, three dollars an ounce on morphine, and twelve dollars a pound on smoking opium. Twelve dollars seems a trifling sum by modern standards, hardly worth the risk of arrest, but in the nineteenth century it was more than most workers earned in a week. Someone who smuggled in fifty pounds of smoking opium in 1895 had gained the equivalent of a year's wages. One knowledgeable authority estimated that when the duty on smoking opium was near its peak, the amount smuggled into the United States was nearly twice that legally imported and taxed. Something similar happened with eighteenth-century tobacco imports to the British Isles. More than a third of the tobacco consumed in England and Scotland circa 1750 had been clandestinely imported in order to avoid a duty of more than five pence per pound. The principle is the same for domestically produced drugs: If taxes are sufficiently onerous, an illegal supply system will spring up. Moonshining existed before and after, as well as during, Prohibition.

The obvious solution is to set taxes at a sufficiently low level to discourage smuggling and illegal manufacturing. But again there is a dilemma. The most important illicit drugs are processed agricultural products that can be grown in several parts of the world by peasant labor. They are not, in other words, intrinsically expensive. Unless they are heavily taxed, legal consumers will be able to acquire them at little cost, less than ten dollars for a gram of cocaine. if drugs are that cheap, to say nothing of being 100 percent pure, the likelihood of a postlegalization epidemic of addiction will be substantially increased. But if taxes are given a stiff boost to enhance revenues and limit consumption, black marketeers will reenter the picture in numbers proportionate to the severity of the tax.

Tax revenues, like drugs themselves, can be addictive. In the twelve years after the repeal of Prohibition, federal liquor tax revenues ballooned from 259 million to 2.3 billion dollars. The government's dependence on this money was one important reason antiliquor forces made so little progress in their attempts to restrict alcohol consumption during World War II. Controlled drug legalization would also bring about a windfall in tax dollars, which in an era of chronic deficits would surely be welcomed and quickly spent. Should addiction rates become too high, a conflict between public health and revenue concerns would inevitably ensue.

When both proponents and opponents of controlled legalization talk about drug taxes, they generally assume a single level of taxation. The assumption is wrong. The nature of the federal system permits state and local governments to levy their own taxes on drugs in addition to the uniform federal customs and excise taxes. This means that total drug taxes, and hence the prices paid by consumers, will vary from place to place. Variation invites interstate smuggling, and if the variation is large enough, the smuggling can be extensive and involve organized crime.

The history of cigarette taxation serves to illustrate this principle. In 1960 state taxes on cigarettes were low, between zero and eight cents per pack, but after 1965 a growing number of states sharply increased cigarette taxes in response to health concerns and as a politically painless way of increasing revenue. Some states, mainly in the Northeast, were considerably more aggressive than others in raising taxes. By 1975 North Carolina purchasers were paying thirty-six cents per pack while New Yorkers paid fifty-four cents. The price was higher still in New York City because of a local levy that reached eight cents per pack (as much as the entire federal tax) at the beginning of 1976.

Thus was born an opportunity to buy cheap and sell dear. Those who bought in volume at North Carolina prices and sold at New York (or Connecticut, or Massachusetts) prices realized a substantial profit, and by the mid-1970s net revenue losses stood at well over three hundred million dollars a year. Much of this went to organized crime. which at one point was bootlegging 25 percent of the cigarettes sold in New York State and *half* of those sold in New York City. The pioneer of the illegal traffic, Anthony Granata, established a trucking company with thirty employees operating vehicles on a six-days-a-week basis. Granata's methods—concealed cargoes, dummy corporations, forged documents, fortresslike warehouses, bribery, hijacking, assault, and homicide—were strikingly similar to those used by illicit drug traffickers and Prohibition bootleggers.

Although high-tax states like Florida or Illinois still lose millions annually to cigarette bootleggers, the 1978 federal Contraband Cigarette Act and stricter law enforcement and accounting procedures have had some success in reducing over-the-road smuggling. But it is relatively easy to detect illegal shipments of cigarettes, which must be smuggled by the truckload to make a substantial amount of money. Cocaine and heroin are more compact, more profitable, and very easy to conceal. Smuggling these drugs to take advantage of state tax differentials would consequently be much more difficult to detect and deter. If, for example, taxed cocaine retailed in Vermont for ten dollars a gram and in New York for twelve dollars a gram, anyone who bought just five kilograms at Vermont prices, transported them, and sold them at New York prices would realize a profit of ten thousand dollars. Five kilograms of cocaine can be concealed in an attache case.

Of course, if all states legalized drugs and taxed them at the same rate, this sort of illegal activity would not exist, but it is constitutionally and politically unfeasible to ensure uniform rates of state taxation. And federalism poses other challenges. Laws against drug use and trafficking have been enacted at the local, state, and federal levels. It is probable that if Congress repeals or modifies the national drug laws, some states will go along with controlled legalization while others will not. Nevada, long in the legalizing habit, might jettison its drug laws, but conservative Mormon-populated Utah might not. Alternately, governments could experiment with varying degrees of legalization. Congress might decide that anything was better than the current mayhem in the capital and legislate a broad legalization program for the District of Columbia. At the same time, Virginia and Maryland might experiment with the decriminalization of marijuana, the least risky legalization option, but retain prohibition of the nonmedical use of other drugs. The result would again be smuggling, whether from Nevada to Utah or, save for marijuana, from the District of Columbia to the surrounding states. It is hard to see how any state that chose to retain laws against drugs could possibly stanch the influx of prohibited drugs from adjacent states that did not. New York City's futile attempts to enforce its strict gun-control laws show how difficult it is to restrict locally that which is elsewhere freely available.

I referred earlier to the legalization debate as an argument about a colossal gamble, whether society should risk an unknown increase in drug abuse and addiction to eliminate the harms of drug prohibition, most of which stem from illicit trafficking. "Take the crime out of it" is the rallying cry of the legalization advocates. After reviewing the larger history of narcotic, alcohol, and tobacco use and regulation, it appears that this debate should be recast. It would be more accurate to ask whether society should risk an unknown but possibly substantial increase in drug abuse and addiction in order to bring about an unknown reduction in illicit trafficking and other costs of drug prohibition. Controlled legalization would take some, but by no means all, of the crime out of it. Just how much and what sort of crime would be eliminated would depend upon which groups were to be denied which drugs, the overall level of taxation, and differences in state tax and legalization policies. If the excluded groups were few and all states legalized all drugs and all governments taxed at uniformly low levels, then the black market would be largely eliminated. But these are precisely the conditions that would be most likely to bring about an unacceptably high level of drug abuse. The same variables that would determine how successful the controlled-legalization policy would be in eliminating the black market would also largely determine how unsuccessful it was in containing drug addiction.

12

Taking Drugs Seriously

John Kaplan

It would be difficult to deny that the efforts and resources expended in our attempt to prevent the production of heroin and cocaine in other countries, and to keep out of the United States those drugs that are produced, have passed the point of diminishing returns. The outcry over drugs in the newspapers and on the political hustings, and a look at what is occurring in many public-housing projects and in the large lower-class black and Hispanic neighborhoods of our central cities, should be enough to convince sober observers that our present drug policies have simply not been successful enough.

Of course, there are politicians who still argue that our drug problems can be substantially improved by further attempts to push the Colombian, Mexican, Burmese, and other governments toward greater efforts. But with the military and internal strength they have at their disposal, they are doing about as well as one could expect.

Nor is the related demand to increase the use of our army or navy to stop drug smuggling a more likely source of improvement. The ingenuity of smugglers, the tremendous volume of legitimate trade, and the huge number of individuals crossing our borders make it impracticable to achieve the kind of increases in the interdiction rate that would make heroin and cocaine significantly less available or more expensive in the United States.

The problem, then, for those who realize that our present efforts have bogged down, is what to do. In this respect, drug policy must proceed by elimination. None of the policy options is attractive. All involve great costs— either in expenditures on law enforcement or in damage to public health.

Reprinted with permission of *The Public Interest,* no. 92 (Summer 1988), pp. 32–50. © 1988 by National Affairs, Inc.

Since no option is without severe disadvantages, we can aim only to choose the policy that is least bad.

At one level, the simplest solution would be simply to get out of the way, legalize heroin and cocaine, and allow their sale as we do alcohol's. Until recently this was rarely advocated in print, though for years one would hear such recommendations in private conversation with intellectuals. Now, however, the legalization movement is becoming respectable, and even popular.

A REPEAL OF DRUG PROHIBITION?

Probably the central problem with the solution of legalization is that it ignores basic pharmacology. There is such a thing as a dangerous drug, and both heroin and cocaine undoubtedly fall into this category. It is here, of course, that the alcohol analogy is usually brought up. The analogy is indeed suggestive, because alcohol is by any standard a dangerous drug as well. And when we repealed Prohibition, we replaced a legal ban on alcohol similar to that now imposed on heroin and cocaine with a system of legal, controlled sale, presumably much like that contemplated for heroin and cocaine. There is no doubt that legalization has attractions. When Prohibition was repealed, the enormous inflow of profits to organized crime and the large-scale corruption of public officials caused by the illegal alcohol traffic dropped sharply. And the large number of civil-liberties violations by Prohibition agents ceased as well.

Several factors, however, made the repeal of Prohibition a much better social decision than would be the case with heroin or cocaine. Hard as it is to believe, the social cost of maintaining Prohibition was not only greater than that which heroin and cocaine currently impose upon us, it was even greater than that imposed by what is now our greatest drug problem—alcohol. Although the addict criminality caused by the high price of heroin and cocaine seems to have had no counterpart in the case of alcohol, the strain on our institutions was far greater. Corruption in the United States during Prohibition approximated that which we now associate with many Third World countries. It is true that the heroin and cocaine trades have corrupted many local police, some prosecutors, and a few local judges. During Prohibition, however, things were much worse. Federal judges, federal and state prosecutors, and countless politicians—from congressmen and state governors to mayors, city councilmen, and chiefs of police—were in the pay of bootleggers.

Part of the difference is due to the passage of time. Wave upon wave of reform has made our government a far more honest one in the last fifty years. Perhaps more important is the fact that both before and during Prohibition, alcohol use was common among all social classes and in virtually every area of the nation, and had a much better "image" than heroin and cocaine do today. A society where many people in all walks of life considered themselves drinkers made this activity far more respectable than the use of "hard drugs" is today. And, of course, when an activity is more socially acceptable, it becomes easier for government agents to accept bribes and favors to allow it to continue.

The strain and social costs attributed to Prohibition were not the only factors justifying the legalization of alcohol. The majority of drinkers enjoyed the use of alcohol without any harm to themselves or society. In a sense, the legalization of alcohol represented the willingness of these drinkers to shoulder their share of the social costs of legalized alcohol.

Nonetheless, the example of alcohol control illustrates a basic rule concerning all attempts to minimize the damage caused by habit-forming and destructive drugs. The principle also applies to a number of consensual (somewhat inaccurately called "victimless") crimes, such as gambling and prostitution. When one of these behaviors is made criminal, its enforcement is not particularly effective; it saddles the criminal-justice system with huge costs; it feeds organized criminal gangs; it causes official corruption; and it leads to large numbers of violations of civil liberties. Finally, the law does not really solve the problems of those engaging in the activity.

On the other hand, the legalization of the behavior produces an increase in the behavior, which can produce a public-health problem of enormous magnitude. Prohibition, for example, despite its faults—including the fact that it was not strictly enforced—did lower the amount of drinking in the United States. The comparative figures for cirrhosis of the liver demonstrate this clearly. With the repeal of Prohibition, both the number of drinkers and their per capita consumption of alcohol gradually but substantially increased leading eventually to one of our major public-health problems— alcoholism. According to most estimates, alcoholism results in somewhere between 50,000 and 200,000 deaths per year. And regardless of whether the yearly social cost of alcoholism amounts to forty billion dollars or one hundred and ten billion dollars (two frequently cited figures), no one would deny that the social cost of alcohol use far exceeds that of all illegal drugs together. The issue then is not whether we were correct in legalizing alcohol or tobacco (I would strongly argue that we were), but what we should do about the drugs that are currently illegal.

A PRESCRIPTION SYSTEM?

Of course, criminalization and legalization are not the only possibilities. We are probably correct in using a prescription system for valium, for example, which is quite a dangerous drug—but also a useful one. When heroin addicts in England consisted overwhelmingly of middle-aged, middle-class men and women who had become addicted during the course of medical treatment, a prescription system was successfully used to dispense the drug. (Sale without a prescription was a rather serious crime.) However, when an increasingly higher percentage of those addicted came to be more like American addicts—lower-class, criminal, and thrill-seeking—the "British system" was abandoned. England stopped using the prescription system for more than a tiny and diminishing number of addicts, adopting instead a legal-control method much like that used in the United States.

In any event, no one seems to be arguing for a prescription system to control our major illegal drugs. If marijuana, cocaine, and heroin have legitimate medical uses (and the possibility that heroin is better than morphine at relieving intractable pain is the subject of heated debate, with most of the evidence apparently arguing against its superiority), then a prescription system seems most suitable. In fact, this is already being done: We allow prescriptions for medical use of cocaine and THC, the major active ingredient in marijuana.

Though we can regard heroin addiction itself as a disease, and hence a possible candidate for a prescription system, the problems in making such a system work seem insurmountable, as the British have discovered. The sizable pool of nonaddicted heroin users forms a ready market for diverted prescribed heroin; the ranks of the addicted would thus swell. (It is impossible for a physician to determine how much heroin an addict really "needs," since this amount varies enormously over time.) Moreover, another drug—methadone—that is available by prescription (although only under certain conditions) is seen, both in the United States and in Britain, as much preferable to heroin for the medical treatment of heroin addiction.

The most important reason, however, why a prescription system for marijuana, cocaine, or heroin is just as inappropriate as it would be for alcohol and tobacco is that people generally use these drugs because they want to, and not to cure their ailments. We may be able to treat them and convince them not to use these drugs, but providing these drugs through prescription is not the way to do it.

If the choice for each of the "recreational" drugs is between criminalization and some kind of legalization, then it must be made on a drug-by-drug basis, as was the case with alcohol and tobacco (and coffee, for that matter), taking into account such variables as the pharmacological makeup of each drug and the cost of attempting to suppress it.

This is not an issue to be decided by John Stuart Mill's "simple principle"—that is, by letting each person decide for himself. No nation in the world follows his rule regarding self-harming conduct, and the rule is probably unworkable in a complex, industrial society—particularly one that is a welfare state. Mill's principle, moreover, seems singularly inappropriate when it is applied to a habit-forming, psychoactive drug that alters the user's perspective as to postponement of gratification and his desire for the drug itself.

No Surrender?

On the other hand, certain arguments against legalization are even less impressive. Mill's principle, after all, is on the whole a rather sensible injunction to government, which tends—almost by reflex—to attempt to forbid any activity that it regards as harmful, immoral, or deviant. Far less sensible is the idea, advanced by Jesse Jackson and echoed by A. M. Rosenthal of the *New York Times,* that "you do not win a war by surrendering." Obviously, surrender is sometimes the better course. We did it with alcohol, and, if we go back further, we did it in many states with tobacco. (And in the international arena both we, in Vietnam, and the Soviet Union, in Afghanistan, seem to have improved our respective positions by abandoning a war.)

The nonpragmatic, no-surrender arguments are often coupled with warnings about the consequences of legalization. Such arguments, however, are insubstantial—particularly when compared with the serious arguments with which we should be grappling. Take Rosenthal's *Times* argument: "How can we continue to fight against alcoholism and tobacco addiction," asks Rosenthal, "if we suddenly say that other drugs—even more dangerous—should be made available?" This is not persuasive. First, virtually every scientist who has looked at the issue would acknowledge that one of the illegal drugs— marijuana—is certainly no more dangerous than alcohol. Second, the argument is a *non sequitur.* Legalizing drugs thought to be more dangerous than alcohol and tobacco might well make it even easier to convince alcohol and tobacco users that legalization does not guarantee that these drugs are safe. The educational message of treating what are patently dangerous drugs the same way we treat alcohol might be valuable for yet another reason. Many people still fail to understand that, by virtually any definition, alcohol is a drug. Treating alcohol the same way we treat cocaine and heroin might help drive this point home to many drinkers.

A similar fallacy lies behind a more common and somewhat more general argument—that legalization of a formerly illegal drug "sends the wrong message" to the public, implying that the drug is safe. The fact is that when Prohibition was enacted alcohol was regarded as dangerous, and Prohibition was not repealed because we changed our minds and decided that alcohol was safe. We all grew up believing that tobacco was habit-forming and stunted one's growth, at the very least. People who chose to drink and smoke did not do so because they believed that no one could be hurt by such behavior or that the government gave them its blessing. The simple increase in availability seems to account for all the increase in drug use when a drug is legalized. After all, those who use dangerous drugs that the public condemns tend not to be highly aware of the nuances of governmental messages.

As a result, the issue boils down to a careful weighing of the costs of criminalization of each drug against the public-health costs we could expect if that drug were to become legally available.

I will not consider the case of marijuana. It is the most used of the three major illegal drugs (although its use has decreased considerably in the last decade); but at present marijuana is also the least socially costly of the illegal drugs, in addition to being the drug that has been most effectively interdicted (because of its relatively large bulk). Finally, marijuana is the drug that promises the lowest public-health costs if legalized.

Various commentators have considered the social costs of marijuana's criminalization and the projected public-health costs of legalization. And though they have been shouted down by parent groups and those who seek their votes, these commentators, by and large, have leaned toward legalization. The report of the National Academy of Sciences Committee on Substance Abuse and Habitual Behavior made a rather conservative recommendation: It merely asserted that "the current policies directed at controlling the supply of marijuana should be seriously reconsidered."

Nor need we devote any attention to LSD, mescaline, PCP, or any number of other illegal drugs here; for the illegal status of these drugs has not created a significant social problem.

Needless to say, this is not the case with heroin and cocaine. The costs of restricting supply of these drugs are substantial. Since space does not permit discussions of both heroin and cocaine, I will discuss only the anticipated costs of legalizing cocaine. First, a reasonable calculation of the public-health costs of heroin legalization, based on our admittedly inadequate information, already exists.[1] Second, since cocaine is far more prevalent than heroin, it imposes greater social costs upon us—from the amount of money flowing into criminal syndicates to the number of users arrested for predatory crimes. Third, there seems to be a widespread public agreement—although it is probably mistaken—that cocaine is the more benign of the two drugs.

THE CASE OF COCAINE

At a minimum, it is clear that anyone advocating the legalization of cocaine would have to make a serious estimate of how many more people would use the drug after it was legalized; how many of these users would become dependent on the drug; and how much harm this would cause them and society. Instead, there has been no serious discussion of all this. Moreover, no one has seriously considered the impact of a "new" drug upon a culture that has yet to develop patterns of self-control with respect to its use; by contrast, we should recall that over many generations our culture has developed a variety of informal controls over alcohol use, which allow most people to lessen the harm that alcohol does both to them in particular and society in general. Societies not accustomed to alcohol, however, such as England prior to the "gin epidemic" of the late seventeenth and early eighteenth centuries, and many Native American and Eskimo cultures, have experienced a public-health catastrophe of huge proportions as a result of the introduction of distilled spirits.

Nor have the advocates of the legalization of cocaine considered how we would be able to prevent teenagers from gaining access to the now legal drug. Many people assume that legalization of a drug would affect only adults, since, as with alcohol, we would make it illegal to sell the drug to minors. The problem, however, is that legal access for adults makes a drug de facto available to the young. This has been the experience with alcohol and tobacco. Cocaine is far less bulky and more concealable than alcohol, and its use does not leave the telltale aroma of smoke; thus it would be even more difficult to keep away from minors.

Yet another problem is the possibility of changes in public consciousness and values. Such changes can make use of a drug less dangerous, but they can also greatly augment its dangers. There are many examples of changes in public consciousness, entirely apart from governmental action, that have influenced drug use. The use of tobacco, alcohol, and marijuana seems to have dropped in the last several years, just as jogging and low-fat diets have increased all as a consequence of the nation's greater fixation on health. Unfortunately, we cannot guarantee that such cultural trends will continue, or even that they will not be reversed, as has often happened in the past.

Youth culture, moreover, seems to be subject to dramatic fluctuations. The rapid changes in styles of dress, hair, music, and entertainment among the young have bewildered their elders for generations; and the appearance of a charismatic proselytizer for cocaine (as Timothy Leary was for LSD and marijuana) could change youth attitudes toward cocaine. Such a cultural change, even if only temporary, could present us with a permanent problem of large numbers of young people who became drug-dependent during the period of the drug's "window of acceptability."

Consider the case of heroin. Though most people have not noticed, the epidemic of heroin use stopped about ten years ago. Each year, the average age of heroin addicts goes up by about a year. Nevertheless, the last heroin epidemic has left us with an endemic problem of about 500,000 addicts who impose large social costs upon us.

THE DANGERS OF COCAINE

This is not to say that problems like these cannot be solved, or that more careful thought and research might not satisfy us. As far as we now know, however, there is no particular cause for comfort. The pharmacological nature of cocaine, in fact, is especially worrisome. We need not list all the serious negative effects cocaine may have on its users, since an impressive list of such effects can be drawn up for any of the psychoactive drugs. The problem is to determine just how prevalent these effects would be if the drug were legalized.

With cocaine, we do not have to consider the relatively rare stoppages of the heart muscle or the incidence of strokes; the common effects of cocaine are the most appropriate reasons for concern. The most important fact about cocaine is that it is an extremely attractive drug. In the 1950s a double-blind experiment on the "enjoyability" of a number of injected drugs was undertaken with twenty normal volunteers. Although fewer than half of the subjects found heroin or morphine euphoric, fully 90 percent liked an amphetamine (which is a pharmacological relative of cocaine), giving it by far the highest "pleasure score."

Probably related to its "pleasure score" is the fact that cocaine is the most "reinforcing" drug known to us. Animal studies corroborate the reports of many human users. Over the past four decades, self-administration equipment has been developed that permits animals to "work" for supplies of a drug and to administer all they want. It turns out that opiates such as heroin lie somewhere between alcohol and cocaine in their reinforcing power. Alcohol seems relatively unattractive; it is quite difficult to get most animals to drink alcohol, and unless they are already addicted, monkeys and many other animals will go to some length to avoid ingesting alcohol. Virtually all monkeys, however, will continue injecting themselves with opiates until they become addicted, and even nonaddicted animals will perform considerable amounts of work to "earn" their injections. But cocaine is the most impressive drug in this respect: animals will do enormous amounts of work to earn their cocaine shots. Indeed, if permitted, they will hit at their levers again and again to gain their reward of cocaine, neglecting food or rest until they die of debilitation.

This problem is exacerbated by several other properties of cocaine. Along with amphetamines, it is one of the few drugs that can improve one's mental and physical performance of a task. In fact, this improvement is limited to performance under conditions of fatigue, and the improvement is only temporary. Nonetheless, there will be many occasions during work, athletics, or studies when an individual will be willing to mortgage his future for a little more energy and mental clarity. Moreover—and in this respect unlike amphetamines—cocaine not only produces an alert high, but also subsequently causes a noticeable low, a kind of depression after its relatively short-term course has been run. This rather unusual effect results in the urge to use the drug again, both to recreate the past enjoyable high and to fight off the present dysphoric low.

The damage wrought by heavy cocaine use in terms of psychiatric symptoms and general debilitation is now widely known. What is less appreciated are the more subtle changes that regular cocaine use can cause. Unlike alcohol and heroin, cocaine use can easily be integrated with everyday activities. Its use can be quite inconspicuous, and, like cigarette smoking, can accompany a host of everyday activities. Cocaine use makes one feel good, then highly competent, then nearly omnipotent. It is easy to see why the use of such a drug would be damaging in a complex, mechanized, and interdependent society such as ours.

Nor should we take much comfort from the fact that most of those who use cocaine today have not become dependent upon the drug. As long as the drug is expensive and relatively difficult to procure, most of its users will be able to avoid dependence. When the drug is easily available, however, we can expect the temptations toward use to increase considerably.

We can see this by doing a quick calculation. Once the nonfinancial cost of cocaine (that is, inconvenience and criminal danger to the user) is greatly reduced by legalization, the drug's financial cost looms as the dominating one. At present, a gram of cocaine sells for about $80–$100. Its cost of production is certainly less than three dollars. Presumably, legalized cocaine would be taxed as heavily as possible, though the cost including tax would have to be sufficiently low, so as to make bootlegging unprofitable. Profits in today's cocaine trade are so huge, though, that it is hard to believe that we could keep the retail price of a gram of cocaine above $20. (Keep in mind that the bootlegger, who tries only to cheat the government out of its tax receipts, is treated much more leniently by both the criminal-justice system and society than is the universally maligned drug pusher.) When one considers that there are about fifty "hits" of cocaine in a gram, one is startled by the realization that at $20 per gram the cost of a hit will be only forty cents—a figure well within the budget of almost all grade-school children. Nor is the specter of very young children destroyed by the use of cocaine in any way unrealistic; there are ten-year-old cocaine addicts on the streets of Bogota today.

It is true that if the number of those dependent upon cocaine merely doubled, we would arguably be well ahead of the game, considering the large costs imposed by treating those users as criminals. But what if there were a fiftyfold increase in the number of those dependent on cocaine? We simply cannot guarantee that such a situation would not come to pass; since we cannot do so, it is the height of irresponsibility to advocate risking the future of the nation.

If all this is not enough to convince reasonably prudent people that legalizing cocaine is too risky a course, we can also consider the consequences of taking the risk and being wrong. After all, if we had legalized cocaine five years ago, we would not have known how easy it is to make cocaine into "crack," universally considered to be a much more habit-forming and dangerous form of the drug. If we legalize cocaine now, how long should we wait before deciding whether we made a mistake? And if we decided that we had, how would we go about recriminalizing the drug? By then, substantial inventories of legal cocaine would have been built up in private hands, and large numbers of new users would have been introduced to the drug. And once a drug has been made legally available, it is very difficult to prohibit it. This consideration helps to explain why Prohibition failed, and also explains why almost no one advocates the criminalization of tobacco.

FINDING A SOLUTION

The problem, then, is what we can do about the present situation. Several factors have made our drug policy politically tolerable up to now. First, it has protected most of middle-class America from the kind of continuous exposure to the use of drugs (and encouragement favoring their use) that are most likely to lead to the problems of drug abuse; such exposure and encouragement characterize the underclass areas in which drug use is endemic. Second, although drug enforcement has been expensive, it would have been even more expensive to do more. Third, we have continued to entertain hopes that we could solve our drug problem on the cheap, either by pressuring other nations to prevent the production of illegal drugs or by keeping drugs from being smuggled into the United States.

If we were to choose to take our drug problem more seriously, it is not clear what we could do. According to public-opinion polls, education is currently the most popular method for dealing with our drug problem. A recent Gallup Poll showed that 47 percent of Americans believe it is the best antidrug strategy. (Thirty-six percent favor interdiction, and 6 percent favor drug treatment.)

Our research shows that it is doubtful that education can do much to lower the level of drug abuse, however. Newspaper advertising campaigns to discourage alcohol abuse and drug use have been shown to be ineffective. We have had experience with temperance campaigns, but as far as we can tell, most young people do not appear to pay much attention to them. Nor do school-based programs seem to be able to reduce alcohol and drug abuse.

This is predictable. Young people are notoriously resistant to their elders' efforts to get them to live less risky, more forward-looking lives. Well into adolescence, they tend to retain what psychiatrists refer to as "remnants of infantile omnipotence." Moreover, entirely apart from the question of risk, young people often take pleasure in things that adults tell them are bad. They are constantly told that they should avoid things (like sex or junk food) that they enjoy. At best they tend to disregard such advice—when they do not actually seek out occasions to disobey their elders' counsel. Indeed, the real mystery is how we have managed to convince significant numbers of youths in inner-city school systems—more than 50 percent of whose students drop out of school, despite a massive publicity campaign to the contrary—to avoid taking drugs, since at least in the beginning they would find drug use so enjoyable.

Nevertheless, one kind of drug education does show some promise. Several small-scale experiments have attempted to use peers to teach young students techniques by which they can refuse cigarettes if they want to. They learn, for instance, what to say when others offer them cigarettes or even exert social pressure on them to smoke; this approach has produced significant decreases in the initiation of cigarette use. Such programs are still quite rare, however, and whether we can duplicate them on a large scale with respect to cocaine and heroin, in the neighborhoods that most need them, is by no means clear. At the very least, we need years of research before we can develop programs that can be trusted to do more good than harm.

The charm of education, nonetheless, is seductive. Compared with other means of coping with illegal drugs, it is cheap and seems humane, because it does not require the coercion of our fellow citizens. In this regard, it is similar to bringing pressure upon foreign nations to prevent the production of illegal drugs. Indeed, education may well become the "crop substitution" of the nineties—that is, the supposed panacea for all drug problems.

Conceivably, we will decide simply to continue our present policies. We can spend a great deal on education programs; we can assign the military the task of sealing our borders against drugs, we can seize yachts or fishing boats when passengers or workers have abandoned marijuana cigarettes on them; we can legislate capital punishment for drug-related killings (as when drug dealers murder one another). But by adopting such a course of action, we would only be making an emphatic statement that we were taking the drug problem seriously; we would not really be acting seriously. For to act in this manner would in effect be to choose to keep putting up with our problem.

For most middle-class Americans, the use of heroin and cocaine is not a major threat. Heroin never was a threat; and although cocaine was very popular with some wealthy users—the conventional wisdom held that they were heavily overrepresented in advertising, entertainment, and professional sports—and its use significantly harmed the lives of many middle-class youths, much of the damage has already been done. Today, cocaine—especially in the form of "crack"—is increasingly becoming a drug of the lower classes. It is true that all of us suffer from the intimate connection between these drugs and predatory crime, and in more indirect ways from the enormous dislocation and damage done to lower-class neighborhoods by the sale and use of these drugs. Nonetheless, we learned to live with problems like these many years ago. Indeed, it seems that the public gets really excited about the drug problem only when someone from the middle class is killed in a gang shootout.

In an ideal world, the best way to reduce the damage done by illegal drugs would be to convince everyone not to use them. In this world, however, we will probably have to reconcile ourselves to using some coercion. On the other hand, once we give up on finding an inexpensive solution, we may take the problem seriously and apply more careful thought and more resources to the job.

SUPPLY-SIDE ENFORCEMENT

So long as we are unable to suppress the sale of drugs, we will be remitting large parts of our cities to the terrorization of innocent people, drug-related killings, and the brutalization that comes from constant exposure to the use of drugs. Perhaps equally demoralizing is the sight of the large number of teenage drug lords who own Jaguars or Ferraris before they are old enough to have driver's licenses. Nonetheless, we can accomplish much more than we have in the past.

Apart from our efforts in other countries and at the borders, the major thrust of enforcement within the United States has been the attempt to break up large-scale drug rings, arrest small-scale dealers when they sell drugs outside the areas in which drug use is endemic, and punish users when they commit other crimes. In recent years local police have stepped up their efforts to restrain street-level selling, and private employers have exerted greater efforts to apprehend their workers' "connection," and to weed out illegal drug users from their work force. The result has been a slow but steady loss of ground for law-enforcement agencies.

One cannot say that careful thought and greatly augmented law-enforcement resources will solve our drug problem. There are large numbers of sellers arranged hierarchically within the United States as part of loose but fairly sizable organizations, taking the drug from its importation into the United States through smaller wholesalers down to the small-scale sellers who provide the drug to users. Unfortunately, we cannot expect to achieve much of a reduction in the number of drug suppliers, even if we jail a sizable percentage of them. The high profits at every level of the drug trade guarantee a huge reservoir of individuals prepared to take the places of those who have been imprisoned. At each level in the distribution scheme there are more than enough competitors; and even at the lowest ranks, those who do minor jobs for the sellers (such as acting as lookouts for the police) seem ready to enter the business.

On the other hand, pressure upon the retailing of heroin and cocaine is not necessarily an unattractive option. In fact, it is probably the major governmental means of restraining drug use in the United States today. The number of locations in which an ordinary middle-class individual can buy heroin and cocaine is not very large. In most of the country, cocaine is not widely available to most people. Heroin is less so. A major task of law-enforcement resources is to increase that area of drug unavailability. At the very least, the police should act immediately to suppress the open-air drug markets that spring up whenever the police are distracted by other duties. In most of our urban areas, greater efforts could drive much of the dealing indoors, where a large percentage of potential customers are afraid to go.

At least for the foreseeable future, it is hard to imagine the police being able to do more than gradually drive the dealing back into the public-housing projects and other relatively small areas in which the police are unable to maintain a presence. Nonetheless, increases in law-enforcement efforts at the retail level may lower the availability of heroin and cocaine to large numbers of people without creating a need to involve ourselves in the most hard-core drug-trafficking areas, in which the police would have to maintain a virtual army of occupation.

Apart from the difficulty of policing the hard-core drug areas, the most important constraint upon our ability to suppress the sale of drugs is the cost of incarceration space. Our prisons and jails are full, and despite a massive and continuing effort to provide the infrastructure to imprison more and more law-breakers, the demand threatens to permanently outrun the supply. Drug sales, moreover, are especially difficult and expensive to restrain through imprisonment. The deterrence we expect from the legal threat is in large part neutralized by the high profits at all levels of the drug trade. And incapacitation, the other major restraint provided by imprisonment, is weakened by the fact that the skills necessary to participate in the drug trade are not at all scarce.

Although we must allocate a large percentage of prison space to the incarceration of drug dealers if we are to make headway, there are other methods that can help. At the higher levels of the drug trade, the forfeiture of assets has proven quite successful. We cannot show that the threat has caused any drug dealers to get out of the business, but at the margin it should have that effect; depriving sellers of working capital makes their reentry into the industry more difficult. At the very least, it assuages our sense of justice, as well as providing additional resources with which to further enforcement. It is likely that we can go a great deal lower in the drug-trade hierarchy before forfeiture is no longer worthwhile. It will require a little more ingenuity by the police and cooperation from the agencies of the criminal-justice system before we can strike at the pocketbook of the small-scale seller, but it can be done—and to good effect.

DEMAND-SIDE ENFORCEMENT

While pressure on the small-scale sale of drugs represents an attempt to influence drug supply, it also has an impact on drug demand—perhaps a greater one. The buyer who does not reside in an area of heavy drug sales must not only come up with the money to pay for the drugs; he may also have to search longer to make a purchase and worry more about the danger of being robbed or assaulted. He may also be more conspicuous to the police. To some extent, we can take advantage of this problem faced by drug buyers by using a relatively inexpensive means of lessening the number of those who are willing to obtain their supplies from the areas of heavy drug dealing. On a few occasions police have seized the automobiles of those who drove them to purchase drugs. This is not only inexpensive, but also far less brutal than imprisoning otherwise law-abiding drug users—and it may have more of an impact. This should be a regular feature of all drug enforcement.

Probably the most important aspect of the attack on drugs is the attempt to lower the amount of predatory crime that drug use engenders. We know, for example, that those who use illegal drugs commit a substantial proportion of our urban burglaries, robberies, and thefts. A number of studies have demonstrated that the criminality rate of those using heroin daily—that is, those who were addicted—was about seven times as great as the criminality rate of the same people when they were using the drug only sporadically or temporarily not using it at all.

Newer studies have shown an even higher correlation between criminality and drug use, and have implicated cocaine as well. Urinalysis of those arrested for crimes in 1986 has revealed that a staggering percentage of those apprehended had recently used cocaine or heroin. In the District of Columbia, 74 percent of non-drug-felony arrestees tested positive for at least one illegal drug other than marijuana. (No one has alleged that marijuana use helps to cause predatory crime, in part because the drug is cheap, in part because it has a tranquilizing effect.) In New York City the figure was 72 percent; in Chicago, 60 percent; and in Los Angeles, 58 percent. It turns out that in large cities about 70 percent of those arrested for robbery, weapons offenses, and larceny tested positive for heroin, cocaine, or (in the few cities where use is common) PCP.

The data on urinalysis suggest an obvious course of action. We must institutionalize routine urinalysis for those arrested for any of the typical crimes arising out of drug use. Then we must act on this information by making maintenance of a urine clean of cocaine, heroin, and PCP a requirement for all those who are released on bail or, after conviction, are placed on probation or released on parole.

A positive urine sample must reliably and immediately mean a return to jail. It is far more important that the enforcement of these rules be consistent than that the jail terms be long. We do not have the jail space that would be needed to provide long terms for this type of offense. And if we try, our efforts will backfire: We will deprive the system of the consistency necessary to get the message through to drug users. But a properly implemented system of imprisonment can make possible a more lasting cure for drug dependency.

This kind of regimen is not without disadvantages. There will inevitably be a dispute over whether we can demand "clean" urine before releasing someone on bail. On the one hand, our jurisprudence tells us that bail is to be used only to guarantee the presence of the accused at judicial proceedings, and there is no firm evidence that drug users are less likely than others to show up in court. On the other hand, more recent precedent seems to allow consideration of the danger to the community if an arrestee is released on bail, and those who use illegal drugs are, on average, much more likely to commit crimes after they have been freed.

Such a system of mandatory urinalysis will also require more money. Parts of the criminal-justice system will simply not give up—even temporarily—the funds they already have and need, even though doing so may help to save money in the long run. The jails are already full, and in many cases under court order not to exceed their present population. Even at two days per failed urinalysis, the increased demand upon those institutions will be substantial. And the maintenance of such a system will require the police to go looking for those who miss urinalysis appointments, a burden that may initially be only partially compensated for by the lower criminality of those now compelled to be drug-free.

Furthermore, the inexpensive urine test, which costs only about $5, but is less than completely accurate, will have to be supplemented by a system in which an arrestee who was confident that he had not used an illegal drug could simply file an affidavit to that effect and be tested by a more expensive but foolproof method (costing about $70). Although there will have to be some sanction for a false affidavit, expensive prosecutions for perjury will not be necessary to deter such conduct (though it is hard to imagine a simpler case to prosecute). The judge, in revoking bail or probation, can simply revoke it for longer.

Then there are the privacy concerns. It should be noted that urinalysis for those who have been arrested involves far fewer restraints on the citizen's right to privacy than the usual attempt to require urinalysis of government employees or members of other large groups, who, as individuals, give us no reason to suspect their drug use. (Nor is it nearly so expensive.) Our statistics on the drug use of those arrested for street crimes already single them out. And apart from the use of urinalysis in the bail decision, there are no real constitutional doubts. If there is a good reason, those arrested for drunken driving, for example, may constitutionally be subjected to blood, urine, or breath analysis, and those released on bail or, after conviction, on probation or parole, forfeit even more of their privacy. They are subject not only to intrusive searches but also to various restrictions on their autonomy. Very few of the restrictions on the privacy and autonomy of defendants in the criminal-justice system make as much practical sense as requiring urinalysis in order to monitor their drug use.

THE PROGNOSIS

What, then, could we expect from the institutionalization of such a regimen? Many of those using drugs will find themselves constantly in and out of jail.

Some would simply decide that enough is enough and clean themselves up. We do know that this can occur when the consequences are immediate and certain enough. Nonetheless, in most cases we will have to rely upon drug treatment to prevent the urinalysis system from becoming a huge, inhumane, and expensive revolving-door operation. While it is true that the most reliable and cost-effective drug treatment—methadone maintenance—is helpful only with heroin addicts, there are other therapies that are more cost-effective than permitting the drug abuser to continue untreated; and it is likely that requiring urinalysis will help persuade drug users to undergo treatment.

Indeed, probably the most foolish aspect of our antidrug posture has been the starvation of drug treatment. In many cities there is a months-long wait for those who want to enter a drug-treatment program; this is a serious problem, considering that the desire to reform is often ephemeral, and disappears if it cannot be acted upon at once. Part of the reluctance to invest in drug treatment stems from the moralistic view that it is wrong to spend resources on making life better for criminals; part stems from the (incorrect) belief that treatment does not work. Treatment is difficult; it is frustrating; and it does not always work. But it is cost-effective—and far more so than its only substitute, imprisonment. A necessary component of any serious effort to lower the social costs of illegal drug use, therefore, is a massive increase in funds for drug treatment.

Another fact about drug treatment is also quite important. Although many believe that compulsory treatment is ineffective, this does not appear to be the case. Virtually everyone undergoing drug treatment is in one way or another forced to do so. Indeed, like many alcoholics, who simply want to become social drinkers again and escape the social, psychological, and physical effects of overindulgence, most drug users do not wish to be abstinent, but rather to return to the early days of their more casual drug use. Nonetheless, one of the effects that those dependent on cocaine and heroin may most wish to escape is the pressure of the criminal-justice system. And a criminal-justice system that makes use of urinalysis will be more effective in driving them into—and keeping them in—treatment.

The approach I am recommending may have another important effect. For years, the drug-producing nations have argued that the United States must share the blame for the drug problem: If they cannot control the production of illegal drugs, neither can we control our consumption. We may now be able to have some success. Those users who are both criminals and drug consumers appear to be not merely a random selection of drug users; they tend, rather, to be the heaviest users. Thus it is likely that these heavy users consume a disproportionate percentage of the illegal drug supply. This should not be surprising: the heaviest-drinking 10 percent of all drinkers drink well over half the total quantity of alcohol—and our evidence, though less conclusive, points in the same direction with regard to illegal drugs.

Indeed, the "J curve" seems to be a constant in human behavior: 15 percent of health-insurance users use 90 percent of the resources; 6 percent of Philadelphia's youths commit over 50 percent of its crimes; and 10 percent of Stanford Law School's students file 90 percent of the petitions to be excused from one requirement or another.

As a result, those users we will be focusing on will be those who do the most to support the illegal market. On average, each seller is supported by three heavy users. If we can bring their use under control—in addition to decreasing the number of predatory crimes—we may finally be able to deal a major blow to the illegal retail-distribution networks. We may also create a sizable cohort of former drug users who can help discourage drug use. If the zeal of the convert in this area is as strong as it seems to be in others—think of ex-smokers, for example—we may reap unanticipated and sizable dividends from our efforts. For decades we have attempted to get at the sellers as a way of preventing use; now we may have the means to get at the users as a means of restraining sales.

I do not mean to suggest that we will be able to solve the problem easily. For the foreseeable future we will have a serious drug problem, but we can lessen it considerably if we have the will. Where will the money necessary to accomplish this come from? The additional resources we need for law enforcement and drug treatment will come from the federal government, or they will not come at all. Whether the resources will come is simply a question of whether we have finally begun to take our drug problem seriously. It will be interesting to find out.

NOTE

1. See my *The Hardest Drug: Heroin and Public Policy* (Chicago: University of Chicago Press, 1983).

13

Don't Legalize Drugs

Morton M. Kondracke

The next time you hear that a drunk driver has slammed into a school bus full of children or that a stoned railroad engineer has killed sixteen people in a train wreck, think about this: If the advocates of legalized drugs have their way, there will be more of this, a lot more. There will also be more unpublicized fatal and maiming crashes, more job accidents, more child neglect, more of almost everything associated with substance abuse: babies born addicted or retarded, teenagers zonked out of their chance for an education, careers destroyed, families wrecked, and people dead of overdoses.

The proponents of drug legalization are right to say that some things will get better. Organized crime will be driven out of the drug business, and there will be a sharp drop in the amount of money (currently about $10 billion per year) that society spends to enforce the drug laws. There will be some reduction in the cost in theft and injury (now about $20 billion) by addicts to get the money to buy prohibited drugs. Internationally, Latin American governments presumably will stop being menaced by drug cartels and will peaceably export cocaine as they now do coffee.

However, this is virtually the limit of the social benefits to be derived from legalization, and they are far outweighed by the costs, which are always underplayed by legalization advocates such as the *Economist,* Princeton scholar Ethan A. Nadelmann,[1] economist Milton Friedman and other libertarians, columnists William F. Buckley and Richard Cohen, and Mayors Keith Schmoke of Baltimore and Marion Barry of Washington, D.C. In lives, money, and human woe, the costs are so high, in fact, that society has no

Originally published in *The New Republic* 198, no. 26 (June 27, 1988). Reprinted by permission of *The New Republic.* © 1988 by The New Republic, Inc.

alternative but to conduct a real war on the drug trade, although perhaps a smarter one than is currently being waged.

Advocates of legalization love to draw parallels between the drug war and Prohibition. Their point, of course, is that this crusade is as doomed to failure as the last one was, and that we ought to surrender now to the inevitable and stop wasting resources. But there are some important differences between drugs and alcohol. Alcohol has been part of Western culture for thousands of years, drugs have been the rage in America only since about 1962. Of the 115 million Americans who consume alcohol, 85 percent rarely become intoxicated; with drugs, intoxication is the whole idea. Alcohol is consistent chemically, even though it's dispensed in different strengths and forms as beer, wine, and "hard" liquor, with drugs there's no limit to the variations. Do we legalize crack along with snortable cocaine, PCPs as well as marijuana, and LSD and "Ecstasy" as well as heroin? If we don't—and almost certainly we won't—we have a black market, and some continued crime.

But Prohibition is a useful historical parallel for measuring the costs of legalization. Almost certainly doctors are not going to want to write prescriptions for recreational use of harmful substances, so if drugs ever are legalized they will be dispensed as alcohol now is—in government-regulated stores with restrictions on the age of buyers, warnings against abuse (and, probably, with added restrictions on amounts, though this also will create a black market).

In the decade before Prohibition went into effect in 1920, alcohol consumption in the United States averaged 2.6 gallons per person per year. It fell to 0.73 gallons during the Prohibition decade, then doubled to 1.5 gallons in the decade after repeal, and is now back to 2.6 gallons. So illegality suppressed usage to a third or a fourth of its former level. At the same time, incidence of cirrhosis of the liver fell by half.

So it seems fair to estimate that use of drugs will at least double, and possibly triple, if the price is cut, supplies are readily available, and society's sanction is lifted. It's widely accepted that there are now 16 million regular users of marijuana, six million of cocaine, a half million of heroin, and another half million of other drugs, totaling 23 million. Dr. Robert DuPont, former director of the National Institutes of Drug Abuse and an anti-legalization crusader, says that the instant pleasure afforded by drugs—superior to that available with alcohol—will increase the number of regular users of marijuana and cocaine to about 50 or 60 million and heroin users to 10 million.

Between 10 percent and 15 percent of all drinkers turn into alcoholics (10 million to 17 million), and these drinkers cost the economy an estimated $117 billion in 1983 ($15 billion for treatment, $89 billion in lost productivity, and $13 billion in accident-related costs). About 200,000 people died last year as a result of alcohol abuse, about 25,000 in auto accidents. How many drug users will turn into addicts, and what will this cost? According to President Reagan's drug abuse policy adviser, Dr. David I. McDonald, studies indicate that marijuana is about as habit-forming as alcohol, but for cocaine, 70 percent of users become addicted, as many as with nicotine.

So it seems reasonable to conclude that at least four to six million people will become potheads if marijuana is legal, and that coke addicts will number somewhere between 8.5 million (if regular usage doubles and 70 percent become addicted) and 42 million (if DuPont's high estimate of use is correct). An optimist would have to conclude that the number of people abusing legalized drugs will come close to those hooked on alcohol. A pessimist would figure the human damage as much greater.

Another way of figuring costs is this: The same study (by the Research Triangle Institute of North Carolina) that put the price of alcoholism at $117 billion in 1983 figured the cost of drug abuse then at $60 billion—$15 billion for law enforcement and crime, and $45 billion in lost productivity, damaged health, and other costs. The updated estimate for 1988 drug abuse is $100 billion. If legalizing drugs would save $30 billion now being spent on law enforcement and crime, a doubling of use and abuse means that other costs will rise to $140 billion or $210 billion. This is no bargain for society.

If 200,000 people die every year from alcohol abuse and 320,000 from tobacco smoking, how many will die from legal drugs? Government estimates are that 4,000 to 5,000 people a year are killed in drug-related auto crashes, but this is surely low because accident victims are not as routinely blood-tested for drugs as for alcohol. Legalization advocates frequently cite figures of 3,600 or 4,100 as the number of drug deaths each year reported by hospitals, but this number, too, is certainly an understatement, based on reports from only seventy-five big hospitals in twenty-seven metropolitan areas.

If legalization pushed the total number of drug addicts to only half the number of alcoholics, 100,000 people a year would die. That's the figure cited by McDonald. DuPont guesses that, given the potency of drugs, the debilitating effects of cocaine, the carcinogenic effects of marijuana, and the AIDS potential of injecting legalized heroin, the number of deaths actually could go as high as 500,000 a year. That's a wide range, but it's clear that legalization of drugs will not benefit human life.

All studies show that those most likely to try drugs, get hooked, and die—as opposed to those who suffer from cirrhosis and lung cancer—are young people, who are susceptible to the lure of quick thrills and are terribly adaptable to messages provided by adult society. Under pressure of the current prohibition, the number of kids who use illegal drugs at least once a month has fallen from 39 percent in the late 1970s to 25 percent in 1987, according to the annual survey of high school seniors conducted by the University of Michigan. The same survey shows that attitudes toward drug use have turned sharply negative. But use of legal drugs is still strong. Thirty-eight percent of high school seniors reported getting drunk within the past two weeks, and 27 percent said they smoke cigarettes every day. Drug prohibition is working with kids; legalization would do them harm.

And, even though legalization would lower direct costs for drug law enforcement, it's unlikely that organized crime would disappear. It might well shift to other fields—prostitution, pornography, gambling or burglaries, extortion, and murders-for-hire—much as it did in the period between the end of Prohibition and the beginning of the drug era. As DuPont puts it, "Organized crime is in the business of giving people the things that society decides in its own interest to prohibit. The only way to get rid of organized crime is to make everything legal." Even legalization advocates such as Ethan Nadelmann admit that some street crimes will continue to occur as a result of drug abuse—especially cocaine paranoia, PCP insanity, and the need of unemployable addicts to get money for drugs. Domestic crime, child abuse, and neglect surely would increase.

Some legalization advocates suggest merely decriminalizing marijuana and retaining sanctions against other drugs. This would certainly be less costly than total legalization, but it would still be no favor to young people, would increase traffic accidents and productivity losses—and would do nothing to curtail the major drug cartels, which make most of their money trafficking in cocaine.

Legalizers also argue that the government could tax legal drug sales and use the money to pay for antidrug education programs and treatment centers. But total taxes collected right now from alcohol sales at the local, state, and federal levels come to only $13.1 billion per year—which is a pittance compared with the damage done to society as a result of alcohol abuse. The same would have to be true for drugs—and any tax that resulted in an official drug price that was higher than the street price would open the way once again for black markets and organized crime.

So, in the name of health, economics, and morality, there seems no alternative but to keep drugs illegal and to fight the animals who traffic in them. Regardless of what legalization advocates say, this is now the overwhelming opinion of the public, the Reagan administration, the prospective candidates for president, and the Congress—not one of whose members has introduced legislation to decriminalize any drug. Congress is on the verge of forcing the administration to raise antidrug spending next year [1989] from $3 billion to $5.5 billion.

There is, though, room to debate how best to wage this war. A consensus is developing that it has to be done both on the supply side (at overseas points of origin, through interdiction at U.S. borders and criminal prosecution of traffickers) and on the demand side (by discouraging use of drugs through education and treatment and/or by arrest and urine testing at workplaces). However, there is a disagreement about which side to emphasize and how to spend resources. Members of Congress, especially Democrats, want to blame foreigners and the Reagan administration for the fact that increasing amounts of cocaine, heroin, and marijuana are entering the country. They want to spend more money on foreign aid, use the U.S. military to seal the borders, and found "nice" treatment and education programs, especially those that give ongoing support to professional social welfare agencies.

Conservatives, on the other hand, want to employ the military to help foreign countries stamp out drug laboratories, use widespread drug testing to identify—and, often, punish—drug users, and spend more on police and prisons. As Education Secretary William Bennett puts it, "How can we surrender when we've never actually fought the war?" Bennett wants to fight it across all fronts, and those who have seen drafts of a forthcoming report of the White House Conference for a Drug-Free America say this will be the approach recommended by the administration, although with muted emphasis on use of the U.S. military, which is reluctant to get involved in what may be another thankless war.

However, DuPont and others, including Jeffrey Eisenach of the Heritage Foundation, make a strong case that primary emphasis ought to be put on the demand side—discouraging use in the United States rather than, almost literally, trying to become the world's policeman. Their argument, bolstered by a study conducted by Peter Reuter of the RAND Corporation, is that major profits in the drug trade are not made abroad (where the price of cocaine triples from farm to airstrip), but within the United States (where the markup from entry point to street corner is twelve times), and that foreign growing fields and processing laboratories are easily replaceable at low cost.

They say that prohibition policy should emphasize routine random urine testing in schools and places of employment, arrests for possession of drugs, and "coercive" treatment programs that compel continued enrollment as a condition of probation and employment. DuPont thinks that corporations have a right to demand that their employees be drug-free because users cause accidents and reduce productivity. He contends that urine testing is no more invasive than the use of metal detectors at airports.

"Liberals have a terrible time with this," says DuPont. "They want to solve every problem by giving people things. They want to love people out of their problems, while conservatives want to punish it out of them. What we want to do is take the profits out of drugs by drying up demand. You do that by raising the social cost of using them to the point where people say, 'I don't want to do this.' This isn't conservative. It's a way to save lives."

It is, and it's directly parallel to the way society is dealing with drunk driving and cigarette smoking—not merely through advertising campaigns and surgeon general's warnings, but through increased penalties, social strictures—and prohibitions. Random testing for every employee in America may be going too far, but testing those holding sensitive jobs or workers involved in accidents surely isn't, nor is arresting users, lifting driver's licenses, and requiring treatment. These are not nosy, moralistic intrusions on people's individual rights, but attempts by society to protect itself from danger.

In the end, they are also humane and moral. There is a chance, with the public and policy-makers aroused to action, that ten years from now drug abuse might be reduced to its pre-1960s levels. Were drugs to be legalized now, we would be establishing a new vice—one that, over time, would end or ruin millions of lives. Worse yet, we would be establishing a pattern of doing the easy thing, surrendering, whenever confronted with a difficult challenge.

NOTE

1. Ethan A. Nadelmann, "Shooting Up," *The New Republic,* June 23,1988.

Part Four

Medical Marijuana: What Counts as Medicine?

14

Federal Foolishness and Marijuana

Jerome P. Kassirer

The advanced stages of many illnesses and their treatments are often accompanied by intractable nausea, vomiting, or pain. Thousands of patients with cancer, AIDS, and other diseases report they have obtained striking relief from these devastating symptoms by smoking marijuana. The alleviation of distress can be so striking that some patients and their families have been willing to risk a jail term to obtain or grow the marijuana.

Despite the desperation of these patients, within weeks after voters in Arizona and California approved propositions [in November 1996] allowing physicians in their states to prescribe marijuana for medical indications, federal officials, including the president, the secretary of Health and Human Services, and the attorney general sprang into action. At a news conference, Secretary Donna E. Shalala gave an organ recital of the parts of the body that she asserted could be harmed by marijuana and warned of the evils of its spreading use. Attorney General Janet Reno announced that physicians in any state who prescribed the drug could lose the privilege of writing prescriptions, be excluded from Medicare and Medicaid reimbursement, and even be prosecuted for a federal crime. General Barry R. McCaffrey, director of the Office of National Drug Control Policy, reiterated his agency's position that marijuana is a dangerous drug and implied that voters in Arizona and California had been duped into voting for these propositions. He indicated that it is always possible to study the effects of any drug, including marijuana, but that the use of marijuana by seriously ill patients would require, at the least, scientifically valid research.

Originally published in *The New England Journal of Medicine* 336, no. 5 (January 30, 1997).

I believe that a federal policy that prohibits physicians from alleviating suffering by prescribing marijuana for seriously ill patients is misguided, heavy-handed, and inhumane. Marijuana may have long-term adverse effects and its use may presage serious addictions, but neither long-term side effects nor addiction is a relevant issue in such patients. It is also hypocritical to forbid physicians to prescribe marijuana while permitting them to use morphine and meperidine* to relieve extreme dyspnea and pain. With both these drugs the difference between the dose that relieves symptoms and the dose that hastens death is very narrow; by contrast, there is no risk of death from smoking marijuana. To demand evidence of therapeutic efficacy is equally hypocritical. The noxious sensations that patients experience are extremely difficult to quantify in controlled experiments. What really counts for a therapy with this kind of safety margin is whether a seriously ill patient feels relief as a result of the intervention, not whether a controlled trial "proves" its efficacy.

Paradoxically, dronabinol, a drug that contains one of the active ingredients in marijuana (tetrahydrocannabinol), has been available by prescription for more than a decade. But it is difficult to titrate the therapeutic dose of this drug, and it is not widely prescribed. By contrast, smoking marijuana produces a rapid increase in the blood level of the active ingredients and is thus more likely to be therapeutic. Needless to say, new drugs such as those that inhibit the nausea associated with chemotherapy may well be more beneficial than smoking marijuana, but their comparative efficacy has never been studied.

Whatever their reasons, federal officials are out of step with the public. Dozens of states have passed laws that ease restrictions on the prescribing of marijuana by physicians, and polls consistently show that the public favors the use of marijuana for such purposes. Federal authorities should rescind their prohibition of the medicinal use of marijuana for seriously ill patients and allow physicians to decide which patients to treat. The government should change marijuana's status from that of a Schedule 1 drug (considered to be potentially addictive and with no current medical use) to that of a Schedule 2 drug (potentially addictive but with some accepted medical use) and regulate it accordingly. To ensure its proper distribution and use, the government could declare itself the only agency sanctioned to provide the marijuana. I believe that such a change in policy would have no adverse effects. The argument that it would be a signal to the young that "marijuana is OK" is, I believe, specious.

This proposal is not new. In 1986, after years of legal wrangling, the Drug Enforcement Administration (DEA) held extensive hearings on the transfer of marijuana to Schedule 2. In 1988, the DEA's own administrative-law judge concluded, "It would be unreasonable, arbitrary, and capricious for

---

*Meperedine hydrochloride is a narcotic, analgesic, sedative, and antispasmodic that may produce physical and psychic dependence. (Ed.)

DEA to continue to stand between those sufferers and the benefits of this substance in light of the evidence in this record."[1] Nonetheless, the DEA overruled the judge's order to transfer marijuana to Schedule 2, and in 1992 it issued a final rejection of all requests for reclassification.[2]

Some physicians will have the courage to challenge the continued proscription of marijuana for the sick. Eventually, their actions will force the courts to adjudicate between the rights of those at death's door and the absolute power of bureaucrats whose decisions are based more on reflexive ideology and political correctness than on compassion.

NOTES

1. F. L. Young, Opinion and recommended ruling, marijuana rescheduling petition. Department of Justice, Drug Enforcement Administration. Docket 86-22, September 6, 1988 (Washington, D.C.: Drug Enforcement Administration).

2. Department of Justice, Drug Enforcement Administration, Marijuana scheduling petition: denial of petition: remand. (Docket No. 86-22.) Fed. Regist. 1992; 57(59): 10489–508.

15

Reefer Madness—
The Federal Response to
California's Medical–Marijuana Law

George J. Annas

Marijuana is unique among illegal drugs in its political symbolism, its safety, and its wide use. More than 65 million Americans have tried marijuana, the use of which is not associated with increased mortality.[1] Since the federal government first tried to tax it out of existence in 1937, at least partly in response to the 1936 film *Reefer Madness,* marijuana has remained at the center of controversy. Now physicians are becoming more actively involved. Most recently, the federal drug policy against any use of marijuana has been challenged by California's attempt to legalize its use by certain patients on the recommendation of their physicians. The federal government responded by threatening California physicians who recommend marijuana to their sick patients with investigation and the loss of their prescription privileges under Drug Enforcement Administration (DEA) regulations.[2]

The editor-in-chief of the [*New England*] *Journal* [*of Medicine*] suggested that prohibiting physicians from helping their suffering patients by suggesting that they use marijuana is "misguided, heavy-handed, and inhumane."[3] He recommended that marijuana be reclassified as a Schedule 2 drug and made available by prescription without the usual requirement of controlled clinical trials. Many states, including Massachusetts, had previously passed laws that permitted their citizens to use marijuana for medicinal purposes under some circumstances.[4] California's law seems to have engendered a uniquely harsh federal response because California is a large, trend-setting state; because its new marijuana law is very broad as compared with others; and because the law was passed by popular referendum. In this article I will discuss the new California law and its implications for physicians.

Originally published in *The New England Journal of Medicine* 337, no. 6 (August 7, 1997).

THE CALIFORNIA PROPOSITION

In the fall of 1996, California voters approved the Medical Marijuana Initiative (Proposition 215) by a vote of 56 to 44 percent. The act is entitled the Compassionate Use Act of 1996, and its purpose is to give Californians the right to possess and cultivate marijuana for medical purposes "where that medical use is deemed appropriate and has been recommended by a physician who has determined that the person's health would benefit from the use of marijuana in the treatment of cancer, anorexia, AIDS, chronic pain, spasticity, glaucoma, arthritis, migraine, or any other illness for which marijuana provides relief."[5] Nothing in the act permits persons using marijuana for medical purposes to engage in conduct that endangers others (such as driving while under its influence), condones "the diversion of marijuana for nonmedical purposes," or permits the buying or selling of marijuana.[6] The two operative sections of the law are as follows:

> Notwithstanding any other provision of law, no physician in this state shall be punished, or denied any right or privilege, for having recommended marijuana to a patient for medical purposes.

> [Existing California law] relating to the possession of marijuana [and the] cultivation of marijuana, shall not apply to a patient, or to a patient's primary caregiver [the person who has consistently assumed responsibility for the patient's housing, health, or safety] who possesses or cultivates marijuana for the personal medical purposes of the patient upon the written or oral recommendation or approval of a physician.[7]

The primary purpose of this law is to provide a specified group of patients with an affirmative defense to the charge of possession or cultivation of marijuana, the defense of medical necessity. To use this defense, the patient must be able to show that his or her physician recommended or approved of the use of marijuana, either orally or in writing. Obviously, a note from a physician is better evidence than a simple assertion that "my doctor said this would be good for me," and most patients will want a written statement to help protect them from problems with the police. Nothing in this law changes current law against buying or selling marijuana or affects federal law; it merely provides that qualified patients and their primary care givers can possess and cultivate their own marijuana for personal medicinal purposes, without violating state drug laws.

COMPASSION AND THE USE OF UNAPPROVED DRUGS

The federal government has been in the business of regulating drugs for almost a century, and few exceptions have ever been made to the basic rules of the Food and Drug Administration (FDA), even for patients with cancer or AIDS. In 1979, for example, the FDA was successful in convincing a unanimous U.S. Supreme Court that Congress intended no exception for terminally ill patients who sought to take laetrile, an unapproved drug, for cancer. The FDA's primary rationale was that the use of this unapproved and useless drug could prevent patients from seeking conventional treatments for cancer that offered them at least some chance of a cure.[8] Under President Ronald Reagan, however, the FDA responded with a great deal more flexibility to the AIDS epidemic and permitted the use and sale of drugs not yet approved (but in use in ongoing clinical trials) if, among other things, "the drug [was] intended to treat a serious or immediately life-threatening disease."[9] More surprisingly, the FDA also permitted individual patients to import unapproved drugs from other countries for their personal, medical use.[10] These regulations were almost purely political, had no scientific basis, and tended to conflate treatment and research and to undermine the very purpose of clinical trials.[11] The theory used to justify these exceptions to federal drug laws was the very one rejected by the Supreme Court: Terminally ill patients have "nothing to lose" and should not be deprived of the hope (even the false hope) that they might escape death.[12]

Given this history, it is not surprising that the advocates of the medicinal use of marijuana concentrate their reform efforts on helping patients with cancer ameliorate the adverse effects of chemotherapy and helping patients with AIDS counteract weight loss and fight their disease. Virtually no one thinks it is reasonable to initiate criminal prosecution of patients with cancer or AIDS who use marijuana on the advice of their physicians to help them through conventional medical treatment for their disease. Anecdotal evidence of the effectiveness of smoked marijuana abounds.[13] Perhaps the most convincing is the account of Harvard professor and author Stephen Jay Gould, one of the world's first survivors of abdominal mesothelioma.* When Gould started intravenous chemotherapy, he writes:

> Absolutely nothing in the available arsenal of antiemetics worked at all. I was miserable and came to dread the frequent treatments with an almost perverse intensity. I had heard that marijuana often worked well against nausea. I was reluctant to try it because I have never smoked any substance habitually (and didn't even know how to inhale). Moreover, I had tried marijuana twice [in the 1960s] . . . and had hated it. . . . Marijuana worked like a charm. . . . The sheer bliss of not experiencing nausea—and not having to fear it for all the days intervening between treatments—was the greatest boost I received in all my year of treatment, and surely the most important effect upon my eventual cure.[14]

---

*Mesothelioma is a rare neoplasm derived from the lining cells of the pleura and peritoneum—also reported in asbestosis. *Stedman's Medical Dictionary.* (Ed.)

Similarly, in patients with AIDS, marijuana has been credited with counteracting such side effects of treatment as severe nausea, vomiting, loss of appetite, and fatigue, as well as with stimulating the appetite to help prevent weight loss.

THE WHITE HOUSE PRESS CONFERENCE

Had the California proposition been limited to the use of marijuana for terminal illnesses such as cancer and AIDS, it would probably have caused much less concern. Arizona passed a much broader initiative that permitted physicians to prescribe any drug on Schedule 1, but in April 1997, the Arizona legislature amended the law to apply only to drugs approved by the FDA, thus effectively repealing it.[15] The California law applies only to marijuana but makes it available for a wide range of medical conditions, including anorexia, pain, spasticity, glaucoma, arthritis, migraine, "or any other illness for which marijuana provides relief."[16] This very broad definition of the potential medicinal uses of marijuana seemed an explicit endorsement of the drug itself, which the Clinton administration and others believed to be sending the wrong message to America's youth. After thinking about the issue for approximately two months, the Clinton administration announced that it would vigorously oppose the implementation of the California proposition and the Arizona law.[17]

Barry McCaffrey, director of the Office of National Drug Control Policy, announced at a White House news conference on December 30, 1996, that "nothing has changed. Federal law is unaffected by these propositions."[18] McCaffrey expressed concern about marijuana as a "gateway drug" and about the potential impact of the law on children. As for the potential medicinal uses of marijuana, he said:

> This is not a medical proposition. This is the legalization of drugs that we're concerned about. Here's what the medical advisor in the state of California saw as the potential uses of marijuana. [Here McCaffrey showed a slide.] . . . It includes recalling forgotten memories, cough suppressants, Parkinson's disease, writer's cramp. This is not medicine. This is a Cheech and Chong show. And now what we are committed to doing is to look in a scientific way at any proposition that would bring a new medicine to the assistance of the American medical establishment.[19]

Secretary of Health and Human Services Donna Shalala said that the initiatives reinforced the growing belief among Americans that marijuana is not harmful, whereas the administration remained "opposed to the legalization of marijuana [because] all available research has concluded that marijuana is dangerous to our health."[20] Nonetheless, she did say that the National Institutes of Health (NIH) would continue to support and review "peer-reviewed" and "scientifically valid" research on "the possible usefulness of smoked marijuana in the limited circumstances where available medications have failed to provide relief for individual patients."[21]

Finally, Attorney General Janet Reno announced that physicians who followed the terms of the California law would be the new targets of federal law enforcement (instead of drug dealers) and threatened physicians with loss of their registrations with the DEA and with exclusion from participation in Medicare and Medicaid. She stated:

> Federal law still applies. . . . U.S. attorneys in both states will continue to review cases for prosecution and DEA officials will review cases as they have to determine whether to revoke the registration of any physician who recommends or prescribes so-called Schedule 1 controlled substances. We will not turn a blind eye toward our responsibility to enforce federal law and to preserve the integrity of medical and scientific process to determine if drugs have medical value before allowing them to be used.[22]

DOCTOR-PATIENT CONVERSATIONS

Two basic issues are raised by the administration's position. One involves government regulation of doctor-patient conversations, and the other the quality of evidence necessary to make marijuana available by prescription. A group of California physicians filed suit against McCaffrey, Reno, and Shalala, arguing that the threats of prosecution against physicians for talking to their patients violate their First Amendment rights and interfere with their ability as physicians to use "their best medical judgment in the context of a bona fide physician-patient relationship."[23]

In the only comparable case to reach the U.S. Supreme Court, the Court narrowly upheld a gag rule related to discussing abortion in a federally funded Title X family-planning clinic.[24] The Court upheld the gag rule because Congress could reasonably limit the types of medical services available at a federally funded facility.[25] The Court was able to sidestep the First Amendment issue because patients (at least in theory) had access to other doctors who had an obligation to furnish them with full information, and the doctor-patient relationship in a Title X clinic was characterized as not "all-encompassing but, rather, as limited only to preconception counseling:

> The Title X program regulations do not significantly impinge upon the doctor-patient relationship. Nothing in them requires a doctor to represent as [his or her] own any opinion that [he or she] does not in fact hold. Nor is the doctor-patient relationship established by expectation on the part of the patient of comprehensive medical advice. The program does not provide post-conception

medical care, and therefore a doctor's silence with regard to abortion cannot reasonably be thought to mislead a client into thinking that the doctor does not consider abortion an appropriate option for her.[26]

Even if one accepts this unconvincing rationale, it is impossible to apply it to California physicians who believe that marijuana would be beneficial for their patients and who are providing their overall health care. Patients receiving care for cancer or AIDS rightfully and reasonably expect and are entitled to full disclosure and discussion of available treatment options. The California physicians are on strong legal ground with their lawsuit, and they should prevail. In early April, U.S. District Court judge Fern M. Smith granted a preliminary injunction prohibiting the DEA from carrying out its threats against California physicians and encouraged the litigants to try to work out a settlement of the dispute.[27]

In response to the lawsuit and the growing opposition to its threats to physicians, the administration issued a clarifying letter, essentially stating that physicians may discuss marijuana with their patients so long as they do not recommend its use.[28] This provides no guidance at all. Of course doctors can talk to patients; the question is what they can tell them. The real subject of dispute remains whether physicians can "recommend" marijuana (and thereby grant their patients immunity from state prosecution), as the California proposition provides. Would, for example, telling a patient with cancer that other physicians have reported that marijuana has given their patients relief from nausea constitute a "recommendation"?

Judge Smith made it clear that the First Amendment protects physician-patient communications and that the government has no authority to determine the content of physicians' speech.[29] She also concluded that the federal statements regarding threatened prosecution were vague and thus could lead to physicians' censuring their own speech to avoid possible federal prosecution. On the other hand, she noted (correctly) that the First Amendment does not protect "speech that is itself criminal because [the speech is] too intertwined with illegal activity."[30] Under federal drug laws, which cannot be affected by legislation in California, it remains a crime for physicians to aid, abet, or conspire—by speech or action— to violate federal criminal statutes. Thus, it is not a violation of the First Amendment for the federal government to prosecute or threaten to prosecute physicians who specifically intend to aid, abet, or conspire with their patients to violate federal drug laws.

Judge Smith could have added that to prevail in such a case the government will have to prove more than simply that the physician recommended marijuana as worth trying for a medical condition. The "more" will include evidence that the physician "associated himself with the venture" of illegally purchasing marijuana as something he wished to bring about and sought by his actions to make succeed."[31] This should require at least that the physician identify a source of the marijuana, and some connection between that source and the physician.[32] It is only speech short of this that the injunction covers. Of course, this formulation still leaves it uncertain exactly how far physicians may go in recommending marijuana use before the federal government is justified in prosecuting them for criminal behavior. Judge Smith concluded with an understatement: "This injunction does not provide physicians with the level of certainty for which they had hoped."[33]

MARIJUANA AS MEDICINE

Attempts to have marijuana reassigned from Schedule 1 to Schedule 2 began almost immediately after Congress passed the Uniform Controlled Substances Act of 1970, which established the current system of drug classification. The following findings must be made to place a drug on Schedule 1: "(A) The drug . . . has a high potential for abuse; (B) The drug . . . has no currently accepted medical use in treatment in the United States; and (C) There is a lack of accepted safety for use of the drug under medical supervision." Part A for Schedule 2 drugs is identical; the other requirements are "(B) The drug . . . has a currently accepted medical use in treatment in the United States . . . and (C) Abuse of the drug . . . may lead to severe psychological or physical dependence."

In 1988, after two years of hearings, DEA administrative-law judge Francis Young recommended shifting marijuana to Schedule 2 on the grounds that it was safe and had a "currently accepted medical use in treatment."[34] Specifically, Judge Young found that "marijuana, in its natural form, is one of the safest therapeutically active substances known to man. . . . At present it is estimated that marijuana's LD-50 [median lethal dose] is around 1:20,000 or 1:40,000. In layman's terms . . . a smoker would theoretically have to consume 20,000 to 40,000 times as much marijuana as is contained in one marijuana cigarette . . . nearly 1500 pounds of marijuana within about fifteen minutes to induce a lethal response." As for medical use, the judge concluded, among other things, that marijuana "has a currently accepted medical use in treatment in the United States for nausea and vomiting resulting from chemotherapy treatments."[35] The administrator of the DEA rejected Young's recommendation, on the basis that there was no scientific evidence showing that marijuana was better than other approved drugs for any specific medical condition. Further attempts to get the courts to reclassify marijuana have been unsuccessful.

Reacting to a DEA suggestion that only a "fringe group" of oncologists accepted marijuana as an antiemetic agent, a survey of a random sample of the members of the American Society of Clinical Oncology was undertaken in 1990.[36] More than one thousand oncologists responded to the survey, and

44 percent of them reported that they had recommended marijuana to at least one patient.[37] Marijuana was believed to be more effective than oral dronabinol (Marinol) by the respondents: of those who believed they had sufficient information to compare the two drugs directly, 44 percent believed marijuana was more effective, and only 13 percent believed dronabinol was more effective.[38] Of course, nothing in the FDA regulations requires a drug to be more effective than an existing one for it to be approved. Nonetheless, in the current anti-marijuana climate, the NIH has consistently refused to fund research on marijuana. In the wake of the California proposition, this position is no longer tenable.

An NIH panel, after a two-day workshop in February [1997], recommended research on marijuana in the areas of wasting associated with AIDS, nausea due to cancer chemotherapy, glaucoma, and neuropathic pain.[39] This list seems reasonable, especially since objective criteria such as weight gain, intraocular pressure, and the frequency of vomiting can be used to determine the drug's effectiveness.

Such research may be difficult to do, but it is possible to compare orally administered dronabinol with smoked marijuana. Some argue that because the symptoms of nausea are so subjective and "extremely difficult to quantify in controlled experiments," marijuana should be available as a prescription drug on a compassionate basis.[40] In fact, current FDA regulations provide the authority for making marijuana available on a compassionate basis while such studies are proceeding. Other support for its compassionate use would appear to come from the Clinton administration's solicitor general, Walter Dellinger, who argued before the Supreme Court less than two weeks after the McCaffrey-Reno press conference that the administration believed that Americans had a weak constitutional right "not to suffer." Although Dellinger said he did not believe this right was broad enough to prohibit the states from making physician-assisted suicide for terminally ill patients a crime, it should certainly be broad enough to prohibit the federal government from denying patients with cancer and AIDS access to drugs that could help them withstand potentially life-saving treatments.

WHAT ABOUT THE CHILDREN?

The final argument that the administration makes against any medical use of marijuana is that this would send the "wrong message" to children, who would then use this "gateway drug" and get hooked on much more harmful substances, such as cocaine and heroin. There are two responses to this argument. The first is provided by *Boston Globe* columnist Ellen Goodman, who asks, "What is the infamous signal being sent to [children]? . . . If you hurry up and get cancer, you, too, can get high?"[41]

The second response relates to the "gateway" issue itself. A 1994 survey found that 17 percent of current marijuana users said they had tried cocaine and only 0.2 percent of those who had not used marijuana had tried cocaine.[42] One way to interpret these data is that children who smoke marijuana are 85 times as likely as others to try cocaine; another is that 83 percent of pot smokers, or five out of six, never try cocaine.[43] Honesty is likely to make a greater and more lasting impression on our children than political posturing and hysteria. Many people want to make marijuana legal for everyone. But opposition to the legalization of marijuana generally is not a good reason to keep it from patients who are suffering. Making marijuana a Schedule 2 drug does not make it widely acceptable or available any more than classifying medicinal cocaine as a Schedule 2 drug made it acceptable or available.

CONCLUSIONS

Doctors are not the enemy in the "war" on drugs; ignorance and hypocrisy are. Research should go on, and while it does, marijuana should be available to all patients who need it to help them undergo treatment for life-threatening illnesses. There is certainly sufficient evidence to reclassify marijuana as a Schedule 2 drug. Unlike quack remedies such as laetrile, marijuana is not claimed to be a treatment in itself; instead, it is used to help patients withstand the effect of accepted treatment that can lead to a cure or amelioration of their condition. As long as a therapy is safe and has not been proved ineffective, seriously ill patients (and their physicians) should have access to whatever they need to fight for their lives.

NOTES

1. S. Sidney, J. E. Beck, I. S. Tekawa, C. P. Quesenberry Jr., and G. D. Friedman, "Marijuana Use and Morality," *American Journal of Public Health* 87 (1997): 585–90.

2. Federal News Service, White House briefing news conference, December 30, 1996.

3. J. P. Kassirer, "Federal Foolishness and Marijuana," *New England Journal of Medicine* 336 (1997): 366–67.

4. Mass. Gen. Laws, Chap. 94D, §2 (West 1996).

5. Cal. Code Sec. 11362.5 (1996).

6. Ibid.

7. Ibid.

8. *United States* v. *Rutherford,* 442 U.S. 544 (1979).

9. Treatment Use of an Investigational New Drug, 21 C.F.R. §312–34.

10. G. J. Annas, "Faith (Healing), Hope and Charity at the FDA: The Politics of AIDS Drugs Trials," *Villanova Law Review* 34 (1989): 771–97.

11. Ibid.

12. *United States* v. *Rutherford*; Annas, "Faith (Healing), Hope and Charity."

13. L. Grinspoon and J. B. Bakalar, *Marihuana: The Forbidden Medicine* (New Haven, Conn.: Yale University Press, 1995).

14. S. J. Gould, "It Worked Like a Charm," *Times,* May 4, 1993.

15. T. Golden, "Medical Use of Marijuana to Stay Illegal in Arizona," *New York Times,* April 17, 1997, p. A14.

16. Cal. Code Sec. 11362.5.

17. Federal News Service, White House briefing conference, December 30, 1996.

18. Ibid.

19. Ibid.

20. Ibid.

21. Ibid.

22. Ibid.

23. *Conant* v. *McCaffrey,* U.S. D.C. No. Cal., No. C97-0139 FMS (1997).

24. *Rust* v. *Sullivan,* 500 U.S. 173 (1991).

25. G. J. Annas, "Restricting Doctor-Patient Conversation in Federally Funded Clinics," *New England Journal of Medicine* 325 (1991): 362–64.

26. *Rust* v. *Sullivan.*

27. T. Golden, "Federal Judge Supports California Doctors on Marijuana Issue," *New York Times,* April 12, 1997, p. 7.

28. S. Stapleton, "Medical Pot: Feds Say Talk Is OK, Just Don't Recommend It," *American Medical News,* March 17, 1997, pp. 1, 33.

29. Ibid.

30. Golden, "Federal Judge Supports California Doctors."

31. *Morei* v. *U.S.,* 127 F.2d. 827 (6 Cir. 1942).

32. *State* v. *Gladstone,* 474 P.2d. 274 (Washington 1970).

33. Golden, "Federal Judge Supports California Doctors."

34. *In the Matter of Marijuana Rescheduling Petition,* U.S. Dept. of Justice, DEA, Docket No. 86-22, September 6, 1988 (Young, J.).

35. Ibid.

36. R. E. Doblin and M. A. Kleiman, "Marijuana as Antiemetic Medicine: A Survey of Oncologists' Experiences and Attitudes," *Journal of Clinical Oncology* 9 (1991): 1314–19.

37. Ibid.

38. Ibid.

39. W. E. Leary, "Panel Urges Study of Medical Marijuana," *New York Times,* February 21, 1997, p. A27.

40. Kassirer, "Medical Foolishness and Marijuana."

41. E. Goodman, "Clear Thinking in the Medical Marijuana Debate," *Boston Globe,* February 2, 1997, p. A27.

42. C. S. Wren, "Phantom Numbers Haunt the War on Drugs," *New York Times,* April 20, 1997, p. 4E.

43. Ibid.

16

Medics in the War on Drugs

Thomas S. Szasz

Drug prohibitionists were alarmed [in] November [1996], when voters in Arizona and California endorsed the initiatives permitting the use of marijuana for "medical purposes."

Opponents of drug prohibition ought to be even more alarmed: The advocates of medical marijuana have embraced a tactic that retards the repeal of drug prohibition and reinforces the moral legitimacy of prevailing drug policies. Instead of steadfastly maintaining that the War on Drugs is an intrinsically evil enterprise, the reformers propose replacing legal sanctions with medical tutelage, a principle destined to further expand the medical control of everyday behavior.

Not surprisingly, the drug prohibition establishment reacted to the passage of the marijuana initiatives as the Vatican might react to an outbreak of heretical schism. Senator Orrin G. Hatch, chairman of the Senate Judiciary Committee, declared: "We can't let this go without a response." Arizona Senator Jon Kyl told the Judiciary Committee: "I am extraordinarily embarrassed," adding that he believed most Arizona voters who supported the initiative "were deceived." Naturally. Only a person who had fallen into error could approve of sin. Too many critics of the War on Drugs continue to refuse to recognize that their adversaries are priests waging a holy war on Satanic chemicals, not statesmen who respect the people and whose sole aim is to give them access to the best possible information concerning the benefits and risks of biologically active substances.

From colonial times until 1914, Americans were the authors of their own drug policy: They decided what substances to avoid or use, controlled the

---

Originally published in *Liberty* magazine 10, no. 4 (March 1997).

drug-using behavior of their children, and assumed responsibility for their personal conduct. Since 1914, the control of, and responsibility for, drug use—by adults as well as children—has been gradually transferred from citizens to agents of the state, principally physicians.

Supporters of the marijuana initiatives portray their policies as acts of compassion "to help the chronically or terminally ill." James E. Copple, president of Community Anti-Drug Coalitions of America, counters: "They are using the AIDS victims and terminally ill as props to promote the use of marijuana." He is right. Former Surgeon General Joycelyn Elders declares: "I think that we can really legalize marijuana." If by "legalizing" she means repealing marijuana prohibition, then she does not know what she is talking about. We have sunk so low in the War on Drugs that, at present, legalizing marijuana in the United States is about as practical as is legalizing Scotch in Saudi Arabia. A 1995 Gallup Poll found that 85 percent of the respondents opposed legalizing illicit drugs.

Supporters of the marijuana initiatives are posturing as advocates of medical "responsibility" toward "sick patients." Physicians complain of being deprived of their right to free speech. It won't work. The government can out-responsible the doctors any day. Physicians have "prescription privileges," a euphemism for what is, in effect, the power to issue patients *ad hoc* licenses to buy certain drugs. This makes doctors major players in the state apparatus denying people their right to drugs, thereby denying them the option of responsible drug use and abdicating their own responsibilities to the government: "We will not turn a blind eye toward our responsibility," declared Attorney General Janet Reno at a news conference on December 30, 1996, where the administration announced "that doctors in California and Arizona who ordered for their patients any drugs like marijuana . . . could lose their prescription privileges and even face criminal charges." I don't blame the doctors for wanting to forget the Satanic pact they have forged with the state, but they should not expect the government not to remind them of it.

The American people as well as their elected representatives support the War on Drugs. The mainstream media address the subject in a language that precludes rational debate: Crimes related to drug prohibition are systematically described as "drug-related." Perhaps most important, Americans in ever-increasing numbers seem to be deeply, almost religiously, committed to a medicalized view of life. Thus, Dennis Peron, the originator of the California marijuana proposition, believes that since relieving stress is beneficial to health, "any adult who uses marijuana does so for medical reasons." Similarly, Ethan Nadelmann, director of the Lindesmith Center (the George Soros think tank for drug policy), states: "The next step is toward arguing for a more rational drug policy," such as distributing hypodermic needles and increasing access to methadone for heroin addicts. These self-declared opponents of the War on Drugs are blind to the fatal compromise entailed in their use of the phrase "rational policy."

If we believe we have a right to a free press, we do not seek a rational book policy or reading policy; on the contrary, we would call such a policy "censorship" and a denial of our First Amendment rights.

If we believe we hare a right to freedom of religion, we do not seek a rational belief policy or religion policy; on the contrary, we would call such a policy "religious persecution" and a denial of the constitutionally mandated separation of church and state.

So long as we do not believe in freedom of, and responsibility for, drug use, we cannot mount an effective opposition to medical-statist drug controls. In a free society, the duty of the government is to protect individuals from others who might harm them; it is not the government's business to protect individuals from harming themselves. Misranking these governmental functions precludes the possibility of repealing our drug laws. Presciently, C. S. Lewis warned against yielding to the temptations of medical tutelage: "Of all the tyrannies a tyranny sincerely exercised for the good of its victims may be the most oppressive. . . . To be 'cured' against one's will and cured of states which we may not regard as disease is to be put on a level with those who have not yet reached the age of reason or those who never will; to be classed with infants, imbeciles, and domestic animals."

Although at present we cannot serve the cause of liberty by repealing the drug laws, we can betray that cause by supporting the fiction that self-medication is a disease, prohibiting it is a public health measure, and punishing it is a treatment.

Part Five

Drug War Metaphors and Addictions: Drugs Are Property

17

The War on Drugs as a
Metaphor in American Culture*

Dwight B. Heath

DECLARATION OF A WAR ON DRUGS

George Bush had been president of the United States for half a year, elected by a landslide victory and inaugurated in a time of welling chauvinism and superficial prosperity. The American people seemed eager to hear his plans when he gave his first televised address in August of 1989. Whatever disappointment there may have been over pressing needs that were not mentioned, his call to arms in the war on drugs struck a responsive chord. During the next several months, the media were full of feature stories, editorials, news reports, and background accounts about "the drug menace," the "war on drugs," and a host of other approaches to drug use and its deadly impact. At one level the imagery of war could be viewed as just a metaphor, a rhetorical device virtually guaranteed to galvanize public opinion, demonstrate the speaker's decisiveness, rally support, and draw a sharp line between "us" and "them." No longer a wimp, as he had earlier been characterized, President Bush had identified a common enemy, announced a firm stand, and promised to take action to "defeat" the other side. Such rhetoric on the part of other presidents had been applauded in connection with the "war on poverty" and the "war on illiteracy," as it had been earlier with the

Originally published in *Drug Policy and Human Nature,* W. K. Bickel and R. J. DeGrandpre, eds. (New York: Plenum Publishing Corporation, 1996). Reprinted by permission of the publisher and author..

*Although some of the ideas herein were used in the author's "U.S. Drug Control Policy: A Cultural Perspective" in *Daedalus: Journal of the American Academy of Arts and Sciences,* and *Proceedings of the American Academy of Arts and Sciences* 121 (1992): 269–91, much has been expanded and updated from the earlier version.

"war against drink" and, probably, in a series of other pseudoevents in American history.

It is an unfortunate characteristic that the United States literally seems to "need" an enemy, as is evidenced in the widespread and vehement spate of Japan-bashing that sprang up as the cold war with the former Soviet Union wound down. Subsequent interventions in Iraq, Rwanda, Somalia, and Haiti, whatever the details given as immediate justification, also fit the longterm pattern. The pervasive imagery of warfare has even permeated our view of health and human biology—the body is characterized as being "attacked" by various kinds of intruding germs or toxins, which are "fought off" by components of the immune system; if the "invading forces" should "overwhelm" them at one point, they are likely to encounter a "second line of defense" in another biochemical process, and eventually be "mopped up." There can be no doubt that war is a powerful metaphor, however reluctant Americans may be to admit to favoring it.

Within a month of President Bush's call to arms, public opinion polls reported that nearly 65 percent of the American people were identifying drugs as "the major issue facing this country," and there appeared to be remarkable consensus in support of a militant agenda against them. A year later, the same pollsters found only 10 percent responding that way, and the number has been diminishing ever since. President Clinton, and, subsequently, even the "new Republicans" have made little mention of any such concern. What was happening on the home front in the war on drugs? This striking change of outlook reflects the complexity and ambivalence of what is often too glibly characterized as a homogenous American culture.

The imagery of war not only caught people's attention and won strong support from the action-oriented media; it also fit with attitudes and values that have deep roots in the U.S. national character. It was perhaps scary, but in a way reassuring, that "the bad guys" who were making huge profits outside of the law, victimizing children and other vulnerable individuals, were mostly foreigners—generally shorter, darker-skinned people with alien names and accents, often operating with apparent impunity in corrupt nations of the Third World. Reports of "drug-related deaths" and other violence mushroomed in number, with the implication being that the few demonstrably innocent victims were more representative than the vast majority who were themselves criminals vying over turf or money.

Even within the United States, those who were "on the other side" in the war on drugs were generally portrayed and perceived as being black or Hispanic, poor (or unjustly rich), unwilling to work, too quick to resort to violence, and in other respects deserving of collective condemnation. Such a stereotype of addicts is regularly contradicted by national surveys of drug use and by enrollment in treatment programs, both of which reveal that regularly employed middle-class whites predominate in number in both categories.

Some social scientists who bring a psychoanalytic perspective to this issue emphasize the tendency of populations to project their fears and vices onto a safely remote and outcast group, unconsciously but effectively pointing to a scapegoat. The suggestion is that we "need" addicts and "drug lords" as vessels for all the negative qualities that we decline to admit within ourselves, seeing them in ways that justify our "waging war" upon them (Stein, 1985). All of those themes were played out as hostile gangs, no longer content to fight among themselves in Los Angeles, were said to be infiltrating smaller cities, and even the previously uncorrupted Midwest. Fidel Castro, who rid Cuba of its traditional drug problem, was accused of trafficking, and General Manuel Noriega—previously an esteemed ally but, in the wake of the Iran-gate trials, branded a "drug lord"—was brought to trial even though the United States had to invade Panama to get him. Evidently the war on drugs, even if it had started as a metaphor, quickly became much more than that.

As if to facilitate the coordination of strategy and to minimize account-ability, a new Office of National Drug-Control Policy was established. Within the White House, it was effectively insulated from influence by the Department of Health and Human Services, the Justice Department, and other agencies in which some administrators already had experience relevant to drug use and its outcomes. First directed by "Drug Czar" William Bennett, whose thinking about drugs was not prejudiced by any previous knowledge on the subject, it rapidly promulgated a policy directed almost exclusively at the supply side. With 70 percent of its generous budget devoted to keeping drugs from entering the United States or from being sold to users, the agency employed a panoply of military hardware and tactics. Large grants were made to the armies and to paramilitary police forces in producing countries, ostensibly to support the office's efforts to eradicate the noxious crops of coca, poppy, and cannabis.

Those who had long been committed to lessening the physical, psychic, and social harm that stems from excessive use of some psychoactive drugs expressed concern that the 30 percent left over for the demand side was grossly inadequate. They deplored the loss of funds for programs of educa-tion, prevention, and treatment that they knew relieved much human suf-fering and that they hoped could immunize the populace against the spread of such problems. When Director Bennett was asked about the insignificant number of deaths that are attributed to "hard drugs" each year and the much larger numbers that are attributed to tobacco and alcohol, he held fast to the idea that legality was the significant boundary, once even recommending the death penalty for drug dealers but exempting legal substances from his policy. As long as the cold war remained an international preoccupation, the Pentagon served as a quiet broker for providing training, supplies, and equip-ment to other countries, but steadfastly declined to become more actively engaged in the war on drugs.

However, as soon as people started talking about how to spend "the peace dividend" that some assumed would flow from progressive disarmament following the collapse of the Soviet Union, the Department of Defense changed its mind and eagerly joined the war on drugs, committing large numbers of planes and ships to constant monitoring of the vast air and sea-traffic by which drugs are brought into the United States. Uniformed soldiers were sent to complement Drug Enforcement Agency operatives as "trainers" and "advisors," and some have already been killed in action in Peru (Morales, 1986; Walker, 1985). Helicopters, jeeps, guns, ammunition, uniforms, radios, and other kinds of military supplies and equipment have been provided so lavishly that, at the second inter-American drug summit, held in early 1992, the presidents of both Bolivia and Colombia declined further assistance. Although they did not say so in public at San Antonio, they made it clear at home that they had become fearful for the security of their own governments in the face of increasingly powerful and corrupt military officers, who appear more often to profit from drug dealers than bring them to justice (MacDonald, 1989).

Farmers in the Andes, who are being paid not to plant coca on old terraces near towns in which it has been the staple crop for centuries, are moving to cultivate it in new areas at a rapid rate (Morales, 1990; Sanabria, 1993). Efforts at interdiction cost far more than the insignificant amounts that are captured, and few traffickers have been caught. The profit margin is so great that smugglers readily abandon planes or boats that are likely to be intercepted, and there is no shortage of personnel at any level in the various stages of production and distribution. The drugs that are banned have probably never been more abundant, less expensive, and of better quality than is the case now, some years after President Bush's dramatic declaration of war on drugs.

Bennett's successor, Lee Brown, was given some symbolic support by having his position added to the president's cabinet while simultaneously seeing his budget and staff both sharply curtailed. He added alcohol to the list of drugs to be dealt with under the national policy but has done nothing to change laws or regulations about alcohol. Meanwhile, the director of the Food and Drug Administration undertook to regulate tobacco products (which had been exempted from its jurisdiction as "agricultural"), on the basis of calling nicotine an addictive drug. During the first half of Clinton's presidency, little else had changed except that the attention devoted by the media and the public to the subject of drugs sharply diminished as concerns about health, the economy, and foreign relations became more dominant.

If it seems paradoxical that, after years of a so-called war on drugs, they are so cheap and readily available, a brief view of the ambivalent love-hate relationship that humankind has had with drugs over time may help us to appreciate some of the factors that are involved.

WHY PEOPLE CARE ABOUT DRUGS:
AN ANTHROPOLOGICAL PERSPECTIVE

Throughout all of recorded history, and probably much earlier according to archeological evidence, psychoactive drugs have been used by humankind. The tendency for people to alter their perceptions deliberately is so old and widespread that Weil (1986) postulated a universal human need for occasional changes in mood and perception, and Siegel (1989) extended that to "the fourth need" for all animals, on the basis of the frequency with which many species of insects, birds, and mammals appear to seek out substances that are psychoactive. What such substances do is alter consciousness, perceptions, moods, and sensations in ways that are closely linked with changes in logical thinking, often resulting in drastic changes in overt behavior. Many of us have noticed that bees or yellow jackets often cannot fly well after having drunk the juice of overripe fruits or berries; bears have been seen to stagger and fall down after eating fermented honey; and birds often crash or fly haphazardly while intoxicated on ethanol that occurs naturally as free-floating microorganisms convert vegetable carbohydrates to sugar. In tropical areas, watching monkeys may have led humans to discover some of the hallucinogenic mushrooms and naturally occurring snuffs that flourish in the jungle. Although some of the psychoactive drugs that are now commercially popular are products of fairly sophisticated chemical technology, others occur naturally, with no human intervention. The glib ideal some people voice of achieving a "drug-free environment" is therefore elusive, if not impossible to achieve.

Although there is still confusion about what constitutes a drug, what drugs may be more harmful or less harmful, and what the costs and benefits of a drug-free workplace are, nevertheless it is altogether feasible for people to exert varying degrees of control over access to and use of such drugs. In most human societies, there are different kinds of social control exercised over those psychoactive substances that are locally recognized, so that not everyone may use them all of the time. Regulation may mean that one drug should be used by males and another by females; that children under a certain age may be discouraged from taking any; and that members of different castes, classes, occupational groups, or other relevant categories may be expected—or forbidden—to indulge. At the same time, there may be social rules defining what is appropriate and what is not in terms of time and place, who else is present, or what one is doing at the same time.

One of the principal reasons why people tend to feel so strongly about psychoactive drugs—whether for or against—is the customary tradition of such social controls, which presumably grew out of ancient observations about the nature of alterations in behavior that accompanied mind alteration. In much of the Western world these days, there are many and severe regulatory and legal restrictions on drugs, including outright prohibition of some, and there appear to be increasing calls for progressively more restrictions, with extremes such as "zero tolerance," a "drug-free workplace," and "Just Say No." At the same time, there has been another strong current of opinion favoring a more libertarian approach to drug use, variously referred to as "legalization," "relegalization" (to emphasize what was legal earlier), or "decriminalization."

These strong countercurrents have resulted in a large and rapidly growing literature, often cast in terms of juxtaposed "pro" and "con" arguments, whether as op-ed essays in newspapers, magazine articles, or paired chapters in books and professional journals. Much of what has been written about drugs lately has been cast in terms of a simplistic "either/or" dialectic: for or against "the war on drugs" or related liberal legal reforms. However accurate, well written, and thoughtful some such efforts have been, most do not address the telling fact that substantive data on the subject are all too scarce. For that matter, it is difficult to imagine what kind of methodologically and ethically sound experiments would really help us weigh these alternatives in a rigorously scientific manner. What we can and should do is go beyond the almost formulaic exchanges that too often present premises as if they were conclusions and represent affect as if it were data.

THE ELUSIVE NATURE OF DRUG PROBLEMS

If we hold to a cultural perspective, we may be able to address the real harm that is done to society as well as individuals and to understand better the probable consequences of various courses of action. By looking at the sociocultural system of the United States in relation to a number of other cultures around the world and in relation to its own historical antecedents, we can muster relevant evidence from a number of "natural experiments." That is, since we cannot easily conduct experiments on large human populations using the classic scientific method of manipulating variables, what we do is refocus our lens and pay attention to those variables as they occur in different combinations around the world. In anthropological terms, such controlled comparison can be said in some measure to do violence to the functional integration and contextual meanings that are sometimes of great significance for certain cultural traits, but more often such strictures are of only minor importance.

Cross-cultural and historical evidence can help us understand the range of psychoactive drug use, its meanings, and its outcomes. As we see that people's views of both drugs and associated problems differ markedly from one population to another, and that such views can change significantly in short periods of time within a given population, it becomes evident that "drug-related problems" are social constructs more than they are objective facts and associations. The natural experiments provided by a cross-cultural perspective also demonstrate the greater value of informal (social and normative) controls over formal (legal and regulatory) controls in shaping individual and collective behavior.

When we take a cross-cultural perspective, some striking facts quickly emerge. One is the great variety of psychoactive drugs that humankind has discovered and invented, some occurring ready-made in nature and others requiring elaborate preparation. Another is the great variety of uses to which they are put, rarely just for relaxation and recreation but more often in close and important association with religious, medical, or other practices. Similarly, there are often fads and fashions, with drugs that have been popular at one time being neglected or even scorned at another time. There are always closely related rules and social norms about who may use a drug, when and where, in the company of whom, in what way, with what utensils or paraphernalia, and even with what result. Such rules and norms are not only clear in prescriptive terms, but they are also usually mirrored by equally strong proscriptions, a list of "Thou shalt not's."

To illustrate, first consider the industrialized nations of North America, which are not generally thought of as being culturally alien. Even in this familiar setting, we find that there is a marked ambivalence toward alcohol and drugs, from strongly favorable to distinctly negative over time, with popular beliefs and attitudes as well as laws and regulations changing to reflect those shifts. Although the view of drugs as "the enemy" has been remarkably persistent, it has been applied to different drugs at different times (Musto, 1989). Similarly, associated restrictions and warnings have been remarkably similar, although the substances targeted have changed. Increase Mather, the quintessentially ascetic Puritan minister of seventeenth-century New England, condemned drunkenness but at the same time celebrated "drink" (a category including distilled spirits as well as beer) as "a good Creature of God" (Mather, 1674). A century later, Declaration of Independence signer and physician Benjamin Rush wrote a book that became a best-seller condemning liquor as a major cause of physical and mental illness (Rush, 1784). By 1840, nearly half of the states had voted their own prohibition laws, but most were repealed in the 1860s (Rorabaugh, 1979). Per capita consumption rose dramatically and saloons—formerly cherished as "the working men's social club"—were targeted as dens of iniquity, sedition, and family breakup. The temperance movement was not a reactionary fringe phenomenon at the time; on the contrary, it tended to be linked closely with such progressive causes as equality of the sexes, child labor laws, and increasing welfare programs. Other ideas that tended to recur regularly with the temperance sentiment have been concerns with fresh air and exercise as wholesome necessities and a preference for loose clothing and "natural" (substantial and unadulterated) foods.

National prohibition (1919–1933) is often derided as a failure because moonshining, speakeasies, and the unprecedented fashionable public drinking by women made a mockery of the law, while criminal gangs gained wealth and power in the illicit trade. After repeal, there was a steady rise in drinking until the 1980s, when a downward trend began and continues. Not only are individuals drinking less—and the beverages themselves are often offered with lowered alcohol content—but the whole meaning of drinking is again being refocused. A highly vocal and effective New Temperance Movement (Heath, 1989), pointing to traffic fatalities, learning disabilities, accelerating health costs, and falling productivity and working through a number of so-called consumer-interest groups is attempting increasingly to restrict the availability of alcoholic beverages, by increasing taxes, limiting hours and outlets of sale, and a variety of other restrictive measures. Although they reject the label of "Neo-Prohibitionists," they were effective in imposing prohibition on anyone under twenty-one years of age; even though the vote, right to marry without parental permission, and other legal perquisites of majority are afforded to eighteen-year-olds. Although it has not yet been enacted into law, we have already seen waiters in restaurants try to enforce prohibition on pregnant women, and U.S. government publications often recommend abstention for women "who might become pregnant"—a sizeable portion of the population—as well as for those "planning to drive or to operate heavy equipment."

If we expand our vision and look beyond North America, we find that all of the psychoactives that are now legal and widely enjoyed were at one time illegal and feared (Brecher, 1972). Coffee and chocolate, which most North Americans now consider innocuous, were viewed with suspicion when they first became available in Europe and the Near East. In terms very similar to those used with reference to "hippy drugs" in the 1960s, they were associated with laziness, sexual license, and political intrigue. In the seventeenth century, just visiting a coffeehouse was a capital offense in what are now Egypt, Saudi Arabia, and Turkey—all places where coffeehouses are now important centers of sociability and business (Hattox, 1985). King James I of England wrote a diatribe against tobacco and would probably have banned it if his advisors had not made so much of its tax value; at various times it was illegal in China, Germany, Persia, Russia, and Turkey, and its use is rapidly being restricted in the United States, after eighty years of unprecedented popularity. Kava was traditionally drunk in ceremonial contexts in much of Melanesia, but it has recently come to be viewed as dangerous when taken with alcohol (Lebot, Merlin, and Lindstrom, 1992). Peyote is a sacrament among various Mexican Indian tribes and in the Native American Church, although its secular use is illegal.

Beer is more important than bread as a staple food in many parts of the world, and may well predate it historically. It was an important offering to the gods in pharonic Egypt, and still is in many African and South American tribes. Hogarth vividly depicted it in his etchings as bringing health, happiness, and prosperity to seventeenth-century London. It was associated with lazy but conniving German socialists in the United States at the beginning of this century, as it is now linked to drunken college students in a noisy "animal house" fraternity or with the brawling "lager louts" who riot after English soccer games.

Marijuana has long been used as an energizer by sugarcane harvesters in Jamaica and by stevedores in Costa Rica. In the United States of the 1920s, it was known but use was virtually limited to poor blacks and jazz musicians. With the repeal of Prohibition, government agents shifted their attention from moonshine to cannabis (Grinspoon, 1977), which they portrayed as leading to the uncontrolled lust of "reefer madness," and, just a few decades later, the diametrically contrasting but equally deplorable "amotivational syndrome." Widely adopted as a relaxant and euphoriant, marijuana was briefly habilitated by many in the medical community. Within less than a decade, the pendulum of opinion swung back, and both physical and mental damage are again often attributed to its use. Many jurisdictions that had decriminalized its sale and use, and more its possession, have rescinded those laws, and the federal government in 1992 banned its use for medical purposes, even under prescription.

The Opium War resulted from British violation of a long-standing ban on opium in China in much the same way that fifty years later, the Chinese were blamed for having forced opium on unsuspecting North Americans (Blum and Associates, 1974). The image of opium, which has been esteemed in the Western world as a stimulant to artistic creativity, became famished late in the nineteenth century, as the association shifted from vague exoticism to utter depravity, part of the Oriental "yellow peril" that was threatening to lure American women into "white slavery" and to erode American will and industriousness.

Coca has been used for nutritive, social, and religious purposes by Andean Indians for millennia, with no evidence of deleterious consequences. In the late 1800s, it and its derivative cocaine were widely regarded as virtual panaceas, supposedly endorsed by famous and successful people including the pope. During World War I, cocaine was rumored to have been a tool of German spies, and in the 1930s the image of the "dope fiend" illustrated how its use supposedly resulted in a kind of amoral and antisocial madness. By the 1970s it had come to be viewed by many, including physicians, as an innocuous "recreational drug," but in the 1990s, it was again deplored as being addictive, a major cause of crime, and a significant threat to the next generation. The smokable derivative "crack" took on an even more sinister image, popularly (but inaccurately) believed to cause "instant addiction." Heroin was initially hailed as a safe alternative to morphine in much the same way that methadone is now used as an addictive but legal substitute for heroin. Tranquilizers that were hailed as a boon in relieving the stresses of the 1960s have evolved, in our thinking, to play an important role in the "multiple dependency" of not only those who use them but also in the "codependency" that supposedly debilitates people who care about such users.

The recent invention and rapid diffusion of glue- and solvent-sniffing as a means of altering consciousness is a fascinating instance of popular inventiveness, adapting familiar industrial products to wholly unforeseen purposes. In that instance, it is apparent that the U.S. mass media played a significant role in rapidly converting what had been harmless tools into dangerous drugs (Brecher, 1972); the same appears to have happened later in Canada (Alexander, 1990).

Much earlier in history and halfway across the world, the Arab culture in which Mohammed was reared valued not only drink but drunkenness; Persian poets waxed eloquent about both in a land that is now officially dry. Similarly, poets and philosophers of ancient China sang the praises of wine and its disinhibiting effects, but prohibition was enacted throughout the empire at various times. Ambivalence is not a new or a Western invention.

For that matter, a visitor from another planet might well be suspicious of Homo sapiens' vaunted preoccupation with positivism and pragmatism, and suggest that it is highly unlikely that the pharmacological action of any given substance, interacting with the physiology of a single species, could result in such diverse effects, whether among different populations at the same time or on the same population at different times. And such a visitor would be justified, inasmuch as many of us earthlings have wondered about the same apparent anomalies.

To a social scientist accustomed to interpreting evidence that is gleaned from natural experiments, the fact that official and popular attitudes toward the use of alcohol and drugs differ not only among various cultures, but that they also shift—often diametrically within a single culture over only a few decades—strongly suggests a few points that appear simple but that may be crucial. First, we must recognize that problems are in no way inherent in an inert substance, but they can emerge in an interaction between it, the user, and the context. As an important corollary of this, we must also recognize that the user is not just a biological organism affected by a chemical, but is also a complex biopsychosocial system. What this means, in specific terms, is that the user also comprises a personality (influenced by expectations, values, and attitudes), a unique life history (influenced by all sorts of teachings and experiences), and a distinctive combination of statuses, many of which imply very different roles (e.g., female, adult, mother, sister, aunt, godmother, professional, etc.) Most of these and other relevant variables have little relationship (of a kind that might be discernible by strict scientific methods) to any psychoactive substance. Nevertheless, they interact in ways that are salient in determining use, quantity and frequency, and even outcomes of use.

The significance of such realizations is that we must also recognize that many of the problems that are said to be caused by or associated with alcohol and drugs can best be viewed as social constructs. Because they have virtually no direct link to the nature of the substance and little linkage to the way those substances interact with the human body, such problems are based instead on clusters of attitudes and associations in the minds of people. In this way, social problems can be seen to reflect opinions and prejudices of the moment, being highly selective among the facts that are available, rather than objectively reflecting actual events or empirical trends.

A striking example is the shift from virtual tolerance of "tipsy" drivers, whose escapades a decade ago were often reported in the press as humorous when no one was hurt, to a rising vengeful clamor to "get the killer-drunks off the road." A sociologist (Gusfield, 1984) effectively documented the process by which drinking and driving so rapidly came to be perceived as a major problem in the United States. A high percentage of traffic crashes are regularly reported as being "alcohol-related," although there is no mention that many are "darkness-related," or "poor road condition-related," because no one has chosen to shape a public definition of such problems. Even some physicians have complained that, "When an adult beats a child, we do not talk about 'physical abuse problem,' and we do not refer to the danger of drowning as the 'deep water problem.' The idea of a drug problem is not necessarily much more coherent."

One of those who early on proclaimed himself a member of the New Temperance Movement in the United States asserted that the major obstacle to broad public support for education, prevention, and treatment of alcoholism was the invisibility of the problem (Beauchamp, 1980). The growth of private and public agencies, the emergence of Mothers Against Drunk Driving and related organizations, and voluminous media coverage are a few illustrations of how quickly that has changed. The sociologist Wiener (1981) has traced not only the emergence of "the alcohol problem" but also the rapidly changing "ownership of it." It is especially ironic that pressures against advertising and in support of higher taxes, shorter hours, and fewer licenses for sale, and a host of other restrictions on the availability of alcohol continue to mount even as consumption has rapidly diminished since 1980, there are fewer cirrhosis deaths, and an increasing number of teetotalers appear in national surveys. Even the National Institute on Alcohol Abuse and Alcoholism, the federal agency that has most to gain from inflated figures on the subject, recently revised its estimates of the economic costs of alcohol abuse. For methodological reasons, the specific numbers are still suspect, but the overall figures are less than half of what they were just a few years earlier. In light of the social construction of alcohol and drug problems, it is little wonder that people often seek a quick and easy solution through prohibition—and that they almost always fail.

PROHIBITION AS A PROBLEM-SOLVING STRATEGY

There is a simple and direct logic that, if something is troublesome, you're better off without it. Presumably this has been at the root of the various bans on different drugs that we have noted around the world. A striking regularity, however, is that all such prohibitions have been circumvented at the time, and almost all were rescinded by administrators who eventually judged the costs to outweigh the benefits.

This often occurs when violations of a prohibition become so common-place that people recognize the discrepancy between law and practice, and challenge the law. If the gap yawns too large, what is challenged may be not only the specific restrictive law of prohibition, but also the rule of law in general. The United States appears to have come close to this kind of anarchy in the waning days of its federal prohibition on alcohol (Levine, 1985). Canada, Finland, Iceland, India, and tsarist Russia all tried to prohibit drinking during this century, but each found that the combined ills of moonshining, bootlegging, poisoning from nonbeverage alcohol, and bribery of police and officials made for a general sense of corruption and lawlessness that outweighed whatever gains there may have been in other respects. Saudi Arabia and Iran are nation-states where prohibition appears to be relatively effective, presumably because it is so firmly imbedded in religious ideology and context.

If we shift our focus from the nation-state to other entities, it is note-worthy that, even after the repeal of federal prohibition, several states in the United States remained officially dry, with Mississippi the last to repeal prohibition laws in 1984. There are many scattered counties and communities that still forbid sale under "local option" laws, and certain places are kept alcohol-free even in otherwise wet jurisdictions (e.g., in cities, state parks, theaters, sports arenas, etc.).

Prohibition applies differently not only to places but also to populations. There are some religious groups, in whatever country, who abstain as an article of faith. The wording of the Koranic injunction about drinking and gambling is equivocal, but most Muslims interpret it as a prohibition (Badri, 1976); similarly, members of the Church of Jesus Christ of Latter Day Saints (Mormons), the Native American Church, and several Protestant churches cite religious justification for avoiding alcohol; some also forbid caffeine.

For that matter, prohibition is usually in effect for at least part of many societies at any given time, although we tend not to phrase it as such. One such selective prohibition is by age; a minimum age for purchase (and sometimes for use) of alcohol was effectively set at twenty-one throughout the United States in response to economic pressures, with the federal government withholding highway fund allocations until states complied. Other jurisdictions have set a minimum age for purchase of tobacco and even glue. In Spain, some bars are closed to those under eighteen—not because of the access to alcohol, but because they contain video games, which are thought to be addictive.

For many years it was illegal to give, sell, or trade alcoholic beverages to Australian Aborigines, Swedish Saami (Lapps), Native Americans, and Alaska Natives. Such bans were "justified" on the basis of a supposed "constitutional weakness" that made drinking more dangerous for those subordinated populations than for members of the politically and economically hegemonic population. It is interesting that, when offered the choice in the 1960s or later, a number of Native American reservations and Alaska Native communities in the United States remained dry. In Canada in recent years, many Native American and Inuit bands and reserves have also opted for prohibition; some Australian communities are experimenting with self-imposed bans on alcohol. The outcome of such local prohibitions has been uneven, with some evidence that they exacerbate rather than relieve problems (*American Indian and Alaska Native Mental Health Research,* 1992; *Contemporary Drug Problems,* 1990).

In other instances, selective prohibition is socially enforced with a variety of attitudes, norms, values, and sanctions, even when it does not carry the weight of law. At the height of the Inca Empire, coca chewing appears to have been the prerogative of the nobility. In Aztec society, only priests and old men were allowed to drink, except on rare religious occasions. Opium smoking was traditionally limited to the aged in many parts of southeastern Asia, as khat-chewing is generally monopolized by men in the Near East (Kennedy, 1987). Within a single village in India, one caste drinks cannabis tea and another drinks liquor, each scorning such barbarous behavior in the other (Carstairs, 1954).

Not only are whole polities, religious groups, and social categories characterized by differential rules about availability, but there is also selective prohibition with respect to place. Within the United States, there are increasing calls for "drug-free workplaces," "drug-free schools," and other zones of prohibition. Even within the workplace, all are not treated equally. Frequent drug testing, supposedly with "zero tolerance," is being promoted for employees in the fields of atomic energy, public transportation, and public administration. The fact that such proposals are phrased in terms of protecting the public interest has not diminished the resentment of discrimination on the part of individuals who hold such jobs.

Context need not be restrictive, however; it can also be permissive. Even Orthodox Jews, world-renowned for their usual sobriety, are exhorted as part of the Purim festival to drink until they can't distinguish the hero from the villain in a biblical story (Snyder, 1958). Drinking is similarly an integral part of saints' days and other fiestas among Roman Catholics throughout Latin America, where drunkenness is eagerly sought as a religious act (Heath, 1982).

Similar illustrations of intrasocietal as well as cross-cultural variability could be cited for most psychoactive drugs and for many of the world's nations and their component societies. The major point is that prohibition, far from being a distinctively North American anomaly, has been an intermittent ancient and widespread phenomenon, usually applied inconsistently on various segments of the population. This very inconsistency strongly suggests that the basis for such controls is not grounded in biochemical, neurophysiological, or even psychosocial effects of use.

BLURRED BATTLE LINES IN THE WAR ON DRUGS

Despite the flurry of concern that followed President Bush's call to arms, media and popular concern flagged early as economic recession worsened, and there was recognition that the highly touted policies were winning few battles and held no promise of winning the war; similar lack of media coverage continues under President Clinton. The General Accounting Office (GAO) and various congressional committees issued authoritative reports that contradicted assertions of the National Office of Drug Control Policy and revealed major methodological and arithmetic flaws in the office's calculations (e.g., U.S. Senate, 1991). People became aware that interdiction could not be effective and that there was not even support for treatment of those addicts who requested it. Ever larger quantities of drugs, at even lower prices, told the lie to a supply side approach. Although few U.S. citizens were aware of it, growing resentment of U.S. drug-related intervention abroad was eroding the patience of some of our allies (Trebach and Zeese, 1990 a, b).

Another aspect of the war on drugs that some prefer to ignore, and others would eagerly change, is the mushrooming rate of prison construction and incarceration. With 455 per 100,000 of the population in jails or prisons, the United States now has the dubious distinction of leading the world—far ahead of South Africa, second with 311. By way of contrast, Japan's rate is only 34. While President Bush's attorney general rated this a sign of success and called for more prison space as the only alternative to more crime, a growing number of critics now view with dismay the expansion that has already occurred and consider it a monument to society's failure in terms of economic opportunities, racial discrimination, education, and other respects.

Although the rhetoric of the "war on drugs" has cooled somewhat and domestic economic and political issues have come to the fore in terms of journalistic attention during Clinton's presidency, there has been little change in governmental policy or police and military actions. More than half of the prison population are still there on drug charges, with blacks and Hispanics disproportionately represented. According to government statistics reported in the 1980s and 1990s issues of *National Crime Survey* and *Jail Inmates*

(U.S. Department of Justice, 1973–, 1983–), federal and state prison populations have increased by 90 percent during the past decade, while the crime rate (adjusted for population) remains virtually unchanged. It is evident that massive incarceration has had little effect in reducing crime. Increased reliance on mandatory sentencing, eliminating parole, and building more jail cells has nothing to do with rehabilitation and apparently accomplishes little in the way of deterrence. Poverty, broken families, and unacculturated immigrants are often cited as important causal factors, but the experience of other countries and the historical precedent in the United States both suggest that other, more fundamental, factors must be involved.

Every major city has had too many incidents in which an innocent bystander was shot, but the majority of drug-related violence is directed against competing drug dealers. In similar fashion, although many addicts resort to theft and a variety of petty deceptive schemes to support their habit, those most frequently victimized by such "hustles" are their friends, family, and acquaintances rather than wealthier strangers (Preble and Casey, 1969; Lex, 1990).

Selective detention may be part of the problem, with a persistent pattern of racial and ethnic prejudice acted out daily, as police harass innocent members of one group and are overly tolerant of another. This is not a universal pattern, but it occurs far too often. Similarly, repeated studies have shown that, although justice can't be bought in a simple straightforward transaction, minority suspects with lower income and education are disproportionately booked by police. In 1989, with blacks comprising 12 percent of the population, 42 percent of drug arrests were of blacks. In the same way, among defendants who are tried, those of minority status with lower income and education are disproportionately sentenced, and their sentences are consistently, and significantly, more severe, even for similar offenses (U.S. Department of Justice, 1930–). To call such discrimination genocidal is polemical overstatement, but to call it normal would be a terrible indictment of our legal system.

In a sense, even those who are not members of the discriminated minorities are being hurt by the heavy involvement that the criminal justice system has in prosecuting the war on drugs. In many jurisdictions the police are so burdened with drug issues that other aspects of their work are often neglected. Courts are incredibly overcrowded, as are jails and prisons. Associated costs add a significant burden to already strained budgets, resulting in escalating taxes that weigh heavily on already overtaxed constituents.

An inner-city individual's occasional "success" (in wealth, prestige, and so forth) associated with drugs is taken by many as evidence that "the system" is failing and that amoral behavior is rewarded. However rare they may be, instances of corruption among police, judges, and other government agents carry the same message. Rightly or wrongly, drugs are associated with the high dropout rate in schools, slow learning, teenage pregnancy, accelerating unemployment, falling productivity, the cost of social welfare, and a host of other aspects of contemporary life that people find annoying and discouraging.

Ironically, some of the problems that can be directly and unequivocally linked with excessive use of drugs—such as the costs of rehabilitation and treatment, and the maintenance of impaired infants—are even more significant than seems to be recognized by many who complain most loudly about drugs and their negative impact on society. This can be taken as another very different kind of evidence in support of the view that public problems are socially constructed. In a social construction, what is left out may be no less important than what is included.

What is being ignored in the dominant image of "the drug problem" in the United States today is the fact that so many of the ills that are cited derive more from the prohibition policies that are in effect than from the use of drugs as such. Nadelmann (1989) succinctly phrased it: "The greatest beneficiaries of the drug laws are organized and unorganized drug traffickers. The criminalization of the drug market effectively imposes a de facto value-added tax that is enforced and occasionally augmented by the law enforcement establishment and collected by the drug traffickers" (p. 941). The same occurred earlier with the prohibition of alcohol in the United States and more recently with strict controls on the availability of alcohol in the former Soviet Union (Heath, 1991).

HOPE FOR AN ARMISTICE

The presumed connections among drugs, crime, violence, and disturbed youth are complex, but the experience that other countries have had with public maintenance of drug-dependent persons, together with the artificially inflated prices that illegality imposes and the politically corrupting influence of the huge sums of money that are involved, all suggest that it is counterproductive to leave monopolistic control of production and distribution of now-illicit drugs in the hands of criminal entrepreneurs.

The fallacy of such action, or inaction, has driven many to contemplate appropriate terms for an armistice in the war on drugs. Specific details can be worked out later, but if we again turn our attention to natural experiments as they occur in cross-cultural experience, the broad outlines of crucial first steps appear clear.

One of the leading nations in the liberalization of drug laws is The Netherlands, in keeping with a governing principle of their public health system: Minimize harm. They still distinguish between "hard" and "soft" drugs and actively restrict traffic in "hard" drugs, but they recognize that those who need hard drugs should not be driven into the underworld in order to survive. Heroin and cocaine are available, at reasonable prices and with hygienic apparatuses, in government clinics. Although the sale of marijuana by unlicensed individuals is still illegal—to curb "pushers" who profit from engaging new users—anyone may buy it in the many coffeeshops that are designated outlets, which are marked by a discreet silhouette of a leaf displayed in a window. The Dutch system is not libertarian, as it is often mislabeled, half of those in prison are there on drug charges. Neither is the country encouraging a generation of dropouts. The Netherlands has become a favorite hangout for expatriates from around the world, but, contrary to dire predictions, its drug policy, in combination with easy availability of treatment, has resulted in a reduction rather than an increase in the number of addicts. The Dutch also have much lower rates of incidence of overdose and of HIV seropositivity in comparison with the United States (Buisman, 1988; Leuw, 1994).

An early experiment with governmental monopoly of "hard drugs" took place in England but was cut short by the Conservative government. On a smaller scale, a program in Liverpool continues to do much to normalize the lives of addicts by making drugs available at a clinic under safe conditions and with the encouragement of self-help group therapy and other treatments, which appear to be enjoying at least as much success as freestanding programs. In such a situation, addicts can hold regular jobs and take part in a wide range of community activities that would be closed to them in a context of prohibition. In a way, the Liverpool alternative is not markedly different from methadone maintenance that is offered at many places in the United States. (The progress of various such programs is chronicled in the *International Journal on Drug Policy.*) No one doubts that methadone is addictive in the sense of creating a regular craving and psychological dependence; users suffer classic withdrawal syndrome if they are deprived of it too long. But it is a legally controlled drug, doled out regularly at clinics around the country and widely accepted as preferable to heroin, which remains prohibited. The dubious logic of this licit-illicit (or "soft"-"hard") drug distinction has been challenged by spokespersons for many minority groups who resent state-supported alternative addiction at a time when they are told that funds for treatment are not available even while facilities have long waiting lists of those who want to rehabilitate themselves.

Legalization of drugs need not be viewed as a single giant step in which all restrictions are abruptly removed, resulting in a chaotic free market. Again, the parallel with the repeal of national prohibition on alcohol is relevant. The federal government retained some oversight over production, quality control, and so forth, and levied a tax on both fermented beverages (wines, beers, ales, and related drinks) and distilled spirits (or "hard liquor"). A remarkable degree of discretion was given to the individual states, some of which further allowed for "local option" at a lower level. Even so, alcohol remains one of the most regulated products available, in terms of licensing, location, time, pricing, advertising, and other respects. Similar liberalization

—with taxation and other regulation—could be tried for other drugs by various states.

In any such program, realistic education about alcohol and drugs and the outcomes of their use should be a cornerstone. The salutary experience of the Framingham, Massachusetts, heart-health study (reported in great detail in a series of books, *The Framingham Study*) and of a related study in Pawtucket, Rhode Island, demonstrates that public education can be immensely effective in promoting salubrious changes in behavior, despite the skepticism voiced by many in the drug field. The discrepancy probably results from a narrow interpretation of education, as if it were restricted to material taught in the classroom, often by individuals who are neither knowledgeable nor particularly interested in the subject. When serious efforts are made to educate an entire community, however, engaging grocery stores, scout groups, civil action organizations, churches, and other institutions as well as schools and the media, abundant knowledge can be effectively communicated in ways that affect attitudes and behavior, which in turn result in significant changes in the incidence and prevalence of various illnesses and other health problems (Anderson, 1988; Downie, Fife, and Tannahil, 1990).

The futility of the drug war in its present mode—both abroad and on the home front—suggests that it is time to call an armistice. Continuing legal prohibition as the major strategy for combating drugs is to attempt the impossible, by means that have already been discredited. Historical and cross-cultural evidence suggests that a wiser course would be to aim for a realistic accommodation, to permit but discourage risky misadventures by means that have already proven their effectiveness. This would not mean "surrender" to "the drug lords," nor would it usher in a period of reckless anarchy. Perhaps it would be less threatening to the narcomilitary complex if we were to speak in terms of "liberalization," rather than legalization, relegalization, or decriminalization. To allow people legal access to a substance does not mean that they need have unrestricted access to unlimited quantities. It might even be feasible for different jurisdictions to set up some natural experiments by adopting different specific regulations within a broad pattern of liberalization. In that way, we could soon expect at least quasiscientific evaluations of the outcomes, valuable information that could eventually serve as substantive data for making more confident choices among alternatives, in terms of public health and social welfare, as well as efficiency and efficacy. Instead of suffering a defeat, it could well be that such actions would, in the long run, signal a major victory for the people who are always the ones to suffer most in any kind of war.

REFERENCES

Alexander, B. (1990). *Peaceful Measures: Canada's Way Out of the War on Drugs.* Toronto: University of Toronto Press.

American Indian and Alaska Native Mental Health Research. (1992). Special issue on prohibition in U.S. Indian reservations, 4 (3).

Anderson, R. (Ed.). (1988). *Health Behavior Research and Health Promotion.* New York: Oxford University Press.

Badri, M. B. (1976). *Islam and Alcoholism: Islam, Alcoholism and the Treatment of Muslim Alcoholics.* Tacoma Park, Md.: American Trust Publications.

Beauchamp, D. E. (1980). *Beyond Alcoholism: Alcohol and Public Health Policy.* Philadelphia: Temple University Press.

Blum, R., and Associates. (1974). *Society and Drugs, Drugs 1: Social and Cultural Observations.* San Francisco: Jossey-Bass.

Brecher, E. (1972). *Licit and Illicit Drugs: The Consumers Union Report on Narcotics, Stimulants, Depressants, Inhalants, Hallucinogens, and Marihuana.* Boston: Little, Brown.

Buisman, W. (1988). *Drug Prevention in The Netherlands.* Utrecht, The Netherlands: National Institute for Alcohol and Drugs.

Carstairs, G. M. (1954). "*Daru* and *Bhang*: Cultural Factors in the Choice of Intoxicant." *Quarterly Journal of Studies on Alcohol* 15: 220–37.

Contemporary Drug Problems. (1990). Special Issue on Alcohol Controls among American Indians 17 (2).

Downie, R., C. Fyfe, and A. Tannahil. (1990). *Health Promotion: Models and Values.* New York: Oxford University Press.

The Framingham Study: An Epidemiological Investigation of Cardiovascular Disease. (1968–). (39 volumes to date.) Bethesda, Md.: National Institutes of Health.

Grinspoon, L. (1977). *Marihuana Reconsidered.* Rev. ed. Cambridge, Mass.: Harvard University Press.

Gusfield, J. (1984). *The Culture of Public Problems: Drinking-Driving and the Symbolic Order.* Chicago: University of Chicago Press.

Hattox, R. S. (1985). *Coffee and Coffeehouses: The Origins of a Social Beverage in the Medieval Near East.* Seattle, Wash.: Near Eastern Studies, University of Washington.

Heath, D. B. (1982). "Historical and Cultural Factors Affecting Alcohol Availability and Consumption in Latin America." In Institute of Medicine (Ed.), *Legislative Approaches to Prevention of Alcohol-Related Problems* (pp. 128–88). Washington, D.C.: National Academy Press.

———. (1989). "The New Temperance Movement: Through the Looking-Glass." *Drugs and Society* 3: 143–68.

———. (1991). "Perestroika vs. Prohibition: A New Soviet Experiment." *Addiction Letter* 7, 5.

International Journal of Drug Policy. (1990–). (Originally bimonthly; quarterly since 1992.)

Kennedy, J. G. (1987). *The Flower of Paradise: The Institutionalized Use of the Drug Qat in North Yemen.* Dordrecht, The Netherlands: D. Reidel.

Lebot, V., M. Merlin, and L. Lindstrom. (1992). *Kava: The Pacific Drug.* New Haven, Conn.: Yale University Press.

Leuw, E. (1994). *Between Prohibition and Legalization: The Dutch Experiment in Drug Policy.* Amsterdam, The Netherlands: Kugler.

Levine, H. G. (1985). "The Birth of American Alcohol Control: Prohibition, the Powerelite, and the Problem of Lawlessness." *Contemporary Drug Problems* 12: 63–115.

Lex, B. W. (1990). "Narcotics Addicts' Hustling Strategies: Creation and Manipulation of Ambiguity." *Journal of Contemporary Ethnography* 18: 388–415.

MacDonald, S. B. (1989). *Mountain High, White Avalanche: Cocaine and Power in the Andean, States and Panama.* Westport., Conn.: Praeger.

Mather, I. (1674). *Wo to Drunkards: Two sermons testifying against the sin of drunkenness, wherein the wofulness of that evil and the misery of all that are addicted to it, is discovered from the Word of God.* Cambridge: Marmaduke Johnson.

Morales, E. (1990). *Cocaine: White Gold Rush in Peru.* Tucson: University of Arizona Press.

———. (Ed.). (1986). *Drugs in Latin America* (Studies in Third World Societies 37). Williamsburg, Va.: College of William and Mary.

Musto, D. (1989). *The American Disease: Origins of Narcotic Control.* Rev. ed. New York: Oxford University Press.

Nadelmann, E. (1989). "Drug Prohibition in the United States: Costs, Consequences, and Alternatives." *Science* 245: 939–47.

Preble, E., and J. Casey. (1969). "Taking Care of Business: The Heroin User's Life on the Streets." *International Journal of the Addictions* 4: 1–24.

Rorabaugh, W. (1979). *The Alcoholic Republic: An American Tradition.* New York: Oxford University Press.

Rush, B. (1784). *An inquiry into the effects of ardent spirits upon the human body and mind: with an account of the means of preventing, and of the remedies for curing them.* Philadelphia: Thomas Bradford.

Sanabria, H. (1993). *The Coca Boom and Rural Social Change in Bolivia.* Ann Arbor: University of Michigan Press.

Siegel, R. (1989). *Intoxication: Life in Pursuit of Artificial Paradise.* New York: E. P. Dutton.

Snyder, C. R. (1958). *Alcohol and the Jews: A Cultural Study of Drinking and Sobriety.* Glencoe, Ill.: Free Press.

Stein, H. (1985). "Alcoholism as Metaphor in American Cultures; Ritual Desecration as Social Integration." *Ethos* 13, 195–234.

Trebach, A., and K. Zeese. (1990a). *Prohibition and the Conscience of Nations.* Washington, D.C.: Drug Policy Foundation.

———. (1990b). *The Great Issues of Drug Policy.* Washington, D.C.: Drug Policy Foundation.

U.S. Department of Justice. (1983–). *Jail Inmates* (annual). Washington, D.C.: Department of Justice.

———. (1973–). *National Crime Survey* (annual). Rockville, Md.: Department of Justice.

———. (1930–). *Uniform Crime Reports* (annual). Rockville, Md.: Department of Justice.

U.S. Senate. (1991). *Committee on the Judiciary Reports on National Drug-Control Policy.* Washington, D.C.: U.S. Government Printing Office.

Walker, W. O. III. (1985). *Drug Control in the Americas.* Albuquerque: University of New Mexico Press.

Weil, A. (1986). *The Natural Mind: An Investigation of Drugs and the Higher Consciousness.* Rev. ed. Boston: Houghton Mifflin.

Wiener, C. L. (1981). *The Politics of Alcohol: Building an Arena around a Social Problem.* New Brunswick, N.J.: Transaction.

18

Curing the Drug-Law Addiction: The Harmful Side Effects of Legal Prohibition

Randy E. Barnett

INTRODUCTION

Some drugs make people feel good. That is why some people use them. Some of these drugs are alleged to have side effects so destructive that many advise against their use. The same may be said about statutes that attempt to prohibit the manufacture, sale, and use of drugs. Using statutes in this way makes some people feel good because they think they are "doing something" about what they believe to be a serious social problem. Others who support these laws are not so altruistically motivated. Employees of law enforcement bureaus and academics who receive government grants to study drug use, for example, may gain financially from drug prohibition. But as with using drugs, using drug laws can have moral and practical side effects so destructive that they argue against ever using legal institutions in this manner.

One might even say—and not altogether metaphorically—that some people become psychologically or economically *addicted*[1] to drug laws. That is, some people continue to support these statutes despite the massive and unavoidable ill effects that result. The psychologically addicted ignore these harms so that they can attain the "good"—their "high"—they perceive that drug laws produce. Other drug-law users ignore the costs of prohibition because of their "economic dependence" on drug laws; these people profit financially from drug laws and are unwilling to undergo the economic "withdrawal" that would be caused by their repeal.

Originally published in *Dealing with Drugs: Consequences of Government Control,* edited by Ronald Hamowy, published by Pacific Research Institute for Public Policy, 1997. Reprinted with permission of Pacific Research Institute for Public Policy.

Both kinds of drug-law addicts may "deny" their addiction by asserting that the side effects are not really so terrible or that they can be kept "under control." The economically dependent drug-law users may also deny their addiction by asserting that (1) noble motivations, rather than economic gain, lead them to support these statutes; (2) they are not unwilling to withstand the painful financial readjustment that ending prohibition would force them to undergo; and (3) they can "quit" their support any time they want to (provided, of course, that they are rationally convinced of its wrongness).

Their denials notwithstanding, both kinds of addicts are detectable by their adamant resistance to rational persuasion. While they eagerly await and devour any new evidence of the destructiveness of drug use, they are almost completely uninterested in any practical or theoretical knowledge of the ill effects of illegalizing such conduct.

Yet in a free society governed by democratic principles, these addicts cannot be compelled to give up their desire to control the consumption patterns of others. Nor can they be forced to support legalization in spite of their desires. In a democratic system, they may voice and vote their opinions about such matters no matter how destructive the consequences of their desires are to themselves, or—more importantly—to others. Only rational persuasion may be employed to wean them from this habit. As part of this process of persuasion, drug-law addicts must be exposed to the destruction their addiction wreaks on drug users, law enforcement, and on the general public. They must be made to understand the inherent limits of using law to accomplish social objectives.

In this chapter, I will not attempt to identify and "weigh" the costs of drug use against the costs of drug laws. Instead, I will focus exclusively on identifying the harmful side effects of drug law enforcement and showing why these effects are unavoidable. Such a "one-sided" treatment is justified for three reasons. First, a cost-benefit or cost-cost analysis may simply be impossible.[2] Second, discussions by persons who support illegalizing drugs usually emphasize only the harmful effects of drug use while largely ignoring the serious costs of such policies. By exclusively relating the other side of the story, this chapter is intended to inject some balance into the normal debate. Third, the effects of drug use will be discussed by other contributors to this volume.

The harmful side effects of drug laws have been noted by a number of commentators,[3] although among the general public the facts are not as well known as they should be. More important, even people who agree about the facts fail to grasp that it is the nature of the means—coercion—chosen to pursue certain ends—the suppression of voluntary consumptive activity—that makes these effects unavoidable. This vital and overlooked connection is the main subject of this chapter.

Clarifying Our Terms

Before we can discuss the destructive effects of drug laws, it is necessary to clarify the nature of (1) the legal approach to social problem-solving and (2) the conduct that is the subject of these particular laws.

The Nature of the Legal Approach

There are two senses in which we regularly use the word law. The term *law* may refer simply to a command that has been enacted according to procedures recognized by a community to be legitimate.[4] In contrast, the same term may also be used to describe a rule or principle that is both duly enacted and sufficiently "right" that it merits at least a prima facie moral duty of obedience.[5] Using the term *law* in the second sense, it may be said that a duly enacted statute or "law" that is unjust is not really a law at all.[6]

This difficulty arises, at least in part, from our using the same word in two ways, where other societies employ two different words.[7] In this discussion, when I use the phrase "drug laws," I am only speaking descriptively about duly enacted statutes regulating drug use. When, however, I speak of the institution of law generally, I mean those rules that are not only duly enacted, but are also in accord with principles of right or justice. I expect that the context will also help clarify this distinction.

Drug laws reflect the decision of some persons that other persons who wish to consume certain substances should not be permitted to act on their preferences. Nor should anyone be permitted to satisfy the desires of drug consumers by making and selling the prohibited drug. For our purposes, the most important characteristic of the legal approach to drug use is that these consumptive and commercial activities are being regulated *by force*.[8] Drug-law users wish to decide what substances others may consume and sell, and they want their decision to be imposed on others by force.

The forcible aspect of the legal approach to drug use is one of two factors that combine to create the serious side effects of drug-law use. The other contributing factor is the nature of the conduct that drug laws attempt to prohibit.

Clarifying the Type of Conduct Under Consideration

Only by understanding the kind of conduct that is the subject of drug laws and how it differs from other kinds of conduct regulated by law can we begin to see why the legal order is the inappropriate sphere in which to pursue our objectives.

No one claims that the conduct sought to be prohibited is of a sort that, if properly conducted, inevitably causes death or even great bodily harm.[9] Smoking tobacco is bad for your health. It may shorten your life considerably. But it does not immediately or invariably kill you. The same is true of smoking marijuana.[10] Of course, prohibited drugs can be improperly administered and cause great harm indeed, but even aspirin can be harmful in certain cases. Further, the conduct that drug laws prohibit is not inevitably addicting.[11] Some users become psychologically or physically dependent on prohibited substances. Others do not.[12]

What then characterizes the conduct being prohibited by statutes illegalizing drugs? It is conduct where persons either introduce certain intoxicating substances into their own bodies, or manufacture or sell these substances to those who wish to use them. The prime motivation for the drug user's behavior is to alter his state of mind—to get "high."[13] The harmful effects of the substances are not normally the effects being sought by the user—thus they are usually termed "*side* effects." People could introduce all sorts of harmful substances into their bodies, but do not generally do so unless they think that it will have a mind-altering effect. Anyone who wishes to ingest substances to cause death or great bodily harm will always have a vast array of choices available to him at the corner hardware store. A widespread black market in poisons has not developed to meet any such demand.

One can speculate about the underlying psyche of those who would engage in such risky behavior. One can argue that such persons must be "self-destructive"—that is, out to harm themselves in some way. It is doubtful, however, that such generalizations are any truer for drug users than they are for alcohol users or cigarette smokers, for whom the adverse health effects may be both more likely and more severe than those of many prohibited substances,[14] or for skydivers or race car drivers—not to mention the millions of people who (for reasons that totally escape me) ardently refuse to wear their seat belts.[15]

We can conclude, then, that the two salient characteristics of drug laws are the *end* or purpose of such laws and the means by which they attempt to fulfill this end. The end of drug laws is to discourage people from engaging in (risky) activity they wish to engage in either because they desire the intoxicating effects they associate with the consumption of a drug or because they desire the profit that can be realized by supplying intoxicating drugs to others. The means that drug laws employ to accomplish this end is to use force against those who would engage in such activities, either to prevent them from doing so or to punish those who nonetheless succeed in doing so.

THE HARMFUL EFFECTS OF DRUG LAWS ON DRUG USERS

At least part[16] of the motivation for drug prohibition is that drug use is thought to harm those who engage in this activity.[17] A perceived benefit of drug prohibition is that fewer people will engage in self-harming conduct than would in the absence of prohibition.[18] While this contention will not be disputed here, there is another dimension of the issue of harm to drug users that may seem obvious to most when pointed out, but nonetheless is generally ignored in policy discussions of drug prohibition. To what degree are the harms of drug use caused not by intoxicating drugs, but by the fact that such drugs are illegal?

Drug Laws Punish Users

The most obvious harm to drug users caused by drug laws is the legal and physical jeopardy in which they are placed. Imprisonment must generally be considered a harm to the person imprisoned or it would hardly be an effective deterrent.[19] To deter certain conduct it is advocated that we punish—in the sense of forcibly inflicting unpleasantness upon—those who engage in this conduct.[20] In so doing it is hoped that people will be discouraged from engaging in the prohibited conduct.

But what about those who are not discouraged and who engage in such conduct anyway? Does the practice of punishing these persons make life better or worse for them? The answer is clear. As harmful as using drugs may be to someone, being imprisoned makes matters much worse.

Normally when considering matters of legality, we are not concerned about whether a law punishes a lawbreaker and makes him worse off. Indeed, normally such punishment is deliberately imposed on the lawbreaker to protect someone else whom we consider to be completely innocent—like the victim (or potential victim) of a rape, robbery, or murder.[21] We are therefore quite willing to harm the lawbreaker to protect the innocent. In other words, the objects of these laws are the victims; the subjects of these laws are the criminal[s].

Drug laws are different in this respect from many other criminal laws. With drug prohibition we are supposed to be concerned with the well-being of prospective drug users. So the object of drug laws—the persons whom drug laws are supposed to "protect"—are often the same persons who are the subject of drug laws. Whenever the object of a law is also its subject, however, a problem arises. The means chosen for benefiting prospective drug users seriously harms those who still use drugs and does so in ways that drugs alone cannot: by punishing drug users over and above the harmful effects of drug use. And the harm done by drug prohibition to drug users goes beyond the direct effects of punishment.

Drug Laws Raise the Price of Drugs to Users

Illegalization makes the prices of drugs rise. By increasing scarcity, the confiscation and destruction of drugs causes the price of the prohibited good to rise. And by increasing the risk to those who manufacture and sell, drug laws raise the cost of production and distribution, necessitating higher prices that reflect a "risk premium." (Price increases will not incur indefinitely, however, because at some level higher prices will induce more production.) Like the threat of punishment, higher prices may very well discourage some from using drugs who would otherwise do so. This is, in fact, the principal rationale for interdiction policies. But higher prices take their toll on those who are not deterred, and these adverse effects are rarely emphasized in discussions of drug laws.

Higher prices require higher income by users. If users cannot earn enough by legal means to pay higher prices, then they may be induced to engage in illegal conduct—theft, burglary, robbery—that they would not otherwise engage in.[22] The increased harm caused to the victims of these crimes will be discussed below as a cost inflicted by drug laws on the general public. Of relevance here is the adverse effects that drug laws have on the life of drug users. By raising the costs of drugs, drug laws breed criminality. They induce some drug users who would not otherwise have contemplated criminal conduct to develop into the kind of people who are willing to commit crimes against others.

Higher prices can also make drug use more hazardous for users. Intravenous injection, for example, is more popular in countries where the high drug prices caused by prohibition give rise to the most "efficient" means of ingesting the drug. In countries where opiates are legal, the principal methods of consumption are inhaling the fumes of heated drugs or snorting.[23] While physical dependence may result from either of these methods, neither is as likely as intravenous injections to result in an overdose. And consumption by injection can cause other health problems as well. For example: "Heroin use causes hepatitis only if injected, and causes collapsed veins and embolisms only if injected intravenously."[24]

Drug Laws Make Drug Users Buy from Criminals

Drug laws attempt to prohibit the use of substances that some people wish to consume. Thus because the legal sale of drugs is prohibited, people who still wish to use drugs are forced to do business with the kind of people who are willing to make and sell drugs in spite of the risk of punishment. Their dealings must be done away from the police. This puts users in great danger of physical harm in two ways.

First, they are likely to be the victims of crime.[25] I would estimate that approximately half the murder cases I prosecuted were "drug related" in the sense that the victim was killed because it was thought he had either drugs or money from the sale of drugs. Crimes are also committed against persons who seek out criminals from whom to purchase prohibited drugs.[26] These kinds of cases are brought to the attention of the authorities when the victim's body is found. A robbery of a drug user or dealer is hardly likely to be reported to the police.

Second, users are forced to rely upon criminals to regulate the quality and strength of the drugs they buy. No matter how carefully they measure their dosages, an unexpectedly potent supply may result in an overdose. And if the drug user is suspected to be a police informant, the dosage may deliberately be made potent by the supplier.

Drug Laws Induce the Invention of New Intoxicating Drugs

Drug laws make some comparatively benign intoxicating drugs—like opiates—artificially scarce and thereby create a powerful (black) market incentive for clandestine chemists to develop alternative "synthetic" drugs that can be made more cheaply and with less risk of detection by law enforcement. The hallucinogen, phencyclidine hydrochloride—or "PCP"—is one drug that falls into this category.[27] Some of these substitute drugs may turn out to be far more dangerous than the substances they replace, both to the user and to others.[28]

Drug Laws Criminalize Users

Prohibition automatically makes drug users into "criminals." While this point would seem too obvious to merit discussion, the effects of criminalization can be subtle and hidden. Criminalized drug users may not be able to obtain legitimate employment. This increases still further the likelihood that the artificially high prices of illicit drugs will lead drug users to engage in criminal conduct to obtain income. It is difficult to overestimate the harm caused by forcing drug users into a life of crime. Once this threshold is crossed, there is often no return. Such a choice would not be nearly so compelling if prohibited substances were legal.

Further, criminalization increases the hold that law enforcement agents have on drug users. This hold permits law enforcement agents to extort illegal payments from users or to coerce them into serving as informants who must necessarily engage in risky activity against others. Thus illegalization both motivates and enables the police to inflict harm on drug users in ways that would be impossible in the absence of the leverage provided by drug laws.

In sum, drug laws harm users of drugs well beyond any harm caused by drug use itself, and this extra harm is an unavoidable consequence of using legal means to prevent people from engaging in activity they deem desirable. While law enforcement efforts typically cause harm to criminals who victimize others, such effects are far more problematic with laws whose stated goals include helping the very people that the legal means succeed in harming. Support for drug laws in the face of these harms is akin to saying that we have to punish, criminalize, poison, rob, and murder drug users to save them from the harmful consequences of using intoxicating drugs.

To avoid these consequences, some have proposed abolishing laws against personal use of certain drugs, while continuing to ban the manufacture and sale of these substances.[29] However, only the first and last of the five adverse consequences of drug prohibition just discussed result directly from punishing and criminalizing users. The other three harms to the user result indirectly from punishing those who manufacture and sell drugs. Decriminalizing the use of drugs would undoubtedly be an improvement over the status quo, but the remaining restrictions on manufacturing and sale would continue to cause serious problems for drug users beyond the problems caused by drug use itself.

As long as force is used to minimize drug use, these harms are unavoidable. They are caused by (1) the use of force (the legal means) to inflict pain on users, thereby directly harming them; and (2) the dangerous and criminalizing black market in drugs that results from efforts to stop some from making and selling a product others wish to consume. There is nothing that more enlightened law enforcement personnel or a more efficient administrative apparatus can do to prevent these effects from occurring. But, as the next section reveals, enlightened law enforcement personnel or an efficient administrative apparatus will not come from employing legal force to prevent adults from engaging in consensual activity.

THE HARMFUL EFFECTS OF DRUG LAWS ON THE GENERAL PUBLIC

The harmful side effects of drug laws are not limited to drug users. This section highlights the various harms that drug laws inflict on the general public. There is an old saying in the criminal courts that is particularly apt here: "What goes around, comes around." In an effort to inflict pain on drug users, drug laws inflict considerable costs on nonusers as well.

Resources Spent on Drug Law Enforcement

The most obvious cost of drug prohibition is the expenditure of scarce resources to enforce drug laws—resources that can thus not be used to enforce other laws or be allocated to other productive activities outside of law enforcement.

Every dollar spent to punish a drug user or seller is a dollar that cannot be spent collecting restitution from a robber. Every hour spent investigating a drug user or seller is an hour that could have been used to find a missing child. Every trial held to prosecute a drug user or seller is court time that could be used to prosecute a rapist in a case that might otherwise have been plea bargained. These and countless other expenditures are the "opportunity costs" of drug prohibition.

Increased Crime

By artificially raising the price of illicit drugs and thereby forcing drug users to obtain large sums of money, drug laws create powerful incentives to commit property and other profitable crimes. And the interaction between drug users and criminally inclined drug sellers presents users with many opportunities to become involved in all types of illegal conduct.

Finally, usually neglected in discussions of drugs and crime are the numerous "drug-related" robberies and murders (sometimes of innocent parties wrongly thought to have drugs) that the constant interaction between users and criminal sellers creates. Drug dealers and buyers are known to carry significant quantities of either cash or valuable substances. They must deliberately operate outside the vision of the police. They can rely only on self-help for personal protection.

Many drug-law users speculate quite freely about the intangible "adverse effects of drug use on a society." They are strangely silent, however, about how the fabric of society is affected by the increase in both property crimes and crimes of violence caused by drug laws.

Harms Resulting from the "Victimless" Character of Drug Use

The best hidden and most overlooked harms to the general public caused by drug prohibition may also be the most significant. These are harms that result from efforts to legally prohibit activity that is "victimless." It was once commonplace to call drug consumption victimless, but not anymore. Therefore, before proceeding, it is very important to explain carefully the very limited concept of "victimless" crime that will be employed in this section.

To appreciate the hidden costs of drug law enforcement, it is not necessary to claim that the sale and use of drugs are "victimless" in the *moral* sense—that is, to claim that such activity harms only consenting parties and therefore that it violates no one's rights and may not justly be prohibited.[30] For this limited purpose it is not necessary to question the contentions that drug users and sellers "harm society" or that drug use violates "the rights of society."

To understand the hidden costs of drug laws, however, it is vitally important to note that drug laws attempt to prohibit conduct that is "victimless" in a strictly *nonmoral* or descriptive sense, that is, there is no victim to complain to the police and to testify at trial. This will be explained at greater length in the next section, and the implications of this dimension of drug law enforcement will then be explored.

The Incentives Created by Crimes without Victims

When a person is robbed, the crime is usually reported to the police by the victim. When the robber is caught, the victim is the principal witness in any trial that might be held. As a practical matter if the crime is never reported, there will normally not be a prosecution because the police will never pursue and catch the robber. From the perspective of the legal system, it will be as though the robbery never took place. So also, if the victim refuses to cooperate with the prosecution after a suspect has been charged, the prosecution of the robber will usually not go forward.[31]

As a theoretical matter, however, the victim of a robbery is not a party to a criminal prosecution.[32] The victim is considered to be a witness—sometimes called a "complaining witness"—to the crime; the government could prosecute the defendant without the cooperation of the victim, as it prosecutes those accused of murder.[33] What special law enforcement problems result from an attempt to prosecute crimes in the absence of a victim (or "complaining witness") who will assist law enforcement officials?

To answer this question, let us imagine that robbery—a crime that undoubtedly has a victim[34]—was instead a "victimless" crime in this very limited sense, and that the police set out to catch, and prosecutors to prosecute, all robbers whose victims refused to report the crime to the police and cooperate with the prosecution. How would the police detect the fact that a crime had occurred? How would they go about identifying and proving who did it? How would the case be prosecuted?

To detect unreported crimes, the police would have to embark on a program of systematic surveillance. Because they could not simply respond to a robbery victim's complaint as they do at present, the police would have to be watching everywhere and always. Robberies perpetrated in "public" places —on public streets or transportation, in public alleys or public parks[35]— might be detected with the aid of sophisticated surveillance equipment located in these public places. Those robberies committed in private places— homes and stores—would require even more intrusive practices.

If the police did detect a robbery, they would be the principal witnesses against the defendant at trial. It would be their word against that of the alleged robber. As a practical matter, it would be within their discretion to go forward with the prosecution or not. There would be no victim pressing them to pursue prosecution and potentially questioning any decision they might make to drop the charges or withhold a criminal complaint.

We can easily imagine the probable results of such a policy of victimless crime enforcement. To the extent that they were doing their job and that money permitted, the police would be omnipresent. One could not do or say anything in public without the chance that police agencies would be watching and recording. The enormous interference with individual liberty that such surveillance would cause is quite obvious. And putting robbery prosecutions entirely in the hands of the police would create lucrative new opportunities for corruption in at least two ways, depending on whether or not a crime had in fact occurred.

When a crime had occurred, if the effective decision of whether or not to prosecute is solely in the hands of the police, police officers would be far more able to overlook a criminal act than they are when a cognizable victim exists. As a result, the opportunities for extortion of bribes and the incentives for robbery suspects to offer bribes are both tremendously increased. When a crime had not occurred, the fact that the courts would be accustomed to relying solely on police testimony in such cases would give the police a greater opportunity to fabricate (or threaten to fabricate) cases to punish individuals they do not like, to coerce someone into becoming an informant, or to extort money from those they think will pay it.

All of the increased opportunity for corruption would result directly from an attempt to prosecute robberies when robbery victims do not come forward to report and prosecute the crime themselves. If robbery were victimless in this way, the natural counterweight to these corrupt practices—the potential outrage of the victim of the robbery and the normal reliance by courts on victim testimony—would be absent.[36]

Of course we know that this is not how robbery victims normally behave. Victims do routinely report instances of robbery, creating a case that the police department must "clear" in some way. And they are usually willing to cooperate with the prosecution, giving the police far less ability to influence the success of a given prosecution.[37] Where a victim exists, the problem of corruption is enormously reduced; this is true even for the crime of murder where the victim cannot be a witness.[38]

Now suppose that in addition to not reporting the crime and not testifying at trial, robbery victims were willing to pay to be robbed; that they actively but secretly sought out robbers, deliberately meeting them in private places so that the crime would be perpetrated without attracting the attention of the police; that billions of dollars in cash were received by robbers in this way.

Such a change in the behavior of robbery victims would dramatically affect law enforcement efforts. First, as will be discussed in the next section, the secrecy engendered by the consensual nature of this "victimless" transaction would make necessary far more intrusive kinds of investigative techniques than we at first supposed. Second, the victims' willingness to pay robbers to be robbed would make robbery more lucrative than it would otherwise be and would thus increase the ability of robbers to bribe the police when they are caught.

Police who are willing to fabricate evidence against someone they knew to be a robber would expect that such a person would probably be able to afford a substantial payoff. Of course, corrupt police officers would be risking detection by honest officers and prosecutors. So we can expect that corrupt officers will attempt to minimize their risk by entering into a regular prepayment arrangement with professional robbers to ensure that they would not be arrested when they commit a robbery. Such an illicit arrangement could be enforced by the corrupt officer's credible threat to prosecute a legitimate case or, if necessary, to fabricate a case.

The sale and use of illicit drugs are like victimless robberies, with the final twist I added. Drug users not only fail to report violations of the drug laws, they actively seek out sellers in ways that are designed to avoid police scrutiny. Drug use is a private act that, unlike most robberies, does not take place in public places. And, because drugs users desire to consume drugs, they are quite willing to pay for the product.

Because drug use and sale are "victimless" in the special descriptive sense employed here, the hypothetical consequences of policing victimless robberies result, all too regularly and unavoidably, from drug law enforcement. The next three sections will discuss some of the more serious of these consequences.

Drug Laws and Invasion of Privacy

The fact that drug use takes place in private, and that drug users and sellers conspire to keep their activities away from the prying eyes of the police, means that surveillance must be extremely intrusive to be effective. It must involve gaining access to private areas to watch for this activity.

One way to accomplish this is for a police officer, or more likely an informant, to pose as a buyer or seller. This means that the police must initiate the illegal activity and run the risk that the crime being prosecuted was one that would not have occurred but for the police instigation.[39] And, since possession alone is also illegal, searches of persons without probable cause might also be necessary to find contraband.

Such illegal conduct by police is to be expected when one seeks to prohibit activity that is deliberately kept away from normal police scrutiny by the efforts of both parties to the transaction. This means that the police must intrude into private areas if they are to detect these acts. The police would be overwhelmed if they actually obtained evidence establishing probable cause for every search for illicit drugs, no matter how small the quantity. But if no constitutional grounds exist for such an intrusion, then a police department and its officers are forced to decide which is more important: the protection of constitutional rights or the failure to get results that will be prominently reported by the local media.

The Weakening of Constitutional Rights

The fact that such privacy-invading conduct by police may be unconstitutional and therefore illegal does not prevent it from occurring. Some of those who are most concerned about the harm caused by drug laws are lawyers who have confronted the massive violations of constitutional rights that drug laws have engendered.[40] Such unconstitutional behavior is particularly likely, given our bizarre approach to policing the police.[41]

At present we attempt to rectify police misconduct mainly by preventing the prosecution from using any illegally seized evidence at trial. While this would generally be enough to scuttle a drug law prosecution, it will not prevent the police from achieving at least some of their objectives. They may be more concerned with successfully making an arrest and confiscating contraband than they are with obtaining a conviction. This is especially true when they would have neither confiscation nor conviction without an unconstitutional search.[42]

In most instances, the success of a suppression motion depends on whether the police tell the truth about their constitutional mistake in their report and at trial. They may not do so if they think that their conduct is illegal. "There is substantial evidence to suggest that police often lie in order to bring their conduct within the limits of the practices sanctioned by judicial decisions."[43] The only person who can usually contradict the police version of the incident is the defendant, and the credibility of defendants does not generally compare favorably with that of police officers.

Those who have committed no crime—who possess no contraband—will have no effective recourse at all. Because no evidence was seized, there is no evidence to exclude from a trial. As a practical matter, then, the police only have to worry about unconstitutional searches if something illicit turns up; but if something turns up and they can confiscate it and make an arrest, they may be better off than if they respect constitutional rights and do nothing at all. Moreover, by encouraging such frequent constitutional violations, the enforcement of drug laws desensitizes the police to constitutional safeguards in other areas as well.

The constitutional rights of the general public are therefore threatened in at least two ways. First, the burden placed on law enforcement officials to enforce possessory laws without victims virtually compels them to engage in wholesale violations of constitutional prohibitions against unreasonable searches and seizures.[44] For every search that produces contraband there are untold scores of searches that do not. And given our present method of deterring police misconduct by excluding evidence of guilt, there is little effective recourse against the police available to those who are innocent of any crime.[45]

Second, the widespread efforts of police and prosecutors to stretch the outer boundaries of legal searches can be expected, over time, to contribute to the eventual loosening up of the rules by the courts. The more cases that police bring against obviously guilty defendants (in drug prosecutions, the evidence being suppressed strongly supports the conclusion that the defendants are guilty), the more opportunities and incentives the appellate courts will have to find a small exception here, a slight expansion there.[46] And instead of prosecuting the police for their illegal conduct, the prosecutor's office becomes an insidious and publicly financed source of political and legal agitation in defense of such illegal conduct.[47]

One point should be made clear. The police are not the heavies in this tale. They are only doing what drug-law users have asked them to do in the only way that such a task may effectively be accomplished. It is the drug-law users who must bear the responsibility for the grave social problems caused by the policies they advocate. By demanding that the police do a job that cannot be done effectively without violating constitutional rights, drug-law users ensure that more constitutional rights will be violated and that the respect of law enforcement personnel for these rights will be weakened.

The Effect of Drug Laws on Corruption

While most people have read about corrupt law-enforcement officials who are supposed to be enforcing drug laws, few people are fully aware how this corruption is caused by the type of laws being enforced. Drug laws allow police to use force to prevent voluntary activities. Unavoidably, the power to prohibit also gives the police a power to (de facto) franchise the manufacture and sale of drugs, in return for a franchise fee.

The increased corruption caused by prohibiting consensual activity is further increased by the ease with which law enforcement officers can assist criminals when there is no complaining victim. As was seen in the discussion of "victimless robberies," without a victim to file an official complaint, it is easier for police to overlook a crime that they might see being committed. When there is no victim to contradict the police version of the event, it is much easier for police to tailor their testimony to achieve the outcome they desire—whether good search/bad search or guilt/innocence. It is usually their word against the defendant's, and in such a contest the defendant usually loses. With no victim pressing for a successful prosecution, the police, prosecutor, or judge may scuttle a prosecution with little fear of public exposure.

Owing to the victimless character of drug offenses (in the limited sense discussed above) and the fact that drug users are willing to pay for drugs, the incentives created by making drug use illegal are quite perverse when compared to a victim crime like robbery. When robbery is made illegal, robbers who take anything but cash must sell their booty at a tremendous discount. In other words, laws against robbery reduce the profit that sellers of illegally obtained goods receive and thereby discourage both robbery and the potential for corruption.[48]

Drug laws have the opposite effect. The actions of drug law enforcement create an artificial scarcity of a desired product. As a result sellers receive a *higher* price than they would without such laws. While it is true that drug prohibition makes it more costly to engage in the activity, this cost is partially or wholly offset by an increased return (higher prices) and by attracting individuals to the activity who are less risk-averse (criminals)—that is, individuals who are less likely to discount their realized cash receipts by their risk of being caught.[49] For such persons, the subjective costs of providing illicit drugs are actually less than they are for more honest persons.

As I have observed elsewhere,[50] the social consequences of the wholesale corruption of our legal system by the large amounts of black-market money to be made in the drug trade have never been adequately appreciated. The extremely lucrative nature of the illicit drug trade makes the increased corruption of police, prosecutors, and judges all but inevitable. And this corruption extends far beyond the enforcement of drug laws.

Since the prohibition of alcohol we have witnessed the creation of a multibillion-dollar industry to supply various prohibited goods and services. The members of this industry are ruthless profit-maximizers whose comparative market advantage is their ability and willingness to rely on violence and corruption to maintain their market share and to enforce their agreements.

The prohibition of alcohol and other drugs has created a criminal subculture that makes little of the distinction between crimes with victims and those without. To make matters worse, to hide the source of their income from tax and other authorities requires these criminals to become heavily involved in "legitimate" or legal businesses so that they may launder their illegally obtained income. They bring to these businesses their brutal tactics, which they employ to drive out the honest entrepreneur.

The fact that law enforcement personnel are corrupted by drug laws should be no more surprising than the fact that many people decide to get high by ingesting certain chemicals. The tragic irony of drug laws is that by attempting to prevent the latter, they make the former far more prevalent. Drug-law users must confront the question of whether the increased systemic corruption that their favored policies unavoidably cause is too high a price to pay for whatever reduction in the numbers of drug users is achieved.

THE INJUSTICE OF DRUG LAWS

In this chapter I have described some people as being "addicted" to drug laws. Just as many people use drugs in spite of the serious harms such conduct can cause, many people advocate the use of drug laws in spite of the savage social and personal harms these laws can inflict. The argument to this point has dwelled exclusively on exposing the hidden costs of drug prohibition—costs that unavoidably result from the fact that drug use is consensual and victimless in a nonmoral or descriptive sense.

There is, however, a more principled or philosophical lesson to be drawn from this discussion of drug laws. How is it that such policies are so popular? True, many of the costs of drug laws are very well hidden and many drug-law supporters directly gain from these policies. Yet the widespread support of such laws may be a symptom of a deeper or more fundamental malady.

We have grown accustomed to thinking that claims of justice are subjective and personal—that such claims are largely extrinsic to "objective" public policy discussions or matters of legality. Some respond to a contention that drug laws are unjust because they violate the *rights* of drug users by characterizing rights claims as "merely assertions. They do not carry any argument with them."[51] To others, any claim about drug laws based on the rights of the drug user is a non sequitur, since they view rights as claims that a legal system will actually respect rather than as claims that a legal system ought to respect.[52] Finally, some would respond to a claim that the drug user's rights render drug laws unjust with the argument that "society" also has rights and that we must look beyond rights to resolve this "conflict between rights."[53]

Each of these commonplace arguments fails to fully grasp the crucial role that moral claims and general principles of justice based on individual rights should play in legal decision making. One can fully appreciate the vital role played by principles of justice only by comparing alternative ways of reaching decisions about such an important issue as which conduct should or should not be illegal. And the main alternative to resolving claims by appealing to rules based on general principles of justice is to resolve claims by determining the specific exigencies of particular policies.

Policy makers, however, are inherently much more limited in their ability to construct good policy than is normally acknowledged. First, policy makers suffer from a pervasive ignorance of consequences.[54] In advance of implementing certain kinds of social programs, it is difficult, if not impossible, to predict the precise effects they will have. The foregoing discussion of the hidden costs of drug laws illustrates that it is often very difficult even to detect and demonstrate the adverse effects of policies that have *already occurred.*

Second, the judgment of policy makers and other "experts" is often influenced by self-interest (as all judgment can be). Careers are often based on an articulated commitment to certain kinds of programs, which then become difficult to reject when the consequences of the programs are not as expected. Jobs will be lost if programs are seen as counterproductive or harmful. In rendering opinions, such influences can be hard (though, of course, not impossible) to resist.

To minimize decisions made in ignorance or out of self-interest, legal policy makers must somehow be constrained. And the most practical way to constrain them is to craft general principles and rules—*laws*—reflecting a conception of individual rights that rests on fundamental principles of justice.[55]

A sound legal system requires a firmer foundation for analyzing questions of legality than ad hoc arguments about the exigencies of particular policies. It requires general principles crafted to minimize—without resorting to an endless series of explicit cost-benefit analyses—the hidden costs of the sort we have identified as attaching to drug laws. It requires principles of general application that can be defended as basically just and right, despite the fact that occasions will arise when adherence to such principles *appears* to be causing harm that a deviation from principle would be able to rectify.

A legal system based on such principles—if such principles can actually be identified—would not be as vulnerable to the shifting winds of opinion and prejudice as are particularistic public-policy discussions. I have discussed the vital social role and the appropriate substance of individual rights at greater length elsewhere and shall not repeat the analysis here.[56] The conclusion of such an analysis when applied to drug laws is that such laws are not only harmful, they are unjust.

Recognizing the rights of individuals to control their external possessions and their bodies—traditionally known as property rights—free from the forcible interference of any other person is the only practical way of facilitating the pursuit of happiness for each individual who chooses to live in a social setting. If the pursuit of happiness is the Good for each person, then property rights are the prerequisites for pursuing that Good while living in close proximity to others. And the social prerequisites of the Good are the tenets of justice that all must live by. To deny these rights is to act unjustly.

The inalienable rights of individuals to live their own lives and to control their own bodies are, according to this analysis essential to human survival and fulfillment in a social setting.[57] Drug laws undermine this control by seeking to subject the bodies of some persons to the forcible control of other persons. Such laws seek forcibly to prevent persons from using their bodies in ways that they desire and that do not interfere with the equal liberty of others.

A proper rights analysis would render most legal cost-benefit calculations superfluous and would avoid tragically wasteful (and often irreversible) social experimentation. The two factors that were seen above to generate the hidden costs of drug laws—the *end* of controlling consensual conduct by forcible *means*—are the very factors that together identify drug laws as violations of individual rights and therefore as unjust interferences with individual liberty.

Just as you do not need to try PCP to know it is, on balance, bad for you, a rights analysis tells us that we do not have to try using drug laws to know they are, on balance, bad for all of us. And this is one important reason why a system of rights is ultimately preferable to a system of ad hoc public-policy determinations. If a system of properly crafted individual rights had been adhered to, we would have avoided incurring these serious harms in the first place.

In his essay *Utilitarianism,* John Stuart Mill provides a defense of the distinction between matters of justice or rights that are properly subject to legal enforcement and matters of morality or vice that are not:

> Justice is a name for certain classes of moral rules, which concern the essentials of human well-being more nearly, and are therefore of more absolute obligation, than any other rules for the guidance of life; and the notion which we have found to be the essence of the idea of justice, that of a right residing in the individual, implies and testifies to this more binding obligation. . . .
>
> The moral rules which forbid mankind to hurt one another (in which we must never forget to include wrongful interference with each other's freedom), are more vital to human well-being than any maxims, however important, which only point out the best mode of managing some department of human affairs.[58]

A rights analysis that shows the fundamentally unjust and misguided nature of drug laws does not deny that persons who use drugs are capable of violating, and do in fact violate, the rights of others. Such rights-violating conduct is, however, properly illegal whether or not one is using drugs at the time.[59] Nor does it deny that drug use can adversely "affect" the lives of others. Many kinds of conduct—from quitting school to having sex with strangers—can adversely affect the lives of those close to the persons who engage in such activity.[60]

Legal institutions are not capable of correcting every ill in the world. On this point most would agree. Serious harm results when legal means are employed to correct harms that are not amenable to legal regulation. An individual rights analysis is a way of distinguishing harms that are properly subject to legal prohibition from those that are not.

Conclusion: Curing the Drug-Law Addiction

An addiction to drug laws is caused by an inadequate understanding of individual rights and the vital role such rights play in deciding matters of legality. As a result, policies are implemented that cause serious harm to the very individuals whom these policies were devised to help and to the general public.

If the rights of individuals to choose how to use their person and possessions are fully respected, there is no guaranty that they will exercise their rights wisely. Some may mistakenly choose the path of finding happiness in a bottle or in a vial. Others may wish to help these people by persuading them of their folly. But we must not give in to the powerful temptation to grant some the power to impose their consumptive preferences on others by force. This power—the "essence" of drug laws—is not only "addictive" once it is tasted, it carries with it one of the few guaranties in life: the guaranty of untold corruption and human misery.

NOTES

1. For those who would object to my use of the word *addiction* here because drug laws cause no physiological dependence, it should be pointed out that, for example, the Illinois statute specifying the criteria to be used to pass upon the legality of a drug nowhere requires that a drug be physiologically addictive. The tendency to induce physiological dependence is just one factor to be used to assess the legality of a drug. Drugs with an accepted medical use may be controlled if they have a potential for abuse, and abuse will lead to "psychological *or* physiological dependence," *Illinois Revised Statutes,* ch. 56½, §1205 (emphasis added). See also, id. §§1207, 1209, 1211. Thus, applying the same standard to drug-law users as they apply to drug users permits us to characterize them as addicts if they are psychologically "dependent" on such laws.

Personally, I would favor limiting the use of the term addiction to physiological dependence. As John Kaplan puts the matter: "While the concept of addiction is relatively specific and subject to careful definition, the concept of psychological dependence, or habituation, often merely reflects the commonsense observation that people who like a drug will continue to use it if they can—so long as they continue to like its effects." John Kaplan, *Marijuana—The New Prohibition* (New York: World, 1970), p. 160. The same might be said about those who like drug laws.

2. I discuss some of the problems with efforts at cost-benefit calculation in Randy E. Barnett, "Public Decisions and Private Rights (Review Essay)," *Criminal Justice Ethics* 4 (Summer/Fall 1984): 50.

3. While there certainly is no consensus on the conclusions that ought to be drawn from the facts of this tragic story, the facts themselves are not unknown in law enforcement or in academia. See, for example, John Kaplan, *The Hardest Drug: Heroin and Public Policy* (Chicago: University of Chicago Press, 1983), and Arthur D. Hellman, *Laws against Marijuana: The Price We Pay* (Champaign: University of Illinois Press, 1975). Nor have they escaped the attention of the popular press. See, for example, the series on "The Drug Trade" in the *Wall Street Journal,* November 27 and 29 and December 3, 1984, p. 1; and the series on "Heroin: The Unwinnable War" in the *Washington Times,* September 24–28, 1984, p. 1A. See also, "Research Suggests That Crime Caused by Drugs Is Less Than Public Believes," *Wall Street Journal,* November 29, 1984, p. 20.

4. The original statement of this view was John Austin's. See John Austin, "The Province of Jurisprudence Determined," in *Lectures in Jurisprudence, or the Philosophy of Positive Law* (1832), vol. 1, ed. Robert Cambell (New York: James Cockcroft, 1875), pp. 3–209. The most famous modern statement of this position, which attempts to correct weaknesses in Austin's approach, is H. L. A. Hart, *The Concept of Law* (Oxford: Oxford University Press, 1961).

5. See, for example, Lon L. Fuller, "Positivism and Fidelity to Law—A Reply to Professor Hart," *Harvard Law Review* 71 (1958): 630–72; George Fletcher, "Two Modes of Legal Thought," *Yale Law Journal* 90 (1981): 970–1003.

6. See, for example, Thomas Aquinas, *Summa Theologica,* as it appears in I. Arthur and W. Shaw, eds., *The Philosophy of Law* (Englewood Cliffs, N.J.: Prentice-Hall, 1984), p. 10: "The force of a law depends upon the extent of its justice. . . . If at any time it departs from the law of nature, it is no longer a law but a perversion of law."

7. See Fletcher, "Two Modes of Legal Thought," pp. 980–84. "Because we have no clear concept of *Right* in English, the single word 'law' does double duty. Until the time of Black-

stone and after, the 'common law' clearly had the connotation of law in the sense of Right. At least since the seventeenth century, however, positivist philosophers have sought to equate the word 'law' with enacted law (*Gesetze*)" (p. 982).

8. See Dale A. Nance, "Legal Theory and the Pivotal Role of the Concept of Coercion," *University of Colorado Law Review* 57 (Fall 1985): 1–43. While force is a neglected element of a proper moral evaluation of law, it may not be a necessary characteristic of law. Some institutions that may be characterized as genuinely legal in nature may do their work without using force. See, for example, Lon Fuller, *The Morality of Law* (New Haven: Yale University Press, 1965), pp. 108–10; *The Principles of Social Order*, ed. Kenneth I. Winston (Durham, N.C.: Duke University Press, 1981), pp. 67–246. What is important here is that the *particular* kind of law advocated by drug-control enthusiasts is that kind that *does* involve the use of force. Therefore, in this chapter I will be using the term "law" in this limited sense, and although I will not repeatedly qualify this use in the manner suggested by Fuller's analysis, such a limited use is intended and should be implied.

9. The State of Illinois classifies or "schedules" controlled substances according to their varying characteristics from most serious (Schedule 1) to least serious (Schedule 5). That drugs can cause death or great bodily harm is not a requirement for prohibition. For drugs under schedules 2–5, potential for causing death or great bodily harm is not even a factor to be considered in determining the classification of a controlled substance. See *Illinois Revised Statutes,* ch. 56½, §§1205, 1207, 1209, 1211 (1984). Schedule 1 drugs are those drugs that have a "high potential for abuse" and have "no currently accepted medical use in treatment in the United States *or* [lack] accepted safety standards for use in treatment under medical supervision," Illinois Revised Statutes, ch. 56½, §§1203 (1984) (emphasis added). In other words, if a drug has no accepted medical use in treatment in the United States, all that is required for it to be scheduled is that it have a "high potential for abuse."

10. In discussing the effects of marijuana, the legislative declaration of the Cannabis Control Act of the State of Illinois states only that "the current state of scientific and medical knowledge concerning the effects of cannabis makes it necessary to acknowledge the physical, psychological and sociological damage incumbent upon its use," *Illinois Revised Statutes* ch. 56½, §701 (1984). But see, for example, Munir A. Khan, Assad Abbas, and Knud Jensen, "Cannabis Usage in Pakistan: A Pilot Study of Long-Term Effects on Social Status and Physical Health," in Vera Rubin, ed., *Cannabis and Culture* (The Hague: Morton Publishers, 1975), pp. 349–50: "The most significant point which emerged was that in a society such as Pakistan where cannabis consumption is socially accepted, habituation does not lead to any undesirable consequences. . . . Our study appears to show that cannabis does not produce any serious long-term effects."

11. "For most heavy users the syndrome of anxiety and restlessness seem to be comparable to that observed when a heavy tobacco smoking American attempts to quit smoking." National Commission on Marijuana and Drug Abuse, *Marijuana: A Signal of Misunderstanding* (Washington, D.C., 1972), p. 43. See also, the President's Commission on Law Enforcement and the Administration of Justice, *The Challenge of Crime in a Free Society* (Washington, D.C., 1967), p. 13 ("Physical dependence does not develop"); Khan, Abbas, and Jensen, "Cannabis Usage in Pakistan," p. 349 ("We have deliberately used the word habituation rather than addiction because we did not find either increased tolerance or withdrawal symptomatology, which are the essential prerequisites for addiction"); and Kaplan, *Marijuana—The New Prohibition,* pp. 157–84.

The Illinois statute prohibiting certain substances exemplifies the fact that drug laws are not aimed exclusively at addictive drugs. The criteria of Schedule 1 drugs, quoted in note 9 above, requires only that the substance have a high potential for abuse. The other schedules make it clear that "abuse" is not the same as potential for "psychological or physiological dependence," by consistently listing them as separate factors that must be found before a drug that does have a legitimate medical usage in the United States may be legally controlled. See *Illinois Revised Statutes,* ch. 56½, §§1203, 1205, 1207, 1209, 1211 (1984).

12. For a recent summary of the latest research on the pharmacology of opiates and their effects on the street user, see Kaplan, *The Hardest Drug,* pp. 3–22.

13. One objection to the definition offered in the text for the subject of drug laws is that it would apply to alcohol and caffeine consumption and for this reason must miss some special purpose of drug laws. On the contrary, the manufacture and sale of alcohol were once made illegal for similar reasons. Only the disastrous consequences that resulted from alcohol prohibition and the social acceptability of both alcohol and coffee have kept both substances legal to date. However, at least with alcohol, regulation and even prohibition is constantly being advocated by some and implemented in certain locales.

14. See John C. Ball and John C. Urbaitis, "Absence of Major Medical Complications among Chronic Opiate Addicts," in *The Encyclopedia of Opiate Addiction in the United States,* pp. 301–306; World Health Organization Special Committee, "Problems Related to Alcohol Consumption: The Changing Situation," *Contemporary Drug Problems* 9 (1981): 185. Since the much heralded appearance of the *Report of the Surgeon General's Advisory Committee on Smoking and Health* (1964), the adverse health effects of tobacco smoking have been much studied and are quite well known.

15. If anything, drug consumption that causes one to get high seems a bit more rational than the unwillingness to use seat belts in that there is a tangible benefit gained in return for the risk incurred. In this respect only it is more difficult to argue against mandatory seat-belt laws than drug laws, for it is unclear what benefit the nonuser of a seat belt gains from the risk that he runs. And yet, because such laws affect nearly everyone, the liberty interest involved is easier to see and more widely trumpeted.

Moreover, for those who may be sanguine about seat-belt laws, the *mixture* of drug laws and mandatory seat-belt laws will create widespread and very potent social side effects of its own. See note 44.

16. The other important motivation for drug prohibition is the perceived effects of drug use on the rest of society. This will be considered below. The countervailing costs imposed on society by drug laws will also be discussed.

17. In its "Legislative declaration," the legislature of the State of Illinois expressed this typical sentiment as its end in passing the "Dangerous Drug Abuse Act" of 1965: "It is the public policy of this State that the human suffering and social and economic loss caused by addiction to controlled substances and the use of cannabis are matters of grave concern to the people of the State. It is imperative that a comprehensive program be established . . . to prevent such addiction and abuse . . . and to provide diagnosis, treatment, care and rehabilitation for controlled substance addicts to the end that these unfortunate individuals may be restored to good health and again become useful citizens in the community" (*Illinois Revised Statutes,* ch. 91½, §§120.2 [1981]).

18. "It is the intent of the General Assembly, recognizing the rising incidence in the abuse of drugs and other dangerous substances and its resultant damage to the peace, health, and welfare of the citizens of Illinois, to provide a system of control over the distribution and use of controlled substances which will more effectively: . . . (2) deter the unlawful and destructive abuse of controlled substances; (3) penalize most heavily the illicit traffickers and profiteers of controlled substances, who propagate and perpetuate the abuse of such substances with reckless disregard for its consumptive consequences upon every element of society" (*Illinois Revised Statutes,* ch. 56½, §§1100 [1984]).

19. Imagine if we told people that if we caught them using drugs, we would send them to the Riviera for a few years, all expenses paid.

20. "Characteristically punishment is unpleasant. It is inflicted on an offender because of an offense he has committed; it is deliberately imposed, not just the natural consequence of a

person's action (like a hangover), and the unpleasantness is essential to it, not an accidental accompaniment to some other treatment (like the pain of a dentist's drill)." Stanley I. Benn "Punishment," in Paul Edwards, ed., *The Encyclopedia of Philosophy* (New York: Macmillan, 1967), 7: 29.

21. Punishment is also favored on the grounds that the lawbreaker deserves to be punished. See, for example, John Hospers, "The Ethics of Punishment," in Randy E. Barnett and John Hagel III, eds., *Assessing the Criminal: Restitution, Retribution, and the Legal Process* (Cambridge, Mass.: Ballinger, 1977), pp. 181–209. For an opposing view, see Walter Kaufmann, "Retribution and the Ethics of Punishment," in ibid., pp. 211–30.

22. The traditional linkage between drug use and crime can be accounted for in three ways. The first way, just suggested in the text, is that the higher prices caused by illegality induce many drug users to commit profitable crimes to pay for the drugs. The second way, presented below, is that the criminalization of drug users can force them out of legitimate employment and into criminal employment. The third way, not mentioned in the text, is that some persons who, for whatever reason, are criminally inclined are just the sort of persons who are also inclined to use drugs. What is important is that even if the third account is true for some (which it undoubtedly is), the first and second will be true for others; this means that drug laws are causing a comparative increase in the number of persons who are criminally inclined—an effect of drug laws that hardly benefits those drug users so affected.

23. "Before the Harrison Act [1914], when opiates were cheap and plentiful, they were rarely injected. Moreover, injection is rare in those Asian countries where opiates are inexpensive and easily available. For instance in Hong Kong until recently, heroin, though illegal, was cheap and relatively available, and the drug was inhaled in smoke rather than injected. In the last few years, however, law enforcement has been able to exert pressure on the supply of the drug, raising its price considerably and resulting in a significant increase in the use of injections" (Kaplan, *The Hardest Drug*, p. 128).

24. Ibid., p. 9. In support of this, Kaplan cites Jerome H. Jaffe, "Drug Addiction and Drug Abuse," in Alfred Goodman Gilman, Louis S. Goodman, and Alfred Gilman, eds., *Goodman and Gilman's The Pharmacological Basis of Therapeutics*, 6th ed. (New York: Macmillan, 1980). Kaplan argues that intravenous injection can also increase dependence by producing strong conditioning effects. See Kaplan, *The Hardest Drug*, p. 44. In support of this he cites Travis Thompson and Roy Pickens, "Drug Enforcement and Conditioning," in Hannah Steinberg, ed., *Scientific Basis of Drug Dependence* (New York: Grune & Stratton, 1969), pp. 177–98. Finally, it should be noted that the spread of AIDS (Acquired Immune Deficiency Syndrome) has been caused in part by the sharing of unsterilized needles by drug users.

25. I make the same observation in Barnett, "Public Decisions and Private Rights," which was a review of John Kaplan's *The Hardest Drug*. In that discussion I mistakenly stated that Kaplan had "missed" this phenomenon in "his otherwise exhaustive treatment" (p. 53). In fact, it was I who missed Kaplan's discussion of this most serious problem for drug sellers and users, which appears at pp. 81–83 of his book.

26. In 1979 I obtained the confessions that were ultimately used in a prosecution involving the savage murder of three young men. See *People* v. *Cabellero*, 102 Ill.2d 23, 464 N.E.2d 223 (1984) (relating the factual details of the case). One of the three had approached four street-gang members to purchase marijuana. When his initial attempt to do business with the gang members was rebuffed, he mistakenly believed that this was due to a lack of trust (rather than a lack of marijuana, which was the case). To ingratiate himself with the gang members, be boasted (falsely) about his gang-affiliated friends and his gang membership. Unfortunately the persons he named were members of a *rival* street gang. The gang members then told him that they could supply marijuana after all and asked the three to accompany them to an alley. There they were held at gun point and eventually stabbed to death. These young men were not members of a street gang. These are drug-*law*-related deaths. Three young men are

dead because drug laws prevented them from buying marijuana cigarettes as safely as they could buy tobacco cigarettes. Smoking either kind of cigarette may be hazardous to their health. Unfortunately that issue is now quite moot. Where and how are their deaths registered in the cost-benefit calculation of drug-law users?

27. Although originally developed by Parke-Davis, "the PCP that is now on the streets is illegally manufactured. Unfortunately, it is very easy and very inexpensive to make, and you don't even need a chemistry background." Oakley Ray, *Drugs, Society, & Human Behavior,* 3d ed. (London: Mosby, 1983), p. 414.

28. Because of the "reefer madness" phenomenon that surrounds early reports by drug-law addicts of the ill effects of drug use, such reports should be heavily discounted until time permits more objective researchers to do more extensive studies. The jury appears to still be out on PCP: "Some reports in the scientific literature associate violence with PCP use. Users, however, do not. . . . When violence occurred it was either against property or a panic reaction to restraint attempts. . . . PCP can appeal to those looking for: euphoria (low dose), a wasted, bodywide anesthetic effect with supersensitivity to sensations—the out-of-the-body stage (a moderate dose); or an incoherent, immobile, conscious state (a high dose). If you're having trouble getting a feel for PCP, you're in good company. Even users can't agree what the experience is like. One-third of PCP users say it's unique, another third say it's like the hallucinogens or marijuana, and the last third isn't sure. When neither the users, the researchers, nor the clinicians can agree on the experience, the mechanisms, or the symptoms, you know that more research is needed." Ray, *Drugs, Society, & Human Behavior,* pp. 415–16.

29. For such a proposal concerning heroin, see for example, Kaplan, *The Hardest Drug,* pp. 189–235.

30. I will discuss later the issue of whether drug laws are just. See below.

31. To enforce his decision of noncooperation, the victim always has available the threat of unhelpful testimony at trial. "I don't remember if that is the man who robbed me" is all the victim need say to end the case—and (notwithstanding the theoretical availability of perjury charges) prosecutors know this.

32. The parties to every criminal case are the government (variously referred to as the State, the Commonwealth, the People, or the United States of America) and the defendant(s).

33. Of course, for this reason murder is one of the hardest of all (victim) crimes to prosecute successfully.

34. I have chosen robbery as my example because I wish in this section to separate the issue of who is affected by a crime (who is and who is not a "victim" in this sense) from the issue of how certain crimes must be enforced in the absence of a cognizable victim-witness-complainant. Robberies undoubtedly "affect" the persons who are robbed—and other persons as well. But notwithstanding these effects, if robberies were "victimless" in the sense used in the text—that is, if there was no victim complaining to the police and testifying at trial—certain unavoidable enforcement problems would develop.

35. Breaking and entering into a home or store when no one is present is most everywhere called a "burglary." When someone is home, the crime is sometimes called "home invasion." The most common form of robbery not committed on streets or trains, in alleys or parks is robbery of businesses.

36. As those who have prosecuted criminal cases know, some percentage of robbery victims are bought off in a similar way. When this occurs, however, it can fairly be said that the robber is, at least in part, satisfying his "debt" to the victim. See Randy E. Barnett, "Restitution: A New Paradigm of Criminal Justice," *Ethics* 87 (1977): 279–301 (discussing a restitutive theory of criminal justice).

37. Even with the presence of victims, police still have an ability to influence the outcome of a prosecution. They might, for example, admit to circumstances that would justify the suppression of vital evidence in a case. We thus see some corruption with almost every category

of crime. The analysis in the text, however, is a comparative one. The point is that, all things being equal, far more corruption is likely to take place in the absence of a victim.

38. With the crime of murder, there may still be occurrence witnesses. If there are no witnesses to the murder, it is the discovery of the body under circumstances indicating foul play—and the normal procedures that then ensue—that gives rise to the investigation and ultimate prosecution. Murder cases, in the absence of occurrence witnesses or a confession, however, remain the toughest cases (with victims) to solve or to prosecute.

39. See, for example, Hellman, *Laws against Marijuana,* pp. 60–88.

40. Ibid., pp. 103–31 ("A large proportion of . . . [marijuana] arrests result from police conduct that violates the spirit if not the letter of the Fourth Amendment's prohibition against unreasonable searches and seizures," p. 103); Kaplan, *The Hardest Drug,* pp. 95–97 ("Many of the techniques used to enforce heroin laws do end up violating the constitutional rights of individuals," p. 96).

41. The discussion that immediately follows in the text is only suggestive of a detailed analysis of this problem and a possible solution I have presented elsewhere. See Randy E. Barnett, "Resolving the Dilemma of the Exclusionary Rule: An Application of Restitutive Principles of Justice," *Emory Law Journal* 32 (1983): 937–85, especially pp. 980–85 where I specifically discuss victimless crimes.

42. "A policeman who is unwilling to lie about probable cause or to conceal a prior illegal search may still be inclined to make an arrest for possession of marijuana, even if he is aware that it will not stand up under judicial scrutiny. At a minimum he will have confiscated a supply of an illegal drug. The defendant will be jailed and have to post bail, and in many cases will have to hire a lawyer; these alone serve as forms of punishment. Finally, there is always the possibility that the defendant will plead guilty to a lesser offense rather than risk a felony conviction." Comment, "Possession of Marijuana in San Mateo County: Some Social Costs of Criminalization," *Stanford Law Review* 22 (1969): 115.

43. Hellman, *Laws against Marijuana,* p. 105.

44. I predict that the current infatuation with mandatory seat-belt laws will, in consort with drug laws, create a new and potent social side effect: Violations of seat-belt laws will supplant taillight and other traffic offenses as the most popular justification—or "probable cause"—for automobile stops that are really made to find drugs and guns. And it takes no great imagination to predict which neighborhoods will bear the brunt of this type of "law" enforcement. (Incidentally, I also predict that automobile accident injuries to those who transport illegal drugs will be greatly reduced, owing to a marked increase of seat belt usage among members of this group who will seek to minimize their risk of being stopped.)

45. See Barnett, "Resolving the Dilemma of the Exclusionary Rule," p. 962.

46. Ibid, pp. 959–65.

47. As I have said elsewhere: "Institutionally, the arm of the government whose function is to prosecute illegal conduct is called upon, in the name of law enforcement, systematically to justify police irregularities. If these arguments are successful, the definition of illegal conduct will be altered. . . . Refusal to consider the long-run effect of this phenomenon on the stability of constitutional protections would be dangerous and unrealistic." Ibid., p. 967. These effects are greatly heightened by the demand that prosecutors successfully prosecute drug laws.

48. Organized burglary and auto theft remain profitable (victim) crimes, in spite of the fact that they are legally prohibited, and the profits earned from thae crimes are used in part to pay for the services of corrupt law-enforcement officials. Note however that—as compared with robbery—these crimes typically occur when the victim is not around, making them effectively "victimless" with respect to having occurrence witnesses available. And property insurance policies greatly cool the victim's enthusiasm to cooperate in the prosecution—another quality of a truly victimless crime.

49. For a discussion of the "time horizons" of criminals that may affect their internal rate

of discount, see Edward C. Banfield, "Present-Orientedness and Crime," in Randy E. Barnett and John Hagel III, eds., *Assessing the Criminal: Restitution, Retribution, and the Legal Process* (Cambridge, Mass.: Ballinger, 1977), pp. 133–42. See also, Gerold P. O'Driscoll Jr., "Professor Banfield on Time Horizon: What Has He Taught Us About Crime," ibid., pp. 143–62; Mario J. Rizzo, "Time Preference, Situational Determinism, and Crime," ibid., pp. 163–77.

50. Barnett, "Public Decisions and Private Rights."

51. Kaplan, *The Hardest Drug*, p. 103.

52. See note 4 above. For a discussion of the reemergence of normative legal philosophy, see Randy E. Barnett, "Contract Scholarship and the Reemergence of Legal Philosophy (book review)," *Harvard Law Review* 97 (1984): 1223–36; Jeffrie G. Murphy and Jules L. Coleman, *The Philosophy of Law: An Introduction to Jurisprudence* (Totowa, N.J.: Rowman & Allanheld, 1984), pp. 7–68.

53. A legal system based on rights cannot knowingly countenance conflicting rights. A theory of rights is adopted as a means of resolving conflicting claims. A claim of a person who has a right prevails when it conflicts with a claim made by a person without a right. A particular system of rights that generated two conflicting but "legitimate" rights would be defective because it would not be capable of resolving the conflicting claims being made by the parties. Such a system would not, then, be truly rights-based, or a "higher" principle that is employed to resolve the dispute would dictate the true legitimate right when this kind of conflict occurs. See Hillel Steiner, "The Structure of a Set of Compossible Rights," *Journal of Philosophy* 74 (1977): 767–75; Randy E. Barnett, "Pursuing Justice in a Free Society: Power v. Liberty," *Criminal Justice Ethics* 4 (Winter/Spring 1985): 58.

54. For an excellent summary of the literature that discusses the "knowledge problem" facing public policy analysts, see Don Lavoie, *National Economic Planning: What Is Left?* (Cambridge, Mass.: Ballinger, 1985). pp. 51–92.

55. See Randy E. Barnett, "Foreword: Why We Need Legal Philosophy," *Harvard Journal of Law and Public Policy* 8 (1985): 6–16.

56. See Barnett, "Pursuing Justice in a Free Society," pp. 56–63.

57. I discuss the distinction between alienable and inalienable rights and the inalienable right one has to one's body in Randy E. Barnett, "Contract Remedies and Inalienable Rights," *Social Philosophy and Policy* 4 (Autumn 1986): 179–202,

58. John Stuart Mill, "Utilitarianism" in *Utilitarianism, Liberty, and Representative Government* (New York: Dutton, 1951), p. 73. The position that the law should not attempt to regulate all vices is, of course, much older than Mill. See, for example, Thomas Aquinas, *Summa Theologica*. There he poses the question, "Whether It Belongs to Human Law to repress All Vices?" and answers in part:

> The same thing is not possible to a child as to a full-grown man, and for which reason the law for children is not the same as for adults, since many things are permitted to children which an adult would be punished by law or at any rate open to blame. In a like manner, many things are permitted to men not perfect in virtue, which would be intolerable in a virtuous man.
>
> Now human law is framed for the multitude of human beings, the majority of whom are not perfect in virtue. Therefore human laws do not forbid all vices, from which the virtuous abstain, but only the more grievous vices, from which it is possible for the majority to abstain; and chiefly those which are *injurious to others, without the prohibition of which human society could not be maintained.* Thus human law prohibits murder, theft and the like.

Ibid., p. 11 (emphasis added). The absence of tangible "injuries to others" led some modern writers to characterize laws regulating matters of vice as "victimless crimes." See, for example,

Edwin M. Schur, *Crimes without Victims* (Englewood Cliffs, N.J.: Prentice-Hall. 1965). pp. 120–80.

59. It is a curious, if not yet again a perverse, offshoot of attitudes toward "good" and "bad" that give rise to a criminal justice system based on punishment, that the use of mind-altering substances while committing a crime can reduce the legal consequences for that act, because it either affects the ability to prove *mens rea* or special statutes have been created to deal with the "addict" offender. The perversity comes from punishing drug users more harshly than alcohol users—in part because of a fear that they will commit crimes—but if they do commit a crime they are not punished at all or may not be punished as severely as other persons who commit the same crime.

60. As Herbert Spencer points out:

> Some may argue that it is not allowable to assume any essential difference between right conduct toward others and right conduct toward self, seeing that what are generally considered private actions do eventually affect others to such a degree as to render them public actions, as witness the collateral effects of *drunkenness* or suicide.
>
> In [this allegation] . . . there is much truth, and it is not to be denied that under a final analysis all such distinctions as those above made must disappear. But it must be borne in mind that similar criticisms may be passed upon all classifications whatever. . . . [Spencer then gives several examples of scientific distinctions.] The same finite power of comprehension which compels us to deal with natural phenomena by separating them into groups and studying each group by itself may also compel us to separate those actions which place a man in direct relationship with his fellows from others which do not so place him, although it may be true that such a separation cannot be strictly maintained.

Herbert Spencer, *Social Statics: The Conditions Essential to Human Happiness Specified and the First of Them Developed* (New York: Robert Schalkenbach Foundation, 1970), pp. 64–65 (emphasis added).

19

Drugs as Property: The Right We Rejected

Thomas S. Szasz

> In its larger and juster meaning, it [property] embraces everything to which a man may attach a value . . . [and includes that] which individuals have in their opinions, their religion, their passions, and their faculties.
> —James Madison[1]

Surely, it would be wrongheaded to contend that drugs do not belong on Madison's foregoing list. In principle, every object in the universe can be treated as property. Two questions thus arise: Whose property is X? And should owning X, qua private property, be legal? X may stand for the shirt on my back or the sidewalk in front of my house, the money I earn as a gardener or the marijuana I grow in my garden. That drugs, like diamonds or dogs, are a form of property no one can deny. Accordingly, we must now ask why the private ownership of drugs should not be just as legal as the private ownership of diamonds or dogs.

THE RIGHT TO PROPERTY

In the English-speaking world, especially since the seventeenth century, the word *freedom* has meant the inalienable right to life, liberty, and property, the first two elements resting squarely on the last. "Though the Earth, and all inferior Creatures be common to all men," wrote John Locke in 1690, "yet every man has a *Property* in his own *Person*. This no Body has any Right to but himself. The *Labour* of his Body and the *Work* of his Hands, we may say, are properly his."[2] More than any other single principle, this idea informed and animated the Framers of the Constitution. "If the United States mean to obtain and deserve the full praise due to wise and just governments," wrote James Madison in 1792, "they will equally respect the rights of property and the property in rights."[3]

The quintessential feature of capitalism as a political-economic system is the security of private property and the free market, that is, the right of every competent adult to trade in goods and services. As Milton Friedman pithily put it, " 'Free markets,' properly understood, are an implication of private property."[4] To ensure such a free social order, the state is obligated to protect people from force and fraud and, to the maximum extent possible, abstain from participating in the production and distribution of goods and services. Of course, no such perfect capitalist order has ever existed or, perhaps, could exist. Still, it is a beacon that lights the way toward respect for persons and social cooperation based on the mutual, noncoercive satisfaction of needs.

The extraordinarily heavy emphasis on the right to property in our Anglo-American tradition does not mean that property is more important than life or liberty, or—as the enemies of individual liberty like to put it—that property is more important than people. It means only that property is "the convention" that best protects life and liberty; that "when life and liberty are at stake, they are already in jeopardy"; and hence that the right to property constitutes "a kind of 'early warning system' to invasions of life and liberty."[5] We ought to heed our loss of the right to drugs as precisely such a warning. Moreover, inasmuch as this alarm was first sounded nearly a century ago, the warning can hardly be said to be early. On the contrary, the sirens have sounded for so long that we no longer hear them: On no other front have the American people been subjected to so relentless a state pressure against their constitutional rights than on the issue of the right to drugs; and on no other front have the American people yielded their rights to encroachments by the federal government so readily, willingly, and indeed eagerly as on this one. I want to show that—because both our bodies and drugs are types of property—producing, trading in, and using drugs are property rights, and drug prohibitions constitute a deprivation of basic constitutional rights.[6]

Negroes and Narcotics: What Counts as Property

My argument that drug prohibitions constitute a deprivation of the constitutional right to property hinges on our accepting drugs as a form of property. Depending on one's values, that may or may not be an obvious proposition. In any case, if the issue of what counts as property affects emotionally charged customs and vested economic interests, then nothing is obvious, and everything is subject to the fiction-making powers of lawmakers—as the precedent of slavery, which holds an important lesson for our problem with drugs, illustrates.

In his classic 1792 essay on "Property," Madison flatly asserted that "government is instituted to protect property of every sort."[7] The legality of slavery rested, of course, on the definition of the Negro as property, a definition that could not be challenged within the slave system. When the judicial system of the United States finally *allowed* it to be challenged, in the celebrated *Dred Scott* case, the formal articulation of the controversy signaled the beginning of the end for slavery.

Dred Scott was an illiterate Negro slave who had been purchased in Missouri, in 1833, by a U.S. Army surgeon named John Emerson. Emerson subsequently traveled with Scott to Illinois, a free state, and then, after a sojourn in Louisiana, took him back to Missouri, a slave state. In 1846, with the help of an anti-slavery lawyer, Scott sued Emerson's brother-in-law John Sandford, who became Scott's owner on Emerson's death, for his freedom (as well as for the freedom of his family, having in the meanwhile married and become the father of a child). The ground for Scott's suit was that his residence in a free state made him a free man. The lower court upheld his claim, but the Missouri Supreme Court ruled against him; the case was subsequently heard by the U.S. Supreme Court. Thus did *Scott v. Sandford* (1857) become one of the most famous and notorious decisions ever rendered by that high court.

The gist of the Court's decision, written by Chief Justice Roger Taney, was that because Scott was property when he was bought and was property when he brought his suit, he had no legal standing to sue; while Sandford, his owner, had a constitutional right to his property—that is, to Dred Scott. I cite a few illustrative lines from Judge Taney's opinion:

> They [Negroes of the African race] are not included, and were not intended to be included, under the word "citizens" in the Constitution. ... He [Scott] was bought and sold, and treated as an ordinary article of merchandise and traffic. ... This opinion was at that time fixed and universal in the civilized portion of the white race. ... No one of that race [black Africans] had ever migrated to the United States voluntarily; all of them had been brought here as articles of merchandise. ... No word can be found in the Constitution which gives Congress a greater power over slave property, or which entitles property of that kind to less protection than property of any other description. The only power conferred is the power coupled with the duty of guarding and protecting the owner of his rights.[8]

Volumes upon volumes have been written on this case, to which I can probably add nothing. Note, however, that Taney specifically cited the fact that the Negroes were bought and sold like property as proof that they were property. What I find remarkable in bringing together the *Dred Scott* case and the Harrison Narcotic Act is that in 1857, American whites had a constitutional right to own American blacks, because Negro slaves constituted property; and that a mere half-century later, in 1914, Americans no longer had a right to own opiates, because Congress declared them to be "narcotics," which could not be bought and sold as "articles of merchandise." From the fiction that Negroes were property and the laws built on it that empowered whites literally to enslave blacks, the nation moved to the fiction that certain drugs (metaphorically) enslaved people and to the legislation built on it that outlawed the slave-holding drugs. *Sic transit infamia mundi.* How terrifyingly right Edmund Burke was when he observed,

> We do not draw the moral lessons we might from history. . . . History consists, for the greater part, of the miseries brought upon the world by pride, ambition, avarice, revenge, lust, sedition, hypocrisy, ungoverned zeal, and all the train of disorderly appetites which shake the public. . . . These vices are the causes of those storms. Religion, morals, laws, prerogatives, privileges, liberties, rights of men, are the pretexts. The pretexts are always found in some specious appearance of a real good.[9]

The Body as Property

The phrase *right to life, liberty, and the pursuit of happiness,* once a vibrantly defiant proclamation, has become meaningless cant, a kind of semantic mummy—the carefully preserved corpse of what only yesterday was a courageous Man. As the preamble to the Declaration of Independence and the Founding Fathers' other writings on political philosophy imply, they saw Man as a being endowed by his Creator with inalienable rights, among them the right to life, liberty, and property. To exercise such rights, Man must be a self-disciplined adult possessing a right anterior to those they enumerated— a right so elementary it never occurred to the Framers that it needed to be named, much less that its protection needed to be specifically safeguarded. They viewed self-ownership thus because, as did Locke, they assumed it precedes all political rights and because, as exemplars of the Protestant Enlightenment, they had a clear view of the distinction between God and state, self and society. Indeed, albeit only in passing, Thomas Jefferson alluded to the crucial importance of bodily self-ownership as a political issue. He mocked would-be statist meddlers into our diets and drugs by reminding his readers that "in France the emetic was once forbidden as a medicine, the potato as an article of food. . . . Was the government to prescribe to us our medicine and diet, our bodies would be in such keeping as our souls are now."[10] But is this not precisely what our government is doing now? Is it not what we expect and demand of it? Foolishly, we embrace the state's "prescrib[ing] to us our medicine and diet" as fulfilling its enlightened duty, guaranteeing us our "right" to health—instead of rejecting it as a crass deprivation of our right to our bodies and to the drugs we want.

It is clear that the Founders took for granted that Jesus' admonition about the soul applied to the body as well, and could be paraphrased thus: What does it profit a man if he gains all the rights politicians are eager to give him, but loses control over the care and feeding of his own body? Mark Twain's following remarks—provoked by the American medical profession's earliest attempts to monopolize the practice of healing—still reflect that point of view:

> The State . . . stands between me and my body, and tells me what kind of a doctor I must employ. When my soul is sick, unlimited spiritual liberty is given me by the State. Now then, it doesn't seem logical that the State shall depart from this great policy . . . and take the other position in the matter of smaller consequences—the health of the body. . . . Whose property is my body? Probably mine. . . . I, not the State. If I choose injudiciously, does the State die? Oh, no.[11]

I contend that, strange as it may sound, we have lost our most important right: the right to our bodies.[12]

How We Lost the Right to Our Bodies

How can a person lose the right to his body? By being deprived of the freedom to care for it and to control it as he sees fit. From the time the Pilgrims first landed until 1914, the American people had the freedom as well as the obligation, the right as well as the duty, to care for and control their bodies, manifested by legally unrestricted access to the medical care and the medicines of their choice. During all those years, the government did not control the market in drugs or the peoples' use.

To follow the critique of the War on Drugs . . . it is crucial that we keep in mind this question: How can a person lose the right to his body? And that we not waver from answering thus: A person can lose the right to his body the same way he can lose the right to his life, liberty, or property—namely, by someone's depriving him of it. When a private person takes away an individual's life, liberty, or property, we call the former a criminal, and the latter a victim. When an agent of the state does such a thing, and does it rightfully, according to law, we regard him as a law enforcement officer carrying out his duties, and regard the person deprived of his rights as a criminal receiving his just punishment. However, when agents of the therapeutic state deprive us of our right to our bodies. we view ourselves neither as victims nor as criminals, but as patients. There is, of course, a third way we can lose our right to property, namely, by taxation.

When a criminal deprives us of property (to enrich himself), we call it "theft." When the criminal justice system deprives us of property (to punish us), we call it a "fine." And when the state deprives us of property (to support itself, ostensibly to serve us), we call it a "tax." Taxation and drug prohibition are both coercive state interventions, and both are justified largely on paternalistic grounds. In the case of taxation, the state lets us buy those things it considers we can manage by ourselves (for example, food and lottery tickets), while it extracts that proportion of our income it deems "socially just," ostensibly to provide us with those things it considers we cannot provide for ourselves (such as health care and postal service). Similarly, in the case of drug controls, the state lets us buy those drugs it considers safe for us to use (over-the-counter drugs), and it removes those drugs it considers unsafe for us to use (prescription drugs and illicit drugs). Then, in the process of taxing us and depriving us of drugs, the state also expropriates sufficient funds to provide politicians and other government parasites with a comfortable living. Surely, it is not an accident of history that only one year separates the enactment of the Sixteenth Amendment, creating the legal authority for the federal income tax (1913). and the passage of the Harrison Narcotic Act (1914), creating the legal authority for the first federal drug prohibition. In short, when the state deprives us of our right to drugs and justifies it as drug controls, we ought to regard ourselves not as patients receiving state protection from illness, but as victims robbed of access to drugs—just as when the state deprives us of our right to property and justifies it as taxing personal income, most of us regard ourselves not as beneficiaries receiving state services for our needs, but as victims robbed of some of our income. Indeed, the deep sense that our property rights are inalienable—that they are not gifts of the government—accounts for the ineradicable streak in the American spirit that continues to regard taxation as legalized robbery.

At this point I want to note briefly that I recognize a need for limiting the free market in drugs, just as I recognize a need for limiting the free market in many other goods. The legitimate place for that limit, however, is where free access to a particular product presents a "clear and present danger" to the safety and security of *others*. On such grounds, the state controls the market in explosives, and on such grounds it may legitimately control the market in plutonium or radioactive chemicals used in medicine. But this is not the basis for our current drug controls.

Since the beginning of this century, through a combination of medical licensure and direct drug-control legislation, the American government has assumed progressively more authority over the drug trade and our drug use. The ostensible aim of these restrictions was to protect people from incompetent doctors and unsafe drugs. The actual result was loss of personal freedom, without the gain of the promised benefits. It is important to keep in mind that our elaborate machinery of drug controls rests largely on prescription drug laws, which, in turn, rest on a medical profession *licensed by the state*. While in *Capitalism and Freedom,* Milton Friedman does not mention drug controls, he addresses the even more sacrosanct subject of medical licensure, and gives it its libertarian due. "The conclusions I shall reach," he writes, "are that liberal principles do not justify licensure even in medicine and that in practice the results of state licensure in medicine have been undesirable."[13] Regardless of their lofty motives, drug controls encourage people to expect politicians and physicians to protect them from themselves—specifically, to protect them from their own inclinations to use or misuse certain drugs. The result is state control of the drug market and an interminable War on Drugs—symptoms of our having, in effect, repealed the Constitution and the Bill of Rights.

The Breached Castle

Consider the following imaginary scenario. Don, a retired widower in his sixties, lives alone in a suburban home. He has many friends, enjoys good health, is economically secure, and has no dependents. His hobby is gardening in the greenhouse attached to his home. A genius at making things grow, Don's home overflows with exotic plants and fresh flowers, and his tomatoes are legendary. Let us imagine further that Don, an adventurous and enterprising person, acquires some marijuana, coca, and poppy seeds, plants them in his greenhouse, nurtures the seedlings into mature plants, harvests them, and produces some marijuana, coca leaves, and raw opium. Much given to privacy, Don does not even let a cleaning person in his home, though he could well afford it. Hence, there is no way for anyone, legally, to know about his miniature drug farm. Finally, let us assume that on an occasional Saturday evening, Don, alone at home, smokes a little marijuana or chews some coca leaves or mixes some opium powder into his midnight tea.

What has Don done, and how does American law—criminal and mental health law—regard him and his behavior? Ownership of land and buildings is a basic property right. Privacy, especially since *Griswold* v. *Connecticut* and *Roe* v. *Wade,* is also a basic right.[14] Thus, Don has simply exercised some of his property and privacy rights: his right to his land, his home, and the fruits of his labor in his own home. He has deprived no one of life, liberty, or property. Conventional wisdom and medical disinformation to the contrary notwithstanding, Don has not harmed himself either. Nevertheless, American criminal law now regards him as guilty of criminal possession and use of controlled and illegal substances, while American mental health law regards him as a psychiatric patient suffering from chemical dependency, substance abuse, personality disorder, and other psychopathological aberrations as yet undiscovered. Moreover, stigmatizing Don as a mentally sick person, criminalizing his behavior as that of an evil-minded lawbreaker, dispossessing him of his home and imposing an astronomical fine on him, and incarcerating him as a dangerous offender—all this is now considered to be perfectly legal and constitutional. At this point, the reader might wonder how legal scholars and justices of the Supreme Court reconcile such seemingly excessive—and hence "cruel and unusual"—punishment with the Constitution.

Justifying Therapeutic Slavery

How can the government of the United States—crafted and considered to possess the most prudently limited powers of any government in the world—prohibit a competent adult from growing or ingesting an ordinary plant, such as coca leaf or hemp? And how can it impose such staggeringly disproportionate punishment—compared, for example, to the punishment imposed on many persons convicted of murder—on an individual who inhales the products of such a plant?[15] The answer is that where there is a political will, supported by popular opinion and powerful factional interest, there is a legal way, paved with the legal fictions necessary to do the job. At the end of the eighteenth century, operating in the context of the old practice of slavery plus the new principle of apportioning congressional seats by population, the manufacturers of legal fictions fabricated the ingenious and ignominious concept of three-fifths persons. Since 1914, the politicians' desire to control the use of certain common plants and their biologically active ingredients, together with the public's fascination with and fear of certain glamorized and scapegoated substances, has led to the fabrication of analogous legal fictions to justify the prohibition of the production, even for private use, of plants or substances deemed dangerous by the government.

The trick to enacting and enforcing crassly hypocritical prohibitions, with the conniving of the victimized population, lies in not saying what you mean and avoiding direct legal rule making. Thus, the Founders did not declare, in so many words, "To justify slavery, in the slave states blacks shall be counted as property; and to apportion more congressional seats to the slave states than they would have on the basis of their white population only, black slaves shall be counted as three-fifths persons." Similarly, our lawmakers do not say, "We shall impose draconian criminal penalties on anyone within the borders of the United States who ingests marijuana he has grown on his own land for his own personal use only." What, then, do they say? Why do legal scholars consider such a prohibition to be constitutional?

The answer to these questions is briefly this. Under the police power, the states can prohibit a wide range of activities regarded as endangering the public welfare, for example, gambling, obscenity, and drugs, notably alcohol. However, Congress has no police power over the nation as a whole. That is why making the sale of alcohol a federal offense required a constitutional amendment. However, there is another route to federal drug prohibition, namely, through the Constitution's Commerce Clause (Article I, section 8, clause 3), which empowers Congress to close the doors of interstate commerce to any unwanted product. Thus, the key subterfuge undergirding the alleged constitutionality of our federal antidrug laws is that their purpose is to protect commerce, not to punish persons for crimes. But where is the commerce in producing a plant for one's own use only? Or in picking a plant found growing in the wild and ingesting it?

Of course, the constitutionality of the drug laws, beginning with the 1906 Food and Drugs Act, was challenged in the courts. Not surprisingly, it was consistently upheld by the Supreme Court, as for example in the 1913 *McDermott* case, where the Court declared,

> [Congress] has the right not only to pass laws which shall regulate legitimate commerce among the States and with foreign nations, but has the full power to keep the channels of such commerce free from the transportation of illicit or harmful articles, to make such as are *injurious to the public health* outlaws of such commerce.[16]

In his scholarly review of the constitutionality of drug laws, Thomas Christopher concludes that "there has been no serious discussion by that body [the Supreme Court] of the over-all constitutional question [of drug regulation]. *It would seem that that issue is too well settled.*"[17] Here we come to the nub of the matter. Under the pretext of the Commerce Clause plus the prevailing medical legerdemain about dangerous drugs, the Supreme Court has, in effect, become the mouthpiece of the Food and Drug Administration and of organized American medicine. Christopher puts it more elegantly. The Court, he writes, "has always shown great respect for the Food and Drug Administration, and for its administrative findings and rulings . . . [d]oubtless [this] is owing to the fact that health matters are involved."[18]

The Commerce Clause as a decoy for the paternalistic-prohibitory purposes of drug laws is a contemporary example of the use of a powerful legal fiction in the service of a popular cause. But the therapeutic state thus engendered is no fiction. The *Wickard* case exemplifies the implausible ends to which the means of Congress's right to regulate commerce may be put in order to justify depriving Americans of their right to manage their own self-regarding, drug-using behavior.

In 1940, pursuant to the Agricultural Adjustment Act of 1938, an Ohio farmer named Roscoe C. Filburn was allotted 11.1 acres for his 1941 wheat crop. He sowed 23 acres. Seeking exemption from the regulations, Filburn filed a civil suit against Secretary of Agriculture Claude Wickard, asking the court to enjoin him from enforcing the act against him. The lower court ruled in Filburn's favor. But in *Wickard* v. *Filburn* the Supreme Court reversed the decision, holding that the act could be applied to Filburn. What was Filburn's violation? Committing "farm marketing excess." What was Filburn's defense? That he used his crop "to feed part to poultry and livestock on the farm . . . some in making flour for home consumption . . . and keep the rest for the following seeding."[19] The Supreme Court ruled against Filburn, declaring:

> The Act includes a definition of "market" and its derivatives so that as related to wheat in addition to its conventional meaning it also means to dispose of "by feeding (in any form) to poultry or livestock which, or the products of which,

are sold, bartered, or exchanged. . . . Hence, marketing quotas . . . so [embrace] what may be consumed on the premises. Penalties do not depend upon whether any part of the wheat . . . is sold or intended to be sold.[20]

Note the Court's redefinition of the word *market* so as to include supplying one's own needs, and its candid admission that such redefinitions may legitimately be manufactured ad hoc—in this case, "as related to wheat." The result of using the Commerce Clause as a pretext for drug prohibition is that, de facto as well as de jure, the American government is empowered to deprive us, as it sees fit, of our ancient freedom to grow—on our own soil, for our own consumption—any crop of its choosing.

Rights: Opportunities vs. Risks

The normal reader, defensive of the rationale of current drug prohibitions, might be inclined to dismiss my hypothetical scenario about "Don" as irrelevant to real life, and might want to change the subject to real problems such as intravenous drug use, AIDS, crack babies, and other assorted horrors. My rejoinder is two-pronged. First, let us remember the adage that hard cases make bad law. Hence there is merit in considering the easiest case first. If such a case suggests that a particular law violates an important political principle, it ought to make us think twice about casually overriding the violation in the name of some temporarily fashionable social cause. Second, let us keep in mind that the essence of freedom is choice, and that choice implies the option to make the wrong choice, that is, to "abuse" freedom and suffer the consequences. Thereby hangs a long tale, with a hopeless quest and many enthusiastic questers as its leitmotif. Like medieval searchers for the Holy Grail, these modern seekers look for the correct answer to an absurd question, namely: How can we reduce or eliminate the risks and undesirable consequences of liberty, while retaining its rewards and benefits? The fact that we cannot do this has not stopped people, especially "democratic socialists" and other optimistic statists from trying. Indeed, the history of modern welfare states is, in part, the history of that self-defeating effort.

Rights entail opportunities as well as risks. This is why some people see the right to property as giving us prosperity and liberty, and others see it as giving us booms and busts; why some see the right to property in land and houses as giving us builders, real estate agents, and landlords who provide us with homes, while others see it as giving us unscrupulous moneylenders and greedy slumlords to exploit people's homelessness. Similarly, we can see the right to drugs as giving us control over our medical and physiological destiny, or as giving us drug abusers and crack babies.

Both images are real. Both are true. And the *choice* is ours. For example, we choose to view the owners and managers of American supermarkets as providing us with the best and most bountiful food and drink in the whole world, not as malefactors determined to make life difficult for troubled anorexics and bulimics. We do not blame the obesity of fat persons on the people who sell them food, but we do blame the drug habits of addicts on the people who sell them drugs. Obviously, the supplier of every good or service is, ipso facto, a potential seducer as well; the only question is whether he is a successful or unsuccessful seducer. The successful seducer becomes a flourishing businessman or entrepreneur; the unsuccessful one goes broke or quits the market. This, in a nutshell, is the free market—the one and only secure foundation of individual liberty. If we try to redefine liberty in such a way that it is not liberty unless its results are individually and collectively "healthy"—which, in the case of drugs, means providing us with effective and affordable treatments for disease *and* protecting us from the abuse of drugs by both patients and doctors—we fool only those foolish enough to believe in miracles. Sometimes, that category includes the majority. We then speak, usually in retrospect of a crowd madness.[21]

THE RIGHT TO DRUGS AS A RIGHT TO PROPERTY

Obviously, viewing the right to drugs as a species of property right presupposes a capitalist conception of the relationship between the individual and the state, incompatible with a socialist conception of that relationship. We are familiar with the fact that capitalism is premised on the right to property. As for socialism, *Webster's* defines it as "a system or condition of society or group living in which there is no private property."[22] Q.E.D.: Drug censorship, like book censorship, is an attack on capitalism and freedom. Psychiatrists either ignore this cardinal connection between the chemicals we call "drugs" and politics, preferring to treat drug use as if it were purely an issue of mental health or psychopathology, or—if they recognize it—treat the relationship with their customary hostility to liberty and property. To illustrate this point, I shall juxtapose the views on liberty and property of two of the most important thinkers of our age: Ludwig von Mises and Sigmund Freud. Although both men lived in Vienna at about the same time and addressed some of the same momentous issues, I have never seen their differing judgments compared and brought to bear on our current views concerning drug controls.

Ludwig von Mises vs. Sigmund Freud

In 1922, Ludwig von Mises—the most unappreciated genius of our century —published a book entitled *Socialism,* establishing his reputation, at least among the cognoscenti. His closing sentences in that work read thus: "Whether Society is good or bad may be a matter of individual judgment; but whoever prefers life to death, happiness to suffering, well-being to misery, must accept . . . without limitation or reserve, private ownership of the means of production."[23]

Seven years later, Sigmund Freud—the most successful charlatan of our century—published *Civilization and Its Discontents,* adding more luster to his already considerable fame especially among the scientistically minded enemies of capitalism and freedom. "I have no concern," declared Freud, "with any economic criticism of the communist system; I cannot inquire into whether the abolition of private property is expeditious or advantageous."[24] Freud's anticapitalist remarks were not isolated comments, tossed off at the spur of the moment. Years before, he greeted the Bolsheviks' declaration of war on private property and religious freedom with a mixture of naiveté and optimism. "At a time when the great nations announce that they expect salvation only from the maintenance of Christian piety," he wrote in 1917, "the revolution in Russia—in spite of all its disagreeable details—seems none the less like the message of a better future."[25] In public, Freud chided the United States for not sharing his disdain for religion; in private, he conducted his business in U.S. dollars only.

Unfortunately, modern liberals continue to focus on human rights rather than on *property* rights. Why? Because it makes them appear socially concerned—"caring" and "compassionate." By splitting off property rights from human rights, liberals have succeeded in giving the former a bad name, undermining the moral legitimacy of all other rights in the process. But property rights are not only just as valid as human rights; they are anterior to, and necessary for, human rights.

Liberty as Choice

Private property is indispensable as an economic base and precondition for forming a government *fit for freedom.* I use this unfamiliar expression to emphasize that no government is, or can be, *committed to freedom.* Only people can be. Government, by its very nature, has a vested interest in enlarging its freedom of action, thereby necessarily reducing the freedom of individuals. At the same fume, the right to private property—as a political-economic concept—is not a sufficient foundation for a government serving the needs and meriting the loyalty of free and responsible persons. It may be worth remembering here that Adam Smith, generally regarded as the father of free-market capitalism, was not an economist (there was no such thing in the eighteenth century). He was a professor of moral philosophy. As such, his brand of economics made no attempt to be value-free. Today, professional economists and observers of the economic scene err in their efforts to make the study of these human affairs into a value-free social "science."

What, then, is the moral merit of the free market? What is good about it, besides its being an efficient mechanism for producing and delivering goods and services? The answer is that the free market is good because it encourages social cooperation (production and trade) and discourages force and fraud (exploitation of the many by a few with the power to coerce), and because it is a legal-moral order that places the value of the person as an individual above that of his value as a member of the community. It is implicit in the idea of the free market that persons who want to enjoy its benefits must assume responsibility, and be held responsible, for their actions; that they look to the principle of caveat emptor—not the paternalistic state—for protection from the risks inherent in the exercise of freedom; and that among the risks with which they must live are those associated with drugs and medical treatments. In short, the fundamental precepts of moral philosophy and political economics cannot be separated: They are symbiotic, the one dependent on the other. "It is . . . illegitimate," Mills warned, "to regard the 'economic' as a definite sphere of human action which can be sharply delimited from other spheres of action. . . . The economic principle applies to all human action."[26]

If we are willing to use our political-economic vocabulary precisely and take its terms seriously, we must conclude that just as the Constitution guarantees us the right to worship whatever gods we choose and read whatever books we choose, so it also guarantees us the right to use whatever drugs we choose. Mises's observation about the characteristic conflict of the twentieth century—which, with welfare-statism in mind, he offered at its beginning—remains true toward its end and applies with special force to the drug problem:

> In the sixteenth and seventeenth centuries religion was the main issue in European political controversies. In the eighteenth and nineteenth centuries in Europe as well as in America the paramount question was representative government versus royal absolutism. Today it is the market economy versus socialism.[27]

Mises never ceased emphasizing that our bloody century is characterized by a struggle between two diametrically opposite types of economic systems: command economies *controlled* by the state, exemplified by socialism (communism), versus free-market economies *regulated* by the supply and demand of individual producers and consumers, exemplified by capitalism (classical liberalism). States based on command economies are inherently despotic—a few superiors issuing orders, and many subordinates obeying them. States based on market economies are inherently democratic—individuals deciding what to produce, sell, and buy and at what prices, producers and consumers alike being free to engage or refrain from engaging in market transactions.

The American Drug Market Today

To clearly understand what has happened to the market in drugs in the United States during the past century, it is necessary, first, to distinguish between consumer goods, which are depleted in use, such as food and clothing, and capital goods, which are used to produce goods, such as machines and tools. This distinction immediately alerts us to the fact that the term *consumer good* has a distinctly individualistic (nonpaternalistic) connotation: It implies that an individual, qua consumer, has an interest in a particular product. After all, not everything a person might be able to consume is—at all times, for all individuals—a consumer good. To qualify, there must be consumers who want it. And the only way we can be certain that a customer really wants a good or service is if he is willing to pay for it. This is what economists call a "demand" for a good. And this is the meaning of the adage "People pay for what they value, and value what they pay for."

Obviously, the presence or absence of demand is an economic and cultural—not a scientific or medical—issue. For example, in the United States today, there is a demand for marijuana, but there is no demand for the powdered horn of the rhinoceros (except perhaps in San Francisco). To be sure, the concept of demand (like the concept of illness) is a manmade category: In each case, the contours of the concept may be redrawn to suit the strategies of the definers; and both "conditions" may be imposed on individuals against their will. Courts now routinely order persons who use illegal drugs to attend drug treatment programs, from which mental health experts and economists conclude that there is a huge demand for drug treatment services in our society. (This creation, by court orders, of drug abusers and a demand for drug treatment services is similar to the creation, by court orders, of mental illnesses and a demand for mental health services. The pathetic and now discredited principles of statist—that is, Soviet—economics thus continue to flourish in our own drug-control and mental-health systems.)

Let us suspend our customary concerns with the drug user's motivations, society's judgments of drug use, and the pharmacological effects of particular drugs. And let us focus instead on the various ways an American who wants to use drugs now actually gains access to them. We can then categorize drugs according to their availability or mode of distribution, as follows:

1. No special government controls limiting sales: for example, coffee, aspirin, laxatives. Produced by private entrepreneurs; distributed through the free market. Product called "food," "beverage," or "over-the-counter drug"; seller, "merchant"; buyer, "customer."
2. Government controls limiting sales:
   a. To adults: for example, alcohol and tobacco. Produced by private entrepreneurs; distributed through the free or state-licensed market. Product called "beer," "wine," "cigarette"; seller, "merchant"; buyer, "customer."

b. To patients: for example, digitalis, penicillin, steroids, Valium. Produced by government-regulated pharmaceutical manufacturers; distributed through state-controlled physicians' prescriptions and pharmacies. Product called "prescription drug"; seller, "pharmacist"; buyer, "patient."

c. To addicts: for example, methadone. Produced by government-regulated pharmaceutical manufacturers; distributed through special federally approved dispensers. No legal sellers or buyers. Product called "drug (abuse) treatment"; distributor, "drug (treatment) program"; recipient, "(certified) addict."

3. Government controls prohibiting sales to everyone: for example, heroin, crack. Produced illegally by private entrepreneurs; distributed illegally through the black market. Product called "dangerous drug" or "illegal drug"; seller, "pusher" or "trafficker"; buyer, "addict" or "drug abuser."

As such a market-oriented perspective on drug distribution shows, we have nothing even remotely resembling a free market in drugs in the United States. Nevertheless, most people mistakenly think of prescription drugs, and even of specifically restricted drugs such as methadone, as "legal."

Although it is a truism, it is perhaps necessary to repeat that the uncorrupted concept of liberty implies no particular result, only the proverbial level playing field where all can play—and win or lose—by the same rules. Despite all the rhetoric to the contrary, no one is, or can be, killed by an illegal drug. If a person dies as a result of using a drug, it is because he *chose* to do something risky: The *drug* he chooses may be cocaine or Cytoxan; the *risk* he chooses to incur may be motivated by the pressure of peers or the pressure of cancer. In either case, the drug may kill him. Some deaths attributed to illegal drug use may thus be accidents (for example, inadvertent overdose); some may be indirect suicides (playing Russian roulette with unknown drugs); and some may be direct suicides (deliberate overdose).

Reforming Drug Policy: Deforming the Market

Because all criticisms of drug-control policies are aimed at the way particular drugs are distributed, proposals for reform correspond to the categories described above. I shall summarize each posture vis-à-vis drug controls by identifying the characteristic strategies of its proponents:

1. Criminalizers ("Do you want more crack babies?"): Keep type 3 substances in category 3; expand categories 3, 2b, and 2c, and constrict categories 1 and 2a; drug offenders are both criminals and patients, who should be punished as well as (coercively) treated.

2. Legalizers ("The war on drugs cannot be won."): Remove certain type 3 substances, such as heroin, from category 3 and transfer them to category 2b or 2c (make the manufacture and sale of heretofore prohibited substances a government monopoly); drug abusers are sick and should be (coercively) treated in government-funded programs.

3. Free marketeers ("Self-medication is a right."): Abolish categories 2b, 2c, and 3, and place all presently restricted substances in category 2a; drug use is personal choice, neither crime nor illness.

I disagree with both the drug criminalizers and the drug legalizers: with the former, because I believe that the criminal law ought to be used to protect us from others, not from ourselves; with the latter, because I believe that behavior, even if it is actually or potentially injurious or self-injurious, is not a disease, and that no behavior should be regulated by sanctions called "treatment."[28]

As we have seen, there are three distinct drug markets in the United States today: (1) the legal (free) market; (2) the medical (prescription) market; and (3) the illegal (black) market. Because the cost of virtually all of the services we call "drug treatment" is borne by parties other than the so-called patient, and because most people submit to such treatment under legal duress, there is virtually no free market at all in drug treatment. Try as we might, we cannot escape the fact that the conception of a demand for goods and services in the free market is totally different from the conception we now employ in reference to drug use and drug treatment. In the free market, a demand is what the customer wants; or as merchandising magnate Marshall Field put it, "The customer is always right." In the prescription drug market, we seem to say, "The doctor is always right": The physician decides what drug the patient should "demand," and that is all he can legally get. Finally, in the psychiatric drug market, we as a society are saying, "The patient is always wrong": The psychiatrist decides what drug the mental patient "needs" and compels him to consume it, by force if necessary.

Merchants thus *advertise*—to create a demand for the goods they want to sell. Tylenol, for example, is advertised to *customers*. Physicians *prescribe* —to open a drug-market otherwise closed to persons and thus make specific drugs available to them. Penicillin, say, is prescribed to *patients*. And psychiatrists *coerce*—to force mental patients to be drugged as they, the doctors, want them to be drugged. Haldol is forcibly injected into *psychotics*.

However, the foregoing generalizations—valid until recently—no longer hold. Drug manufacturers have begun to advertise prescription drugs to the public. While this practice reveals the hitherto concealed hypocrisy of prescription laws, it introduces increasingly serious distortions into the drug market. For example, tobacco—a legal product—cannot be advertised on television, but Nicorette—an illegal product—can be. (Nicorette is a nicotine-containing chewing gum available by prescription only.) Here are some other current examples of prescription drug advertisements aimed at the public:

For Estraderm, an estrogen patch for women: "Now the change of life doesn't have to change yours."[29]

For Minitran, a transdermal form of nitroglycerin: "Everything you asked for in a patch . . . for less."[30]

For Seldane, an antihistamine: "You've tried just about everything for your hay fever. . . . Have you tried your doctor?"[31]

For Rogaine, an anti-baldness drug: "The earlier you use Rogaine, the better your chances of growing hair."[32]

The advertisement for Rogaine goes beyond simply alerting the customer to the availability of a prescription drug about which he might not be aware: It offers him cash for going to see a doctor and demanding the drug. In a coupon at the bottom of the page, a smaller caption tells the reader: "Fill this in now. Then, start to fill in your hair loss." The coupon is worth $10 "as an incentive" to see a doctor. Because many of the prescription drugs advertised to the public are very expensive, the logic of this practice suggests that drug companies may be tempted to offer increasingly large sums to would-be patients, in effect to bribe them to solicit a prescription from their physician.

Naturally, drug companies defend the practice. "The ads," they say, "help educate patients and give consumers a chance to become more involved in choosing the medication they want."[33] But that laudable goal could be better served by a free market in drugs. In my opinion, the practice of advertising prescription drugs to the public fulfills a more odious function, namely, to further infantilize the layman and, at the same time, undermine the physician's medical authority. The policy puts physicians in an obvious bind. Prescription laws give doctors monopolistic privilege to provide certain drugs to certain persons, or withhold such drugs from them. However, the advertising of prescription drugs encourages people to pressure their physicians to prescribe the drugs they *want,* rather than the drugs the physicians believe they *need.* If a doctor does not comply, the patient is likely to take his business elsewhere. A professor of medicine at Columbia University tells *Time* magazine, "There is no question that certain physicians are being influenced to issue prescriptions that they would not otherwise write."[34] Missing is any recognition of the way this practice reinforces the role of the patient as helpless child, and of the doctor as providing/withholding parent. After all, we know why certain breakfast food advertisements are aimed at young children: Because while they cannot buy these foods for themselves, they can pressure their parents to buy the advertised cereals for them. Similarly, the American people cannot buy prescription drugs, but they can pressure their doctors to prescribe the advertised drugs for them.

The Fiction of Drug Abuse Services

American law, medicine, and public opinion regard not only involuntary confinement in a mental hospital but also involuntary confinement in a drug treatment program as bona fide medical treatments: "Civil commitment is frequently used with addicts who are arrested for criminal activity; with criminal charges pending, the addict can be coerced into treatment and retained long enough to receive the benefits of a treatment program."[35] Thus, perhaps the most important function of our fashionable drug-treatment rhetoric is to distract us from the fact that the drug user wants the drug of his choice, not the drug treatment the authorities choose for him. We are flooded with news stories about addicts robbing people to get money to pay for drugs. But who has ever heard of an addict robbing a person to get money to pay for drug treatment? Q.E.D.

If we were to view the whole package of illegal drug use plus legally coerced drug treatment from a free-market perspective, we would see the drug abuser's behavior as his existential and economic demand for the drug of his choice—and the drug prohibitionist's so-called services as deceptive and coercive meddling deliberately mislabeled as "therapy." Indeed, so long as the drug counselor (or whatever he is called) acts as a paid agent of the state (or some other third party in conflict with the self-defined interests of the drug user), we would have to define his intervention as interference not only in the life of his nominal client, but in the free market in drugs as well. All this, and more, Frederic Bastiat had warned against in the early nineteenth century. "To rob the public," he observed, "it is necessary to deceive it. To deceive it, it is necessary to persuade it that it is being robbed for its own benefit, and to induce it to accept, in exchange for its property, services that are fictitious or often even worse."[36]

If ever there were services that are fictitious or even worse, they are our current publicly financed drug-treatment services. The wisdom of our language reveals the truth and supports the cogency of these reflections. We do not call convicts "consumers of prison services," or conscripts "consumers of military services"; but we call committed mental patients "consumers of mental health services," and paroled addicts "consumers of drug-treatment services." We might as well call drug traffickers—conscripted by the former drug czar William Bennett for beheading—"consumers of guillotine services." After all, Dr. Guillotin was a doctor, and Mr. Bennett used to teach ethics.

To be sure, persons drafted as convicts, conscripts, and "chemically dependent persons" all receive certain services, such as food, shelter, clothing, and antidrug propaganda. The provision of such "services" is then used to mask the fact that the beneficiaries would prefer being left alone by their benefactors. Like the mythologizing of personal problems as mental diseases, so the mythologizing of illegal drug use as a disease has been overwhelmingly successful. In 1991, the federal government [spent] *more than $1 billion on drug treatment research.** Enthusiasm for such "research" is not diminished by the fact that, according to a General Accounting Office report

---

*According to the Office of National Drug Control Strategy, President Clinton requested $2,908,700,000 from Congress for drug-abuse treatment for fiscal year 1997. (Ed.)

released in September 1990, "researchers know little more about the best way to treat various drug addictions than they did ten years ago."[37]

THE WAR ON DRUGS AS A WAR ON PROPERTY

Although it is obvious that the American drug market is now completely state controlled, most people seem at once unaware of this fact and pleased with it, except when they want a drug they cannot get. Then they complain about the unavailability of that particular drug: For example, cancer patients complain that they cannot get Laetrile; AIDS patients, that they cannot get unapproved anti-AIDS drugs; women, that they cannot get unapproved chemical abortifacients; terminally ill patients in pain, that they cannot get heroin; and so on. It seems to me that just as the Soviet people [suffered] the consequences of their war on private property, we shall have to suffer still more wrenching personal and national tragedies as the consequences of our War on Drugs.

Sadly, the very concept of a closure of the free market in drugs is likely to ring vague and abstract to most people today. But the personal and social consequences of a policy based on such a concept are anything but abstract or vague. Every aspect of our life that brings us into contact with the manufacture, sale, or use of substances of pharmacological interest to people has been utterly corrupted. The result is that, in all the complex human situations we call "drug abuse" and "drug abuse treatment," the voluntary coming together of honest and responsible citizens trading with one another in mutual trust and respect has been replaced by the deceitful and coercive manipulation of infantilized people by corrupt and paternalistic authorities, and vice versa. The principal role of medical, and especially psychiatric, professionals in the administration and enforcement of this system of chemical statism is to act as double agents—helping politicians to impose their will on the people by defining self-medication as a disease, and helping the people to bear their privations by supplying them with drugs. This is a major national tragedy whose very existence has so far remained unrecognized.

The War on Drugs has many grave consequences. In this discussion I can touch on only a few of them. Perhaps the most obvious consequences of drug prohibition are the explosive increase in crimes against persons and property and the corresponding increase in our prison population. Both phenomena are typically attributed to "drugs," a misleading locution for which the media bear an especially heavy responsibility. I shall not belabor the fact that drugs do not—indeed, cannot—cause crime. Suffice it to repeat that crime is an act; that the criminal actor, like all actors, has motives; and that drug prohibition provides powerful economic incentives for both the trade in prohibited drugs and crimes against persons and property.

The United States vs. Drug-Tainted Property

One of the most ominous and least publicized consequences of the War on Drugs is the government's use of the Internal Revenue Service and of the international banking system to detect and apprehend persons engaged in the drug trade, along with its practice of confiscating property from persons accused of drug offenses even when they are innocent. These measures illustrate that the War on Drugs is, *literally*, a war on property—waged by the U.S. government with the enthusiastic support of the Supreme Court. The leading Supreme Court decision supporting the charade of the so-called civil forfeiture procedure—legitimizing the government's seizure of the property even of innocent persons connected to drug-related offenses—merits brief mention.

In 1971, the Pearson Yacht Leasing Company of Puerto Rico (called the "appellee" in the decision) rented a yacht to two Puerto Rican residents. Subsequently, the police found *one marijuana cigarette* on board the yacht, charged the lessees with violation of the Controlled Substances Act of Puerto Rico, and seized the yacht.[38] The lessor (the yacht-leasing company) sued to recover its vessel. The case reached the Supreme Court, which held that, even though the lessor was innocent, the seizure was legal. I will briefly summarize how the Court reached this remarkable conclusion.

The Court acknowledged that the "appellee was in no way . . . involved in the criminal enterprise carried on by [the] lessee and had no knowledge that its property was being used in connection with or in violation of [Puerto Rican law]."[39] Nevertheless, the Court—led by Justice William Brennan, one of its leading liberals—ruled against the yacht company, holding that "statutory forfeiture schemes are not rendered unconstitutional because of their applicability to the property interests of innocents, and here the Puerto Rican statutes, which further punitive and deterrent purposes, were validly applied to appellee's yacht."[40]

Justice William O. Douglas dissented—not on principle, but because he felt the punishment was disproportionate to the (nonexisting) crime:

> Only one marihuana cigarette was found on the yacht. We deal here with trivia where harsh judge-made law should be tempered with justice. I realize that the ancient law is founded on the fiction that the inanimate object itself is guilty of wrongdoing. But that traditional forfeiture doctrine cannot at times be reconciled with the requirements of the Fifth Amendment.[41]

Note that Justice Douglas cavalierly sidesteps the legitimacy of the core issue, namely, the prohibition of marijuana. Instead of engaging in a principled argument, he magnanimously offers to return the yacht to its rightful owners.

A closely related case, in which the Supreme Court ruled unanimously that the government could dispossess a person of his property *even after he had been acquitted* on a related criminal charge (of gun law, rather than drug law, violation), deserves to be mentioned in this connection. In 1977, Patrick Mulcahey was apprehended by agents of the Bureau of Alcohol, Tobacco, and Firearms and charged with dealing in firearms without a license. Although Mulcahey had no license, a jury acquitted him, perhaps because it felt that he had been entrapped. Following Mulcahey's acquittal, the United States moved to "forfeiture of the seized firearms."[42] The Court held that

> an acquittal on criminal charges does not prove that the defendant is innocent; it merely proves the existence of reasonable doubt as to his guilt. . . . [T]he substantive criminal provision under which Mulcahey was prosecuted, does not render unlawful an *intention* to engage in the business of dealing in firearms without a license; only the completed act of engaging in the prohibited business is made a crime. . . . Because the par. 924(d) forfeiture proceeding brought against Mulcahey's firearms is not a criminal proceeding, it is not barred by the Double Jeopardy Clause.[43]

The crux of the matter is Congress's power to define punishment as a "remedial act." With the transforming of de facto punishments into sanctions de jure "intended to be civil and remedial, rather than criminal and punitive,"[44] our rights to liberty and property vanish. Mental patients have, of course, long been the beneficiaries of such remedial sanctions, being incarcerated though innocent of crime. Civil commitment skirts the prohibition against *preventive detention* by permitting "mental patients," accused of being "dangerous," to be deprived of their liberty. This is accomplished by calling the legal procedure for incarcerating the victim "civil," and the place of confinement a "hospital."[45] In the same way, the federal forfeiture laws skirt the prohibition against *punishing innocent persons* by permitting "drug criminals," *accused* of "having used or intending to use" their property to commit or facilitate a drug law violation, to be deprived of their property.

The Fourth Amendment protection against unreasonable searches and seizures is thus neatly nullified by calling the legal procedure for confiscating the property "civil," and the economic loss imposed on the victim a "storage fee." People suspected of drug-related offenses have thus been deprived of their boats, cars, houses, and money, which they may or may not be able to regain after they prove their innocence, by which time the effort may be counterproductive. One victim of this civil deprivation-of-property procedure, whose boat worth $7,600 was seized and kept for three and a half months, got it back "upon payment of $4,000 in storage and maintenance charges."[46] Another had his brand-new $140,000 fishing boat seized after Customs Service agents found 1.7 grams of marijuana in a crewman's jacket pocket. "Customs officials admitted that Mr. Hogan [the owner] knew nothing about the marijuana. But they held his boat long enough for him to miss the halibut season (a $30,000 loss), and at first demanded that he pay a

$10,000 fine for failing to keep drugs off his vessel."[47] Similar horror stories abound.[48]

During the past half-dozen years, civil forfeiture has become a huge federal business, and a huge federal boondoggle. According to a 1991 report of the General Accounting Office, the inventory of property seized by the Federal Marshalls Service "grew from 2,555 items at the start of the 1985 fiscal year, to 31,110 by December 31, 1990"—by which time the service was "mismanaging more than $1.4 billion in commercial property seized from drug dealers."[49] Although not offered in connection with the drug laws and their enforcement, a remark made by Jefferson scholar Forrest McDonald is apposite here: "The Government of the United States [now] interferes on a level in ordinary people's lives in a way they [the Founding Fathers] would have regarded as the most vicious form of tyranny imaginable. George the Third and all of his ministers could not have imagined a government this big, this intrusive."[50]

Every Man Has a Right to Eat as He Pleases

In 1884, protesting the arguments of (alcohol) prohibitionists, Dio Lewis—a physician and temperance reformer—declared, "Every man has a right to eat and drink, dress and exercise as he pleases. I do not mean moral right, but legal right."[51] The profound truth of this simple statement is reflected, I believe, in an important inference that we ought to—but never do—draw from the Prohibition Amendment.

The men who drafted the Volstead Act, which provided for enforcement of the Eighteenth Amendment, wanted to prohibit the consumption of alcohol; however, they did not outlaw it. They were not interested in whether people transported bottles of chemicals from one place to another, yet *that* is what they outlawed. I infer from this that, deep in their hearts, they and their constituents realized that a competent adult in the Land of the Free has an inalienable right to ingest whatever he wants. It should be unnecessary to add (but our current drug scapegoating justifies my adding) that there was no question, during Prohibition, of randomly testing people to determine if there was any ethanol in their system, or of searching their homes for alcohol, or of imprisoning them for possessing alcohol, or of involuntarily treating them for the disease of unsanctioned alcohol use.

DRUG CONTROLS AS CHEMICAL STATISM

The contemporary legal justification of drug controls rests heavily on the traditional Judeo-Christian equation of murder and suicide as two species of *homicide,* combined with the modern and peculiarly Western tendency to view both as due to abnormal mental states. Although murder and suicide both result in death (as do many other human behaviors), they are as different from one another as rape and masturbation. The one someone else does *to* you; the other you do *for* yourself. Drug abuse, like food or sex abuse, can injure or kill only the abuser; and of course it rarely does that. However, drug-law abuse—the criminalization of the free market in drugs—injures and kills users and so-called abusers alike. Many have already been killed by impure drugs, the adulteration of a criminalized product ("dope"); by bullets fired, in the course of gang wars, for instance, by persons engaged in the illegal trade in drugs ("pushers"); and by AIDS, owing to the absence of a free market in clean hypodermic syringes and needles ("drug paraphernalia"). Many more will surely be killed in the name of this holy war that promises to purify America and make it drug-free.

The Fable of the Bees vs. the Medical Model

The close connection we now tend to draw between suicide and murder, between drug abuse as harm to self and harm to others, is a manifestation of what is often called the "medical model": the viewing of behavior—especially socially disturbing behavior—as if it were a disease or the product of a disease. This absurd but nonetheless popular perspective on bad habits—on which our drug controls and much else in our contemporary struggle with lack of self-discipline and self-responsibility rest—is, in effect, an inversion of our traditionally moral perspective on behavior. The latter perspective Hobbes stated, simply and forcefully, when he declared; "Of the voluntary acts of every man, the object is some *good to himself.*"[52] Indeed, what else could be their object? Yet it pains us now to acknowledge this.

Try as we might to hide from ourselves the bitter truth about the influence of our societal perspective on behavior in these matters, we shall have to rediscover it or perish. Such painful learning by collective experience seems to be a characteristic feature of the free market and of the nearly reflexive human revolt, born out of an innate combination of dependency and paternalism, against it. However, overcoming our predicament with respect to the market in drugs will require just such relearning.

In this connection, consider the illuminating title of Bernard de Mandeville's epoch-making work *The Fable of the Bees: Or Private Vices, Publick Benefits.*[53] By cannily characterizing the market as a mechanism for turning private vices into public virtues—benefits, as he put it—Mandeville (1670–1733), a Dutch-born British physician-satirist, succeeded not only in giving a satisfactory account of its psychosocial underpinnings, but also in making it socially acceptable. Mutatis mutandis, abolishing the free market—in drugs or other goods or services deemed "dangerous" or "sinful"—reverses the process Mandeville described. Replacing personal efforts at self-control with impersonal laws coercing others, sumptuary laws prohibiting private pleasures create a mechanism for turning *private virtues into public vices.* This is precisely the lesson we draw from what communism has wrought in the Soviet Union, and is the lesson we ought to draw—but so far have stubbornly refused to draw—from what drug controls have wrought in the United States.

The Case for Chemical and Economic Statisms

Our individualist-libertarian and collectivist-redemptionist impulses—each robust in our political traditions—are, of course, at odds with one another and need to be constantly reconciled. In 1917 this ambivalence emerged as the principal ideological conflict of our age, pitting the United States and the Soviet Union against one another in a bitter antagonism. While the intensity of this conflict as an international struggle for power now appears diminished, its future as a domestic conflict within the American soul remains unpredictable. What is clear is that our justificatory images for chemical statism (command pharmacology) and for economic statism (command economy) are much the same, as the following schematic syllogisms illustrate.

> *Under conditions of economic insecurity,* inexorable under capitalist exploitation, freedom is a meaningless concept. The precondition of true freedom is economic security, which can be assured only by government ownership of the means of production and state control of the market in goods and services. Ergo, only in a communist society, based on command economy, can there be true freedom.

> *Under conditions of chemical insecurity,* inexorable under narcoterrorism, freedom is a meaningless concept. The precondition of true freedom is pharmacological security, which can be assured only by government ownership of pharmaceutical production and state control of the market in drugs. Ergo, only in a therapeutic state, based on command pharmacology, can there be true freedom.

These are marvelously persuasive arguments. If the first were not, fewer people would accept it in communist countries as providing moral and political legitimacy for the policy of state control of the market in goods and services; and if the second were not, fewer would accept it in the United States as providing legitimacy for the control of the market in pharmaceutical goods and services. There is only one thing wrong with these arguments, namely, that they are erroneous. Nothing can alter the fact that, like disease and death, insecurity and risk are intrinsic to the human condition. The state cannot protect us from any of them. The most the state can do is provide us with a social environment in which we can protect ourselves from the various risks that life poses. We, in turn, must learn to protect ourselves and others we care for, by cultivating our intelligence, prudence, and self-discipline.

Although the state cannot protect us from the risks of life, it can easily create an economic and legal environment in which we are deprived of the goods and drugs we crave. Perfect economic and pharmacological security is not to be had in this world. However, states whose citizens acquiesce in policies ostensibly aimed at protecting them from their own antisocial and/or unhealthy dispositions can easily bring about crushing economic and pharmacological deprivation for all but a corrupt elite.

Toward Politics qua Therapy

In recent years, there has been no shortage of critics of big government, on both sides of the rusted Iron Curtain. But words are cheap. Mikhail Gorbachev criticize[d] communism but continue[d] to practice it where it count[ed], maintaining state control of the means of production. Similarly, George Bush criticize[d] opponents of the free market but continue[d] to practice state interventionism where it count[ed], maintaining and even intensifying state control of medicine and especially the trade in drugs. And sadly, there seems to be little recognition of this, even within the ranks of anti-statists. Paul Johnson, for example, writes of the disenchantment with messianic politics and asks, "Was it possible to hope that the 'age of politics,' like the 'age of religion' before it, was now drawing to a close?"[54]

But so long as human nature remains what it is, neither religion nor politics will disappear. Hence, Johnson's question is poorly framed. We might better ask, "Is it possible to hope that the 'age of politics qua nationalism,' like the 'age of politics qua religion' before it, is now drawing to a close?" To which I would answer, The "age of politics qua nationalism" is already past, having been replaced by the "age of politics qua therapy."

When all is said and done, what has made the United States a safe haven for the weak and the oppressed? Due process—a lofty tradition of according *persons* genuine legal protection against accusations of wrongdoing. But the American political system accords no similar legal protection to *drugs*. The state may call a person dangerous, but it cannot deprive him of liberty unless it can prove him guilty of a crime (or incriminate him as mentally ill). Similarly, the state may—and can—call a drug dangerous and remove it from the market, and there is nothing any of us can do about it. Thus, all that the therapeutic demagogues need to do is declare a particular drug to be the embodiment of transcendent disease-producing evil and, presto, we have the perfect modern medicomythological scapegoat. This *pharmakos* (Greek for scapegoat) is not a person, so why should it have any rights? It is an ominous threat, causing deadly dangerous diseases, so what rational person would come to its defense?

In 1889, Emile Zola aroused the world when he cried, "*J'accuse!*" But Dreyfus was a man, a human being for whom people could feel compassion. Today, the orchestrators of universal sympathy feel compassion for animals, plants, the ecosystem, the whole universe. But who can feel compassion for "crack"?

NOTES

1. J. Madison, "Property," *National Gazette,* March 29, 1792, reprinted in *The Writings of James Madison,* vol. 6, ed. Gaillard Hunt (New York: G. P. Putnam's Sons), p. 101.

2. J. Locke, "The Second Treatise of Government," bk. 2, ch. 5, sec. 27, in *Two Treatises of Government,* 1690, reprint, ed. Peter Laslett (New York: Mentor Books, 1965), pp. 328–29.

3. Madison, "Property," p. 103; for a more sustained analysis of this theme, see S. M. Szasz, "Resurfacing the Road to Serfdom," *Freeman* 41 (February 1991): 46–49.

4. M. Friedman, "Private Property," *National Review* (November 5, 1990): 55–56; quote at p. 56.

5. E. J. Erler, "The Great Fence to Liberty: The Right to Property in the American Founding," in E. H. Paul and H. Dickman, eds., *Liberty, Property, and the Foundations of the American Constitution* (Albany: State University of New York Press, 1989), pp. 43, 56.

6. See R. E. Barnett, ed., *The Rights Retained by the People* (Fairfax, Va.: George Mason University Press, 1989).

7. Madison, "Property," p. 105; see also J. Nedelsky, *Private Property and the Limits of American Constitutionalism* (Chicago: University of Chicago Press, 1990), esp. pp. 16–66.

8. *Scott* v. *Sandford,* 60 U.S. (19 How.) 393 (1857), cited in V. G. Rosenblum and A. D. Castberg, eds., *Cases on Constitutional Law* (Homewood, Ill.: Dorsey Press, 1973), pp. 73–85; quote at pp. 74–79.

9. E. Burke, *Reflections on the Revolution in France,* 1790, reprint, ed. Conor Cruise O'Brien (London: Penguin, 1986), pp. 247–48.

10. T. Jefferson, "Notes on the State of Virginia," 1781, reprinted in A. Koch and W. Peden, eds., *The Life and Selected Writings of Thomas Jefferson* (New York: Modern Library, 1944), p. 275.

11. M. Twain, "Osteopathy," 1901, quoted in C. T. Harnsberger, ed., *Mark Twain at Your Fingertips* (New York: Beechhurst Press, 1948), pp. 341–42.

12. See T. S. Szasz, "The Ethics of Birth Control—Or: Who Owns Your Body?" *Humanist* 20 (November/December 1960): 332–36.

13. M. Friedman, *Capitalism and Freedom* (Chicago: University of Chicago Press, 1962), p. 138.

14. See *Griswold* v. *Connecticut,* 381 U.S. 479 (1965), and *Roe* v. *Wade,* 410 U.S. 113 (1973).

15. See, for example, " 'Grass' Could Cost a Rancher His Land," *Syracuse Herald-Journal,* March 19, 1991.

16. *McDermott* v. *Wisconsin,* 228 U.S. 115 (1913); emphasis added.

17. T. W. Christopher, *Constitutional Questions in Food and Drug Laws* (Chicago: Commerce Clearinghouse, 1960), p. 3; emphasis added.

18. Ibid., pp. 3–4.

19. *Wickard* v. *Filburn,* 317 U.S. 111 (1942), p. 84.

20. Ibid., p. 86. I wish to thank Arthur Spitzer, legal director of the ACLU's Washington, D.C., office, for kindly calling my attention to this case. The interpretation I advance is solely my responsibility.

21. C. Mackay, *Extraordinary Popular Delusions and the Madness of Crowds,* 1841, 1852, reprint (New York: Noonday Press, 1962).

22. *Webster's Third New International Dictionary,* unabridged (Springfield, Mass.: G&C Merriam, 1961), p. 2162.

23. L. von Mises, *Socialism,* 1922, reprint, trans. from the 2nd German edition by J. Kahane (Indianapolis, Ind.: Liberty Classics, 1981), p. 469.

24. S. Freud, *Civilization and Its Discontents,* 1929, reprint in SE, vol. 21, p. 113.

25. S. Freud, *The Introductory Lectures on Psychoanalysis,* 1916–17, reprint in SE, vol. 16, p. 389.

26. Mises, *Socialism,* p. 107.

27. L. von Mises, *Human Action* (New Haven, Conn.: Yale University Press, 1949), p. 874.

28. Even many libertarians do not support a free market in drugs—a market uncontaminated by the presumption that drug (ab)use is a disease. Among those who do, see, for example, M. N. Rothbard, *For a New Liberty* (New York: Collier 1973), pp. 111–12; C. N. Mitchell, *The Drug Solution* (Ottawa, Canada: Carleton University Press, 1990); and R. M. Ebeling, "The Economics of the Drug War," *Freedom Daily* 1 (April 1990): 6–10.

29. *Lear's* (March 1990).

30. *TV Guide* (May 19–25, 1990).

31. *People* (May 21, 1990).

32. *Time* (December 17, 1990): 19.

33. A. Purvis, "Just What the Patient Ordered," *Time* (May 28, 1990): 42.

34. Ibid.

35. M. D. Anglin and Y. Hser, "Legal Coercion and Drug Abuse Treatment: Research Findings and Social Policy Implications," in J. A. Inciardi and J. R. Biden Jr., eds., *Handbook of Drug Control in the United States* (Westport, Conn.: Greenwood Press, 1990), pp. 151–76; quote at p. 152.

36. F. Bastiat, *Economic Sophisms,* 1845/1848, reprint, trans. Arthur Goddard (Princeton, N.J.: Van Nostrand, 1964), pp. 125–26.

37. L. Jones, "Evaluation of Drug Treatment Research Urged," *American Medical News* (October 26, 1990): 4.

38. *Calero-Toledo v. Pearson Yacht Leasing Co.,* 416 U.S. 663 (1974).

39. Ibid., p. 665.

40. Ibid., p. 663.

41. Ibid., p. 695.

42. *United States v. One Assortment of 89 Firearms,* 465 U.S. 354 (1974), p. 356.

43. Ibid.

44. Ibid.

45. See, for example, T. S. Szasz, *Law, Liberty, and Psychiatry,* 1963, reprint (Syracuse, N.Y.: Syracuse University Press, 1989) and *Psychiatric Justice,* 1965, reprint (Syracuse, N.Y.: Syracuse University Press, 1988).

46. See S. B. Herpel, *"United States v. One Assortment of 89 Firearms,"* *Reason* (May 1990): 3–36

47. J. Dillin, "Nation's Liberties at Risk," *Christian Science Monitor,* February 2, 1990.

48. For example, see J. B. Treaster, "Agents Arrest Car Dealers in Sales to Drug Traffickers," *New York Times,* October 4, 1990.

49. "Marshalls Faulted on Drug Property Report Says Mismanagement of Seized Real Estate Has Cost the U.S. Millions," *New York Times,* April 21, 1991.

50. F. McDonald, quoted in L. M. Werner, "If Jefferson et al. Could See Us Now," *New York Times,* February 12, 1987

51. D. Lewis, "Prohibition and Persuasion," *North American Review* 139 (August 1884): 188–99, quote at p. 194, reprinted in C. Watner, "Foreword," in L. Spooner, *Vices Are Not Crimes: A Vindication of Moral Liberty* 1875, reprint (Cupertino, Calif.: Tanstaafl, 1977), pp viii–ix.

52. T. Hobbes, *Leviathan,* 1651, reprint, ed. Michael Oakeshott (New York: Collier Macmillan, 1962), p 105

53. B. Mandeville, *The Fable of the Bees,* 1732, reprint, F. B. Kaye edition, 2 vols. (Indianapolis, Ind.: Liberty Press, 1988); see also R. Hunter and I. Macalpine, eds, *Three Hundred Years of Psychiatry, 1535–1860* (London: Oxford University Press, 1963), p. 296.

It may be of interest to note that Bernard de Mandeville was also a pioneer in psychiatry (psychotherapy)—an enterprise closely related to economics, albeit this connection is no longer officially recognized. Mandeville's medical practice was limited to patients suffering from what the alienists called "nerve and stomach disorders" or, as he called them, the "hypochondriack and hysterick passions." In 1711 he published *A Treatise of the Hypochondriack and Hysterick Passions,* written explicitly "by way of Information to Patients [rather] than to teach other Practitioners." Although Mandeville's books went through numerous printings and he was one of the most famous and influential figures of his age, his name is now rarely mentioned except by libertarian writers

54. P. Johnson, *Modern Times* (New York: Harper & Row, 1983), p. 728.

20

There's No Justice in the War on Drugs

Milton Friedman

Twenty-five years ago, President Richard M. Nixon announced a "War on Drugs." I criticized the action on both moral and expediential grounds in my *Newsweek* column of May 1, 1972, "Prohibition and Drugs":

> On ethical grounds, do we have the right to use the machinery of government to prevent an individual from becoming an alcoholic or a drug addict? For children, almost everyone would answer at least a qualified yes. But for responsible adults, I, for one, would answer no. Reason with the potential addict, yes. Tell him the consequences, yes. Pray for and with him, yes. But I believe that we have no right to use force, directly or indirectly, to prevent a fellow man from committing suicide, let alone from drinking alcohol or taking drugs.

That basic ethical flaw has inevitably generated specific evils during the past quarter century, just as it did during our earlier attempt at alcohol prohibition.

1. The use of informers. Informers are not needed in crimes like robbery and murder because the victims of those crimes have a strong incentive to report the crime. In the drug trade, the crime consists of a transaction between a willing buyer and willing seller. Neither has any incentive to report a violation of law. On the contrary, it is in the self-interest of both that the crime not be reported. That is why informers are needed. The use of informers and the immense sums of money at stake inevitably generate corruption—as they did during Prohibition. They also lead to violations of the civil rights of innocent people, to the shameful practices of forcible entry and forfeiture of property without due process.

As I wrote in 1972: ". . . addicts and pushers are not the only ones corrupted. Immense sums are at stake. It is inevitable that some realtively low-paid police and other government officials—and some high-paid ones as well—will succumb the temptation to pick up easy money.

2. Filling the prisons. In 1970, 200,000 people were in prison. Today, 1.6 million people are. Eight times as many in absolute number, six times as many relative to the increased population. In addition, 2.3 million are on probation and parole. The attempt to prohibit drugs is by far the major source of the horrendous growth in the prison population.

There is no light at the end of that tunnel. How many of our citizens do we want to turn into criminals before we yell "enough"?

3. Disproportionate imprisonment of blacks. Sher Hosonko, at the time Connecticut's director of addiction services, stressed this effect of drug prohibition in a talk given in June 1995:

> Today in this country, we incarcerate 3,109 black men for every 100,000 of them in the population. Just to give you an idea of the drama in this number, our closest competitor for incarcerating black men is South Africa. South Africa—and this is pre-Nelson Mandela and under an overt public policy of apartheid—incarcerated 723 black men for every 100,000. Figure this out: In the land of the Bill of Rights, we jail over four times as many black men as the only country in the world that advertised a political policy of apartheid.

4. Destruction of inner cities. Drug prohibition is one of the most important factors that have combined to reduce our inner cities to their present state. The crowded inner cities have a comparative advantage for selling drugs. Though most customers do not live in the inner cities, most sellers do. Young boys and girls view the swaggering, affluent drug dealers as role models. Compared with the returns from a traditional career of study and hard work, returns from dealing drugs are tempting to young and old alike. And many, especially the young, are not dissuaded by the bullets that fly so freely in disputes between competing drug dealers—bullets that fly only because dealing drugs is illegal. Al Capone epitomizes our earlier attempt at Prohibition; the Crips and Bloods epitomize this one.

5. Compounding the harm to users. Prohibition makes drugs exorbitantly expensive and highly uncertain in quality. A user must associate with criminals to get the drugs, and many are driven to become criminals themselves to finance the habit. Needles, which are hard to get, are often shared, with the predictable effect of spreading disease. Finally, an addict who seeks treatment must confess to being a criminal in order to qualify for a treatment program. Alternatively, professionals who treat addicts must become informers or criminals themselves.

6. Undertreatment of chronic pain. The Federal Department of Health and Human Services has issued reports showing that two thirds of all ter-

minal cancer patients do not receive adequate pain medication, and the numbers are surely higher in nonterminally ill patients. Such serious undertreatment of chronic pain is a direct result of the Drug Enforcement Agency's pressures on physicians who prescribe narcotics.

7. Harming foreign countries. Our drug policy has led to thousands of deaths and enormous loss of wealth in countries like Colombia, Peru, and Mexico, and has undermined the stability of their governments. All because we cannot enforce our laws at home. If we did, there would be no market for imported drugs. There would be no Cali cartel. The foreign countries would not have to suffer the loss of sovereignty involved in letting our "advisers" and troops operate on their soil, search their vessels, and encourage local militaries to shoot down their planes. They could run their own affairs, and we, in turn, could avoid the diversion of military forces from their proper function.

Can any policy, however high-minded, be moral if it leads to widespread corruption, imprisons so many, has so racist an effect, destroys our inner cities, wreaks havoc on misguided and vulnerable individuals, and brings death and destruction to foreign countries?

Part Six

Addiction Is a Behavior:
The Myth of Loss of Control

21

Defining "Addiction"*

Bruce K. Alexander and Anton R. F. Schweighofer

The word "addiction" has too many meanings. This is partly because it contains a fundamental ambiguity. For centuries, "addiction" referred to the state of being "given over" or intensely involved with any activity. The ambiguity lay in the value attached to this state; addiction could be either tragic or enviable, or somewhere in between. As well, a second meaning emerged in the nineteenth century, and now coexists with the earlier one. The new meaning is more restrictive than the traditional one in three ways; it links addiction to *harmful* involvements with *drugs* that produce *withdrawal symptoms or tolerance*.

Ambiguity in such a basic term confuses the study of psychology, and of drug issues in particular. We believe the confusion can be dispelled by abandoning the restrictive meaning, which does not fit with the realities of addiction, and by clarifying the ambiguity in the traditional meaning.

In the first section of this article, historical studies are used to show that the restrictive meaning did not grow from scientific or medical discoveries, but from the rhetoric of the temperance and anti-opium movements of the nineteenth century. In the second section, contemporary research is used to show that the traditional concept describes the clinical realities of addiction far better than the restrictive concept does. In the third section, new interview data on university students are used to show how the traditional concept also describes the dependent and addictive patterns of nondiagnosed people better than the restrictive concept does.

Originally published in *Canadian Psychology* 29 (1988). Copyright 1988 Canadian Psychological Association. Reprinted with permission.

*This project was supported by the Steel Fund, Simon Fraser University. Valuable help was provided by Patricia Holborn, E. Wyn Roberts, Howard Gabert, Maureen Okun, and Kim Bartholomew.

The conclusion of this article argues that the restrictive meaning should be discarded because it artificially limits addiction to a special case. Although fixation on this special case reflects social concern, the restrictive definition has proven not to consistently identify the types of addiction that are harmful. Glasser's distinction between "positive" and "negative" addiction, with some refinement, adds a socially critical distinction to the traditional definition of addiction. Finally, the potential for increased understanding that grows from critically examining the meanings of "addiction" is explored.

HISTORY OF THE WORD "ADDICTION"

The Latin verb *addico* signifies "giving over" either in a negative or a positive sense. In Roman law, for example, an *addictus* was a person given over as a bond slave to a creditor. In its positive uses, *addico* suggested devotion, as in *senatus, cui me semper addixi* ("the senate, to which I am always devoted") or *agros omnes addixit deae* ("he dedicated the fields entirely to the goddess) (Lewis and Short, 1879).

The traditional English meaning of "addiction" is similar. The 1933 *Oxford English Dictionary* defines addiction as: ". . . a formal giving over or delivery by sentence of court. Hence, a surrender or dedication of any one to a master. . . . The state of being (self-) addicted or given to a habit or pursuit: devotion" (Murray, Bradley, Cragie, and Onions, 1933, p. 104). A similar definition appears in Webster's original American dictionary (Webster, 1898/1970).

Uses of "addiction" over several centuries compiled in the *Oxford English Dictionary* show that, as in Latin, "addiction" could be used in a favorable sense ("His own proper Industry and Addiction to Books") and an unfavorable sense ("A man who causes grief to his family by his addiction to bad habits"). Our reading of the uses of "addiction" in Shakespeare, Hobbes, and Gibbon suggests that the unfavorable sense was less common than favorable or neutral usage.

Prior to the nineteenth century, "addiction" was rarely associated with drugs. Although opium had been well known from earliest recorded history. references connecting it to addiction, or any synonym for addiction, were unusual prior to the nineteenth century (Parssinen and Kerner, 1980). In prenineteenth century Europe, opium was usually referred to as a medicine (Sonnedecker, 1962). The word was generally not applied to alcohol use either. Sometimes, though rarely, habitual drunkards were said to be "addicted to intemperance" (Levine, 1978).

The restrictive usage of "addiction" emerged in language of the nineteenth-century temperance and anti-opium movements (Berridge and Edwards, 1981, chap. 13; Levine, 1978; 1984; Sonnedecker, 1963, pp. 30–31).

"Addiction" came to replace terms like "intemperance" or "inebriety" for excessive alcohol and opium use. In the process, the traditional meaning of "addiction" was narrowed in at least three ways. The new usage linked "addiction" tightly to drugs, especially alcohol and opium, gave addiction an invariably harmful connotation as an illness or vice, and identified addiction with the presence of withdrawal symptoms and tolerance.

The nineteenth century use of "addiction" is sometimes seen as a medical or scientific achievement—an enlightened replacement for an earlier moralistic view of drunkenness. However, it was not scientific, it was only incidentally medical, and, in the end, it was harsher than the view of addiction it replaced (Alexander, in 1987).

Prior to the nineteenth century, at least in the United States, habitual alcohol use was not generally viewed as a sin but as a matter of choice, with relatively little ultimate significance (Levine, 1978). The restrictive definition first appeared in the doctrine of the Temperance Movement where it was part of the rhetoric used to change the image of chronic heavy drinking from an indulgence that might be laughed at, ignored, or possibly punished, to something necessarily sick or evil (Levine, 1978; Shaffer, 1985, p. 67). The application of "addiction," in its restrictive sense, to habitual alcohol use was *not* ". . . an independent medical or scientific discovery, but . . . part of a transformation in social thought grounded in fundamental changes in social life—in the structure of society" (Levine, 1978, pp. 165–66).

The restrictive use of "addiction" served diverse motives. It was used by anti-opium reformers in the United States apparently to frighten people into abstinence by linking opium with horrifying (and greatly exaggerated) descriptions of withdrawal symptoms (Musto, 1973, chap. 4). Later in the nineteenth century, the Chinese empress mounted an antiopium drive and Theodore Roosevelt seized the opportunity to attack opium, partly to curry favor in the "China Market." The American government supported Chinese opium prohibition at international conferences, pressured other nations to prohibit opium use, and pushed the American Congress to lead the way with national opium prohibition laws. Part of this effort to win public support for opium prohibition entailed dramatizing the concept of addiction (see Musto, 1973, p. 33).

In nineteenth-century England, public health concerns over excessive opium use were inflamed by health professionals who wished to construe opium-eating as an addictive disease that fell within their professional domains (Berridge and Edwards, 1981). This was part of a process of medicalizing various forms of deviance that eventually expanded the domain of the medical profession (Parssinen and Kerner, 1980).

This was also a period of class tension and the English middle classes apparently needed conceptually simple bases for condemning restive segments of the lower class. One basis was created by exaggerating the evils associated with widespread lower class opium use, labeling users as addicts and addiction as something evil or sick (Berridge and Edwards, 1981).

The interplay of motives in England has been summarized this way:

> Addiction is now defined as an illness because doctors have categorized it thus. . . . It was a process which had its origins in the last quarter of the nineteenth century . . . but such views were never, however, scientifically autonomous. Their putative objectivity disguised class and moral concerns which precluded an understanding of the social and cultural roots of opium use. (Berridge and Edwards, 1981, p. 150)

Manipulating the meaning of "addiction" has continued into the present, with still other motivations:

> Images of addiction are in fact consistently and relentlessly marketed—in the nineteenth century to make opium the property of the medical profession. In the twentieth century to justify the position of enforcement agencies or the international control apparatus, or to win tomorrow's research budget. Images compete, and in the process the marketing becomes even more aggressive. The medical and scientific images feed and change the public, administrative and political view, and in return these perceptions give the doctors and scientists the needed support. . . . (Berridge and Edwards, 1981, p. 250).

Although the restrictive definition of addiction flourished, the traditional definition was deeply rooted and never entirely displaced. The consequent co-existence of two dissonant meanings, each with its variations (plus a trivial usage, meaning an ordinary habit), became so confusing that some authorities began to urge abandoning the word altogether (LeDain, 1973: Paton, 1969; Zinberg and Robertson, 1972). In fact, some major scholars have adroitly managed to excise the term entirely from discussions of compulsive drug use (American Psychiatric Association, 1980; Edwards, Arif, and Hodgson, 1982; Vaillant, 1983).

But the word "addiction" has refused to be expunged from the language. The traditional meaning is still widely applied, both in its positive sense (Glasser, 1976; Land, 1971) and its negative sense (Hatterer, 1980; Peele, 1985). Likewise, the restricted meaning can be found in popular literature (Kline, 1985; Gold, 1984) and scientific contexts (Dole and Nyswander, 1980; Smart, 1983). Modern dictionaries generally give both meanings or try to combine them.

Why has this fractured, embattled word survived? Perhaps because it designates, however imperfectly, an important human state that requires a name. Perhaps because proposed substitutes, like "psychological dependence," "physical dependence," "drug abuse," and "substance abuse" introduce new ambiguities (Blackwell, 1985; Peele, 1977; Zinberg, Harding, and Apsler, 1978).

Although the word "addiction" has proved hardy, its ambiguity has almost destroyed its usefulness. The confusion can best be cleared by abandoning the restrictive meaning and addressing the ambiguity in the traditional meaning.

In the next section, a brief literature review will introduce the evidence that the restrictive definition does not fit well with the reality of addiction. In the subsequent section, new interview data will show that addiction in a non-diagnosed population fits with the traditional sense of "addiction" better than with the restrictive sense. The interview data also document the ambiguity in the traditional definition.

RECENT ADDICTION RESEARCH

Recent research on addiction will be used to evaluate the three major ways that the restrictive usage narrowed the traditional meaning of "addiction," i.e., linking it to drugs, to harmfulness, and to withdrawal symptoms.

Is Addiction Limited to Drug Use?

Contrary to the restrictive definition, there is no basis for linking the word "addiction" primarily or exclusively to drug habits. Nor is there a basis for assuming that the most severe addictions necessarily involve drugs.

This has been demonstrated in many ways. For example, severely compulsive love relationships have been found to be as intense, irrational, and ultimately self-destructive as intense heroin addiction. A review of "crimes of passion" in the news might suggest that the potential for tragedy is at least as severe among "love addicts" as among drug addicts. Differences that popular wisdom might assert between the two kinds of addiction disappear once the distorted media view of heroin addiction is discounted and the two addictions are compared on the same basis (Peele and Brodsky, 1975).

Other authors have likewise shown that severe drug addictions closely resemble destructive involvements with: gambling (Orford, 1985), exercise (Morgan, 1979), accumulating money (Slater, 1980), childish fantasy (Alexander, 1982), television-viewing (Winn, 1977), working (Oates, 1971), pentecostal religion (Womack, 1980), and numerous other activities and substances (Hodgson and Miller, 1982; Orford, 1985; Peele, 1985). Compulsive involvements with any of these can consume a person's entire existence and can have tragic consequences. Therefore, linking the term "addiction" solely to drugs creates an artificial distinction that strips the language of a term for the same condition when drugs are not involved.

Those who have not actually had clinical experience with patients addicted to activities other than using drugs, or who have not read a number of case studies, may not fully believe that severe addictions to activities can *really* be as serious as addictions to heroin or cocaine. However, the observations of numerous professionals who have had the opportunity to observe people addicted to both drugs and other activities cannot be easily dismissed.

The similarity between severe addictions to drugs and other activities may be partly obscured by everyday experience. Whereas it is easy to observe people with nonharmful involvements in everyday activities, most of the available information on illicit drugs comes from dramatic presentations of severe addictions. In addition, the criminality associated with the use of illicit drugs exacerbates the harm done by addiction to these substances. However, more systematic observations have now shown that the potential for tragically destructive addiction is not peculiar to drugs.

Is Addiction Always Harmful?

Addiction can be a devastating, ultimately fatal condition, but it can also be harmless or even beneficial. The distinguished scientist Edwin Land (1971) provided a personal account of beneficial addiction in a *Science* article entitled "Addiction as a necessity and opportunity." Land described his own life as an alternation between a state in which he was in touch with people and the environment and one in which he was given over to his work. Land correctly identified this second state as addiction and described it as temporary and beneficial. In his words:

> You want to be undisturbed. You want to be free to think not for an hour at a time, or three hours at a time, but for two days or two weeks, if possible, without interruption. You don't want to drive the family car or go to parties. You wish people would just go away and leave you alone while you get something straight. Then, you get it straight and you embody it, and during that period of embodiment you have a feeling of almost divine guidance. Then it is done, and, suddenly, you are alone, and you have a need to go back to your friends and the world around you, and to all history, to be refreshed, to feel alive and human once again. (Land, 1971, pp. 151–52)

It may be harder to acknowledge addiction as sometimes beneficial for people who use drugs, rather than engage in scientific contemplation. However, the evidence is just as clear. Khantzian, Mack, and Schatzberg (1974) presented five brief case studies of male American heroin addicts who would fit both the traditional or the restrictive definitions. Several vital functions that heroin addiction may serve were identified, including: calming the user; controlling premature ejaculation; "keeping him going"; helping the user feel better when angry, nervous, or depressed; eliminating migraine headaches; reducing fear; providing a feeling of belonging to the society of drug takers; controlling homesickness; and creating detachment from bad news.

It seems quite likely from this account that there were extended periods for each man during which the benefits of addictive heroin use outweighed the costs. In the researchers' words:

> Addicts' use of opiates represents a unique and characteristic way of dealing with a range of human problems involving emotional pain, stress, and dysphoria . . . addicts take advantage of the powerful action of the drug to mute and extinguish their emotions and to solve, at least in the short run, problems associated with interpersonal relationships. In addition . . . the transaction and practices of the pseudoculture in which the addict immerses himself also play a part in filling his social vacuum. . . . (Khantzian et al., 1974, p. 110)

Extensive contact with current and former heroin addicts in Vancouver over several years [has] convinced us that this unexpectedly favorable cost/benefit ratio is not uncommon.

This is not to say that addiction cannot be disastrous. But particular people in particular circumstances may conscientiously find addiction, even to drugs, to be the most adaptive way they can live, at least for a time. In extreme cases, addiction may save them from debilitation or suicide. Similar observations have been elaborated by many scholars (e.g., Chein, Gerard. Lee, and Rosenfeld, 1964; Kaplan and Wieder, 1974; Marlatt, 1985; Peele, 1985; Shaffer and Burglass, 1981; Wishnie, 1977; Wurmser, 1978). Others, who do not grant that addiction can be actually beneficial, nevertheless note that it is not always harmful, contrary to the restrictive meaning (Edwards, Arif, and Hodgson, 1982, p. 10; Westermeyer, 1982).

ARE WITHDRAWAL SYMPTOMS AND TOLERANCE LINKED TO ADDICTION?

There is extensive evidence and growing recognition that withdrawal symptoms and tolerance only sometimes accompany addiction and are rarely its cause (Alexander, 1984; Edwards, Arif, and Hodgson, 1982; Goldstein, 1983; Jaffe, 1980). For example, by carefully interviewing addicts, Cummings, Gordon, and Marlatt (1980) found that "relapses involving opiates do not occur primarily in response to somatic discomfort" (p. 305). Chaney, Roszell, and Cummings (1982) found that only 16 percent of the relapses of methadone patients "involved coping with physiological states associated with prior substances use" (p. 294).

Another strong indication that withdrawal symptoms and addiction are not always linked is that profound addictions often occur without withdrawal symptoms. For example, many researchers have found that a significant proportion of people who live the devastating lives of street junkies do not have withdrawal symptoms when heroin supplies are interrupted or when they are pharmacologically deprived by a "naloxone challenge" (e.g., Glasser, 1974; O'Brien, 1976; Peachy and Franklin, 1985).

In contrast, some drugs that produce withdrawal symptoms are not used compulsively, for example imipramine, a drug prescribed for depression (Jaffe, Peterson, and Hodgson, 1980, p. 1). Finally, tolerance develops to the sedative effects of the phenothiazenes (chlorpromazine, etc.) and to other drugs that are not addicting by either the traditional or restrictive definition (Recta and Moore, 1971, pp. 299–301). Although withdrawal symptoms and tolerance are frequently associated with addiction to the opiates, they are neither necessary nor sufficient to cause compulsive drug use, nor invariably concomitant with it.

SELF-REPORT DATA FROM UNIVERSITY STUDENTS

For several years we have interviewed university students about their drug use, dependencies, and addictions. The students' self-descriptions conform more closely to the traditional definition than to the restrictive definition on the key differences between the two. The methods and findings are summarized here.

Methods

Sampling

Three sets of students at Simon Fraser University were chosen arbitrarily and an attempt was made to interview all the students in each set. The three sets comprised sixty students who worked in the University Center Building, forty-nine students enrolled in fourth-year psychology courses, and thirty students enrolled in the campus karate club. Every potential subject but one was eventually interviewed in each set (total $N = 136$). For our purposes the advantages of the minimal self-selection obtained in this manner outweighed the loss of a random sample of the entire student body (See Schachter, 1982).

The interviewers were student members of the subpopulation they interviewed. Prior to actual collection of data they received extensive training and supervised practice on the interview. We also observed some actual data collection by each interviewer, to maintain standardization.

Interview Terminology

The interview was based on drug-use categories (see Table 21.1) derived from Jaffe's (1980) concept of a *continuum of involvement* with drugs, from "exper-

---

Table 21.1: Involvement Definitions

1. (Abstention). Did not use at all.
2. (Experimental Use). Used on no more than a few occasions out of curiosity, or to conform to a group.
3. (Circumstantial Use). Used only in specific circumstances when effects were helpful, e.g., unusual fatigue, illness, pain, etc.
4. (Casual Use). Used infrequently for its pleasurable effects.
5. (Regular Use). Used regularly for pleasurable effects.
6. (Dependence). Used regularly, without medical necessity; effects felt as needed for continued well-being; probably would continue use in spite of adverse medical or social effect.
7. (Positive and Neutral Addiction). Overwhelmingly involved with using and/or obtaining it; pervades total life activity and controls behavior in a wide range of circumstances; high tendency to resume use after stopping.
8. (Negative Addiction). (This category was scored if the subject chose category 7 *and* gave a negative response to both followup questions: "Did you like being that involved with _____?" Did you feel good about yourself when you were that involved with _____?")
9. (Withdrawal Symptoms). Continued use is necessary to prevent a syndrome which could include headaches, nausea, diarrhea, chill, cramps, mental imbalance, etc. (At least one physical manifestation, i.e., other than "mental imbalance" must be mentioned.)

Notes.

Subjects were recorded as "Quitting" if they reported that they were involved in trying to terminate their use of a drug or activity.

Subjects were scored as fitting the *Traditional Definition* if they chose category 7 or 8.

Subjects were scored as fitting the *Restrictive Definition* if they chose category 9.

Category 9 could be double scored with categories 3, 5, 6, 7, or 8.

Subjects were not shown the material in parentheses.

---

imental use" to "addiction." Jaffe's definition of "addiction" is very close to the traditional meaning; it is an "overwhelming involvement" neither intrinsically linked to illness and vice, nor to withdrawal symptoms and tolerance.

In pilot interviews, hundreds of students were asked if they could apply Jaffe's definitions to their own behavior. In the process, the definitions gradually reached their forms in Table 21.1, which retain Jaffe's original conceptions but are more readily comprehensible to students. Two categories were added to accommodate distinctions that many students felt important. Jaffe's "casual or recreational use" was divided into "casual use" (category 4) and "regular use" (category 5). Jaffe's "addiction" was supplemented with "negative addiction" (category 8) to separate out the subset of addictions that were intensely aversive to the students from those that were not.

Responses that fit Jaffe's definition of addiction (category 7) were reclassified as "negative addiction" (category 8) if students reported unequivocally *both* that they did not enjoy being overwhelmingly involved with the drug or activity and that they did not like themselves at the time of the involvement. When students described themselves in this way it was often with visible emotion or concern. Because instances of negative addiction were put into category 8, category 7 is referred to as "positive and neutral addiction."

Categories 7 and 8 combined served as a definition of addiction in the traditional sense.

Jaffe's (1980) description of withdrawal symptoms was adapted to serve as an operational definition of addiction in the restrictive sense (category 9). Withdrawal symptoms were not part of Jaffe's continuum of involvement, but rather an effect of past use. Therefore, students who reported withdrawal symptoms were asked to choose one of the involvement categories as well, and students who indicated any kind of regular use (categories 3, 5, 6, 7, 8) were asked if they also had withdrawal symptoms. All students were able to understand the logic of double-scoring category 9.

A comprehensive list of types of psychoactive drugs was taken from a drug physiology text (Julien, 1981) and modified by adding locally popular drugs and drug names. A list of nondrug activities popular with students was accumulated during the pilot interviews and expanded once as the actual study progressed. The students were asked the same questions about the drugs and nondrug activities.

Interview Procedure

Students were invited to participate in an interview on "their involvement with drugs and other activities." Interviewers did not use the words "addiction" or "dependence," but referred by number to the definitions in Table 21.1 (without the parenthesized labels), which the students had before them throughout the interview. Subjects were informed that their confidentiality would be scrupulously respected. Interviews lasted forty-five to ninety minutes.

The subjects were encouraged to actively help in accurately translating their complex life experiences into numbers. They responded comfortably in that collaborative atmosphere. In fact, many spontaneously commented that they enjoyed the interview because it gave them the opportunity to evaluate themselves in new terms.

To maximize accuracy and consistency, the interviewers offered to review the categories' meanings before the interview. They also queried the subjects from time to time about each category to be sure the subjects had understood it correctly, had considered all parts of it, and were applying it uniformly to their use of various drugs and activities. When this was not the case, subjects were asked to reconsider their choices, but the final choice was always theirs.

The interviewer first asked subjects to "describe their level of current involvement" with each drug and activity by indicating an involvement category. Next, they asked subjects to report the number of days they had used each drug or activity in the previous thirty. They next asked the category of the subjects' "highest ever" involvement with each drug or activity.

After responding to all the drugs and activities on the list, subjects were asked if there were other drugs or activities that they used, and to categorize these in the same ways. Finally, subjects were asked if they were attempting to terminate their involvement with any drug or activity. If they were, "quitting" was recorded.

Subjects were encouraged not to select an involvement category unless one really fit. When none did, verbal descriptions were transcribed but for quantitative purposes the code "can't answer" was recorded. There were few "can't answer" responses in the involvement categories: less than 3 percent for all drugs and activities except nicotine, sex, and love, where there were between 4 and 6 percent "can't answers."

Since the involvement categories were originally taken from a pharmacology text, their wording is more suitable for drugs than for other activities. In particular, the verb "use" was awkward for many subjects when categorizing their involvement with nondrug activities. For example, it is awkward to say that one "uses" love or children. Therefore subjects were asked to mentally substitute an appropriate verb, but to otherwise apply the definitions literally, as they had with the drug items.

Since addiction is a sensitive topic some underreporting seemed inevitable. On the other hand a number of investigators have found that interview subjects accurately describe their own addictions, if the interviews are carefully conceived and conducted (See Vaillant, 1983 pp. 31–32; Westermeyer, 1982, p. 83; Zinberg, 1984, pp. 64–68). Zinberg (1984) has described the positive results of an elaborate cross-checking scheme on the self-reports of heroin users.

Results and Discussion

On the key issues of whether addiction is linked to drugs, to harm, and to withdrawal symptoms, the data supported the traditional definition. However, these data describe only a subset of a university student population. Further research is obviously required to determine their generality.

**Table 21.2: Drug Involvements =
Percentage of Total Involvements**

Type of Involvement	Percentage of Type That Involved Drugs
Addiction: Traditional Definition	
(Categories 7 + 8)	7.3
Positive and Neutral Addiction (7)	4.5
Negative Definition (8)	19.3
Restrictive Definition (9)	54.8
Dependence (6)	23.1
Regular Use (5)	29.2
"Quitting"	60.5

Note: The numbers following each definition refer to the involvement definitions from Table 21.1.

Is Addiction Restricted to Drug Habits?

As Table 21.2 shows, addiction is not restricted to drugs, *by any definition.* By the traditional definition (i.e., categories 7 and 8 combined), only 7.3 percent of the students' addictions were to drugs (See Table 21.2). The most common addictions were to love, sports, work, sex, school, self-reflection, etc. The most common drug addiction, by the traditional definition, was to nicotine, which was thirteenth on the list with twelve students reporting addiction to it at some time in their lives. The next most frequent drugs of addiction were cannabis (16th), alcohol (21st), and caffeine (22nd). Drug addictions were also a minority of all addictions when positive and neutral addiction (category 7) and negative addiction (category 8) were considered separately (Table 21.2 is based on current and past addictions combined. Data on current addictions show a similar pattern of results, although the totals in all categories are lower).

Less than 20 percent of the reported instances of negative addiction—the addictions that the students found intensely aversive—involved drugs. The most frequently reported negative addictions were to love and food, reported by fifteen and seven of the students respectively. The most commonly reported negative addiction to a drug was to nicotine, reported by six of the students. The most commonly mentioned illicit drug was cannabis, reported by four students.

By the restrictive definition (category 9), the most frequent addictions were to nicotine, caffeine, love, and sports, in that order. About 45 percent of the addictions were to activities, rather than drugs, even though withdrawal

**Table 21.3: "Negative Addictions" and
"Positive or Neutral Addictions" to Drugs and Activities**

		Current	Highest Ever
Drugs	Positive or Neutral Addiction (7)	0	17
	Negative Addiction (8)	8	17
Activities	Positive or Neutral Addiction (7)	174	361
	Negative Addiction (8)	6	62

symptoms were not recorded unless the subject reported a definite physical symptom, not merely "mental imbalance" (Table 21.2).

Three other categories could be interpreted as suggesting addiction in weaker senses of the term: "dependence," "regular use," and "negative involvement." For each category, drugs are involved less often than nondrug activities (Table 21.2).

The highest ratio of drug addictions to total addictions was for "quitting." Sixty percent of the habits that students reported having tried to quit were drug habits. The most frequently mentioned habits were nicotine, food, alcohol, and an "other activities" category. But even if "quitting" were taken as the definition of addiction, 40 percent of the reported addictions were to nondrug activities.

Obviously, the percentage of addictions that involve drugs depends on how the term is defined. But addictions were not limited to drugs by any definition. By the most severe definition of addiction, negative addiction, drug habits comprised less than 20 percent of total addictions.

Is Addiction Necessarily Harmful?

The students were not specifically asked about the harmfulness of their involvements, but their interviews did provide relevant information. If it is fair to assume that people eventually develop a strong aversion toward habits that harm them, even when they cannot quit, then the ratio of negative addiction to positive and neutral addiction approximates the ratio of harmful addiction to harmless or beneficial addictions. These data appear in Table 21.3.

For nondrug activities, only a small minority of the reported addictions were negative addictions. For drugs, the proportion was higher. In fact, there was some support for the restrictive definition in that all eight of the current drug addictions were categorized as negative addictions. However, only seventeen of the thirty-four "highest ever" drug addictions (which includes both current and past addictions) were categorized as negative addictions. Some of the drug addictions that were not categorized as negative addictions were addictions of

Table 21.4: Withdrawal Symptoms Accompanying Dependence, Positive and Neutral Addiction, and Negative Addiction	Drugs		Activities	
	No	Yes	No	Yes
Dependence (6)	93	9	377	2
Positive and Neutral Addiction (7)	11	6	346	15
Negative Addiction (8)	13	4	61	1

short duration, usually occurring in summers during which students and their friends had been overwhelmingly involved with marijuana, alcohol, or LSD and had enjoyed the experience, both at the time and looking back.

Of course, it may be that the students' temporary periods of drug addiction were harmful, regardless of how they remembered them, but this is a risky assumption. Adventurous or rebellious adolescents often develop extravagant passions for dangerous sports, forbidden loves, drug subcultures, etc. Although such youthful involvements may offend the larger society, they may serve important functions, as rites of passage or first tries at adult autonomy (Erikson, 1950). They might also serve to teach young people that they cannot long escape adult responsibilities with addictive pursuits. These hypothetical beneficial functions seem to us as plausible as the assumption that all drug addictions are inevitably harmful, even when the formerly addicted person says they were not.

Are Withdrawal Symptoms Linked to Addiction?

This question was explored by determining the number of addictions that were accompanied by withdrawal symptoms. The three most compulsive forms of drug involvement included in the interview were "dependence," "positive and neutral addiction" and "negative addiction." Whenever students chose one of these descriptions they were asked if category 9 (withdrawal symptoms) also applied. Table 21.4 presents these data.

Contrary to the restrictive definition, Table 21.4 shows that withdrawal symptoms were not typically concomitant with compulsive use, either for drugs or nondrug involvements, even in the case of negative addiction. The majority of reported dependencies, addictions, and negative addictions did not involve withdrawal symptoms.

Even though a clear somatic manifestation was required for withdrawal symptoms to be recorded, withdrawal symptoms followed the cessation of some nondrug habits, e.g., love and sports, as well as some drug habits. This fact suggests that withdrawal symptoms are not a purely pharmacological phenomenon although they were associated with a higher percentage of drug habits than of other involvements.

CONCLUSIONS AND HYPOTHESES

The restrictive concept of addiction is a relic of nineteenth-century temperance doctrine that penetrated the twentieth-century dressed up as medical or scientific knowledge. Its origins are neither medical nor scientific and it does not mesh well with contemporary knowledge. The restrictive usage reduces the complex phenomenon of addiction to nothing more than a disease of excessive drug consumption accompanied by withdrawal symptoms and tolerance. By implication, it denies other manifestations of addiction, such as harmful addictions to nondrug activities and positive or neutral addictions.

Discarding the restrictive definition should make it possible to think more precisely about addiction and drug problems. Moreover, scholars can stop seeking substitutes for a useful term that designates an important aspect of human existence.

Obviously, restoring the traditional definition does not, in itself, answer the difficult questions. Instead it eliminates pseudo-answers, so real understanding can be sought. Why, for example, is addiction sometimes miserable and destructive but sometimes beneficial and enjoyable? The restrictive definition suggests a facile, but spurious answer—addiction is harmful only when it involves drugs. Abandoning this spurious answer reveals the need to identify the real differences in the dynamics of the two kinds of addiction.

We hypothesize that the difference between positive and negative addiction lies in the effect of the addiction on the *organization* of a person's life. In beneficial addictions, people may become "given over" or "overwhelmingly involved" in a way that integrates the vital components of their lives. For many people, addiction to religious ideals, scientific inquiry, physical exercise, or even a drug may serve such a purpose. Their life is not narrowed by addiction, but organized. Family, friends, work, entertainment, etc., are all centered by the addiction. Such an addiction can be thought of as "centripetal" or integrative—it organizes the elements of life by drawing them to a center.

Many harmful addictions may be thought of as "centrifugal"—addictions that force most of the normal components of life to the periphery. However, even centrifugal addictions may be beneficial *if they are temporary*: In the quotation cited earlier, Edwin Land described a way of giving himself over to his work in a centrifugal sense. His life was not impoverished by this practice because he interspersed periods of centrifugal addiction with long periods of nonaddiction. Students who told our interviewers of summers given over to a drug-using circle of friends and drug-centered social events may have been describing another type of beneficial, centrifugal addiction, one that may occur only once in a lifetime.

The genuinely destructive addictions may be those that are both *prolonged and centrifugal.* For example, not everyone who is addicted to religious, scientific, or physical ideals can be described in the positive terms used above. When these addictions are prolonged and centrifugal, they can devastate the addicted person's life and alienate their family and community.

In a sense, this formulation of the difference between beneficial and destructive addictions merely moves the essential issue back one step. *Why* do some people develop and maintain addictive involvements that rule out most of what makes life satisfying to others? The complex issue of causation has been taken up in another article (Alexander, 1990).

There is also the question of what habits have the greatest addictive potential. Obviously the most publicized and feared addictions are to illicit drugs like heroin and cocaine, and the restrictive meaning of addiction would imply that drugs pose the major danger of negative addiction. However, our student data suggest that more negative addictions may be associated with nondrug activities than with drugs, and more with legal drugs than with illegal ones. Of course, such conclusions cannot be generalized from a small student population without further research. But if this conclusion turns out to be true even of students in general, it would suggest that helpful information for this group should be directed more at avoiding negative addictions than at avoiding illicit drugs.

What are the drawbacks of choosing the traditional definition over the restrictive one? The traditional definition might be criticized because it is not a useful diagnostic category, but this is not a weighty criticism. We suspect the traditional definition is not a diagnostic category because addiction *is simply not a disease.* Moreover, the restrictive definition is not a useful diagnostic category either. Many people with serious problems of compulsive drug use do not fit the restrictive definition, e.g., heroin or cocaine addicts who do not have withdrawal symptoms. On the other hand, many people who do fit the traditional definition, such as heavy coffee drinkers with tolerance to caffeine and painful withdrawal symptoms, do not appear to warrant treatment or incarceration.

If the restrictive meaning of addiction is to be abandoned, a term is needed for the subset of addictions that are seriously harmful to the individual and to society. The DSM-III definitions (American Psychiatric Association, 1980) of "substance abuse" and "substance dependence" do not serve well, because they are burdened with logic carried over from the restrictive definition. For example, to be classified as "substance dependent," the most severe "substance use disorder," a patient must show withdrawal symptoms or tolerance, although this is pointless in view of the evidence reviewed above. Moreover, the DSM-III definitions are different for different drugs, so no overriding concept is generated. The term "negative addiction" as originally popularized by Glasser (1976) has a similar limitation; like the restrictive definition it is tied to the object of the addiction, drugs and alcohol, more than the nature of the addiction.

However, if Glasser's analysis is revised and negative addiction is defined simply as those addictions that individuals and society eventually recognize as harmful, regardless of what drug or activity is involved, then the term becomes useful. Moreover, such a simple concept invites the development of more definite criteria such as, perhaps, the concept of "prolonged, centrifugal addictions" suggested above.

An objection to discarding the restrictive meaning might be that the two views can somehow be combined. The desire to compromise seems to be manifested in the early definitions of the World Health Organization and many other formal definitions or in the acceptance of the disease concept of addiction as a "metaphor" . . . proposed by Shaffer (1985). Shaffer provides an important reminder that the disease concept of addiction, which is intertwined with the restrictive meaning, is used in the lifesaving work of Alcoholics Anonymous and in other therapeutic relationships.

Nevertheless, we think combining the two views is neither helpful nor necessary. Fortunately, people who are busy saving lives do not need academic approbation for their definitions. They will not, and should not, be distracted from their way of using the term addiction unless more effective therapeutic techniques emerge from new thinking. On the other hand, the fact that a doctrine is a useful way to think in some therapeutic contexts does not prove that it must be integrated into scholarly theory outside of those milieux. Useful theory and social policy require unambiguous concepts, not diplomatic accommodations between ideas. We believe this is partially recognized in the current World Health Association definition of "drug dependence" which moves quite far toward the traditional meaning. "Drug dependence" is defined as follows: "a syndrome manifested by a behavioral pattern in which the use of a given psychoactive drug, or class of drugs, is given a much higher priority than other behaviors that once had higher value" (Edwards, Arif and Hodgson, 1989, p. 10). The outmoded criteria of withdrawal symptoms and tolerance are left behind, as they should be.

Can rigorous scholarship be satisfied with the ordinary language definitions for "addiction" and "negative addiction" that are proposed in this chapter? Are concepts like "given over," "overwhelmingly involved," "higher priority" and "harmful to the individual and society" precise enough? For the present, the ordinary English language seems superior to the medicalized restrictive definition, and far superior to the continued confusion of conflicting definitions.

This is not a case where a scientific definition clarified ordinary language, but one where a concept from a social movement confused ordinary language and should now be withdrawn. Once the restrictive definition is abandoned, research can deepen the understanding of addiction to the point that definitions that improve traditional language can emerge.

In the end, addiction is too important to be oversimplified by the restrictive definition. Addiction is one of the proclivities that gives human existence its intensity and mystery. Addiction has to do with the triumph of devotion and the horrors of compulsion. It is something that must be faced in its fullest sense, if we are to know ourselves.

REFERENCES

Alexander, B. K. (1982). "James M. Barrie and the Expanding Definition of Addiction." *Journal of Drug Issues* 11: 77–91.

———. (1984). "When Experimental Psychology Is Not Empirical Enough: The Case of the Exposure Orientation." *Canadian Psychology* 25: 84–95.

———. (1987). "Disease and Adaptive Models of Addiction: A Framework Evaluation." *Journal of Drug Issues* 17: 47–66.

———. (1990). "Empirical and Theoretical Bases for an Adaptive Model of Addiction." *Journal of Drug Issues* 20: 37–66.

American Psychiatric Association. (1980). *Diagnostic and Statistical Manual of Mental Disorders.* 3d ed. Washington, D.C.: Author.

Berridge, V., and G. Edwards. (1981). *Opium and the People: Opiate Use in Nineteenth-Century England.* London: Allan Lane.

Blackwell, J. S. (1985). "Opiate Dependence as a Psychophysical Event: Users' Reports of Subjective Experiences." *Contemporary Drug Problems* 12: 331–50.

Chaney, E. F., D. K. Roszell, and C. Cummings. (1982). "Relapse in Opiate Addicts: A Behavioral Analysis. *Addictive Behaviors* 7: 291–97.

Chein, I., D. L. Gerard, R. S. Lee, and E. Rosenfeld. (1964). *The Road to H: Narcotics, Delinquency, and Social Policy.* New York: Basic Books.

Cummings, C., J. R. Gordon, and G. A. Marlatt. (1980). "Relapse: Prevention and Prediction" (1980). In W. R. Miller, ed., *The Addictive Behaviors* (pp. 291–321). Oxford: Pergamon.

Dole, V. P., and M. E. Nyswander. (1980). "Methadone Maintenance: A Theoretical Perspective." In D. J. Lettieri, M. Sayers, and H. W. Pearson, eds., *Theories on Drug Abuse: Selected Contemporary Perspectives* (pp. 256–61). NIDA Research Monograph 30. Washington, D.C.: U.S. Government Printing Office.

Edwards. G., A. Arif, and R. Hodgson. (1982). "Nomenclature and Classification of Drug- and Alcohol-Related Problems: A Shortened Version of a WHO Memorandum." *British Journal of Addiction* 77: 3–20.

Erikson, E. (1950). *Childhood and Society.* New York: Norton.

Glasser, F. B. (1974). "Psychologic vs. Pharmacologic Heroin Dependence." *New England Journal of Medicine* 290: 231.

Glasser, W. (1976). *Positive Addiction.* New York: Basic Books.

Gold, M. S. (1984). *800-Cocaine.* New York: Bantam Books.

Goldstein, A. (1983). "Some Thoughts about Endogenous Opioids and Addiction." *Drug and Alcohol Dependence* 11: 11–14.

Hanerer, L. J. (1980). *The Pleasure Addicts: The Addictive Process—Food, Sex, Drugs, Alcohol, Work, and More.* South Brunswick: A. S. Barnes.

Hodgson, R., and P. Miller. (1982). *Self-Watching: Addictions, Habits, Compulsions: What to Do about Them.* London: Century.

Julien, R. M. (1981). *A Primer of Drug Action.* 3d ed. San Francisco: Freeman.

Jaffe, J. (1980). "Drug Addiction and Drug Abuse." In A. G. Gilman, L. S. Goodman, and A. Gilman, eds., *Goodman and Gilman's the Pharmacological Basis of Therapeutics.* 6th ed., pp. 535–84. New York: Macmillan.

Jaffe, J. H., R. Peterson, and R. Hodgson. (1980). *Addiction: Issues and Answers.* New York: Harper & Row.

Kaplan, E. H., and H. Wieder. (1974). *Drugs Don't Take People, People Take Drugs.* Secaucus, N.J.: Lyle Stuart.

Khantzian, E. J., J. E. Mack, and A. F. Schatzberg. (1974). "Heroin Use as an Attempt to Cope: Clinical Observations." *American Journal of Psychiatry* 131: 160–64.

Kline, D. (1985). "The Anatomy of Addiction." *Equinox* 4 (23): 77–86.

Land, E. H. (1971). "Addiction as a Necessity and Opportunity." *Science* 171: 151–53.

LeDain, G. (1973). *Final Report of the Commission of Inquiry into the Medical and Nonmedical Use of Drugs.* Ottawa: Information Canada. (Catalogue No. H21-5370/2).

Levine, H. G. (1978). "The Discovery of Addiction: Changing Conceptions of Habitual Drunkenness in America." *Journal of Studies on Alcohol* 39: 143–74.

———. (1984). "The Alcohol Problem in America: From Temperance to Alcoholism." *British Journal of Addiction* 79: 109–19.

Lewis, C. T., and C. Short. (1879). *A Latin Dictionary: Founded on Andrews Edition of Freund's Latin Dictionary.* Oxford: Oxford University Press.

Marlatt, G. A. (1985). "Coping and Substance Abuse: Implications for Research, Prevention, and Treatment." In S. Shiffman and T. A. Wills, eds., *Coping and Substance Use* (pp. 367–86). New York: Academic Press.

Morgan, W. (1979). "Negative Addiction in Runners." *The Physician and Sportsmedicine* 7: 56–69.

Murray, J. A. H., H. Bradley, W. A. Craigie, and C. T. Onions. (1933). *The Oxford English Dictionary.* Oxford: Oxford University Press.

Musto, D. F. (1973). *The American Disease: Origins of Narcotic Control.* New Haven: Yale University Press.

O'Brien, C. P. (1976). "Experimental Analysis of Conditioning Factors in Human Narcotic Addiction." *Pharmacological Review* 27: 533–43.

Oates, W. (1971). *Confessions of a Workaholic: The Facts about Work Addiction.* New York: World.

Orford, J. (1985). *Excessive Appetites: A Psychological View of Addictions.* Chichester, England: Wiley.

Parssinen, T. M., and K. Kerner. (1980). "Development of the Disease Model of Drug Addiction in Britain, 1870–1926." *Medical History* 24: 275–96.

Paton, W. M. D. (1969). "A Pharmacological Approach to Drug Dependence and Drug Tolerance." In H. Steinberg, ed., *Scientific Basis of Drug Dependence* (pp. 31–48). London: Churchill.

Peachy, J. E., and T. Franklin. (1985). "Methadone Treatment of Opiate Dependence in Canada." *British Journal of Addiction* 80: 291–99.

Peele, S. (1977). "Redefining Addiction: 1. Making Addiction a Scientifically and Socially Useful Concept." *International Journal of Health Sciences* 7: 103–24.

———. (1985). *The Meaning of Addiction: Compulsive Experience and Its Interpretation.* Lexington, Mass.: D. C. Health.

Peele, S., and A. Brodsky. (1975). *Love and Addiction.* Scarborough, Ontario: New American Library of Canada.

Rech, R. H., and K. E. Moore. (1971). *An Introduction to Psychopharmacology.* New York: Raven Press.

Schachter, S. (1982). "Recidivism and Self-Cure of Smoking and Obesity." *American Psychologist* 37: 436–44.

Shaffer, H. J. (1985). "The Disease Controversy: Metaphors, Maps, and Menus." *Journal of Psychoactive Drugs* 17: 65–76.

Shaffer, H. J., and Burglass, M. E. (1981). "Epilogue: Reflections and Perspectives of the History and Future of Addictions." In H. J. Shaffer and M. E. Burglass, eds., *Classic Contributions in the Addictions* (pp. 481–96). New York: Brunner/Mazel.

Slater, P. (1980). *Wealth Addiction.* New York: Dutton.

Smart, R. G. (1983). *Forbidden Highs: The Nature, Treatment, and Prevention of Illicit Drug Abuse.* Toronto: Addiction Research Foundation.

Sonnedecker, G. (1962). "Emergence of the Concept of Opiate Addiction." *Journal Mondial de Pharmacie* 3: 275–90.

———. (1963). "Emergence of the Concept of Opiate Addiction." *Journal Mondial de Pharmacie* 1: 27–34.

Vaillant, G. E. (1983). *The Natural History of Alcoholism.* Cambridge, Mass.: Harvard University Press.

Westermeyer, J. (1982). *Poppies, Pipes and People: Opium and Its Use in Laos.* Berkeley and Los Angeles: University of California Press.

Winn, M. (1977). *The Plug-In Drug.* New York: Bantam Books.

Wishnie, H. (1977). *The Impulsive Personality.* New York: Plenum.

Webster, N. (1828/1970). *An American Dictionary of the English Language.* New York: Johnson Reprint Company.

Wurmser, L. (1978). *The Hidden Dimension: Psychodynamics in Compulsive Drug Use.* New York: Jason Aarsonson.

Zinberg, N. E. (1984). *Drug, Set, and Setting: The Basis for Controlled Intoxicant Use.* New Haven: Yale University Press.

Zinberg, N. E., W. M. Harding, and R. Apsler. (1978). "What Is Drug Abuse?" *Journal of Drug Issues* 8: 9–35.

Zinberg, N. E., and J. A. Robertson. (1972). *Drugs and the Public.* New York: Simon & Schuster.

22

Drugs and Free Will

Jeffrey A. Schaler

"That was the disease talking . . . I was a victim." So declared Marion Barry, fifty-four, mayor of the District of Columbia. Drug addiction is the disease. Fourteen charges were lodged against him by the U.S. attorney's office, including three counts of perjury, a felony offense for lying about drug use before a grand jury; ten counts of cocaine possession, a misdemeanor; and one count of conspiracy to possess cocaine.

Barry considered legal but settled for moral sanctuary in what has come to be known as the disease-model defense. He maintained that he "was addicted to alcohol and had a chemical dependency on Valium and Xanax." These are diseases, he asserted, "similar to cancer, heart disease and diabetes." The implication: It is as unfair to hold him responsible for drug-related criminal behavior as it is to hold a diabetic responsible for diabetes.

The suggestion was that his disease of addiction forced him to use drugs, which in turn eroded his volition and judgment. He did not voluntarily break the law. According to Barry, "the best defense to a lie is truth," and the truth, he contended, is that he was powerless in relation to drugs, his life unmanageable and "out of control." His behaviors or acts were purportedly the result, that is, symptomatic, of his disease. And jail, say those who agree with him, is not the answer to the "product of an illness."

This disease alibi has become a popular defense. Baseball's Pete Rose broke through his "denial" to admit he has a "gambling disease." Football's Dexter Manley claimed his drug use was caused by addiction disease. Addiction treatment professionals diagnosed televangelist Jimmy Swaggart as having "lost control" of his behavior and as being "addicted to the chemical released in his brain from orgasm." They assert that Barry, Rose, Manley, and Swaggart all need "twelve-step treatment" for addiction, the putative disease that, claims the multimillion-dollar addiction treatment industry, is reaching epidemic proportions and requires medical treatment. To view addiction-related behaviors as a function of free will, they often say, is cruel, stigmatizing, and moralistic, an indication that one does not really understand the disease.

Others are more reluctant to swallow the disease model. After testing positive for cocaine in 1987, Mets pitcher Dwight Gooden said he could moderate his use of the drug and was not addicted. This is heresy according to disease-model proponents, a sign of denial, the salient symptom of the disease of addiction and considered by some to be a disease itself. There is no such thing as responsible drug taking or controlled drinking for an addict or an alcoholic, they assert.

The tendency to view unusual or questionable behavior as part of a disease process is now being extended, along with the characteristic theory of "loss of control," to include all sorts of "addictive" behaviors. We are currently experiencing the "diseasing of America," as social-clinical psychologist Stanton Peele describes it in his recent book of the same name (1989). The disease model is being applied to any socially unacceptable behavior as a means of absolving people of responsibility for their actions, criminal or otherwise. The practice is justified on this basis: Drug use constitutes an addiction. Addiction is a disease. Acts stemming from the disease are called symptoms. Since the symptoms of a disease are involuntary, the symptoms of drug addiction disease are likewise involuntary. Addicts are thus not responsible for their actions.

Is this analogizing of drug addiction to real diseases like diabetes, heart disease, and cancer scientifically valid? Or is the word "disease" simply a misused metaphor? Does drug use truly equal addiction? Are the symptoms of drug addiction really involuntary?

LOSS OF CONTROL

At the heart of the idea that drug use equals addiction is a theory known as "loss of control." This theory may have originated among members of Alcoholics Anonymous "to denote," as described by researcher E. M. Jellinek in his book *The Disease Concept of Alcoholism* (1960), "that stage in the development of [alcoholics'] drinking history when the ingestion of one alcoholic drink sets up a chain reaction so that they are unable to adhere to their intention to 'have one or two drinks only' but continue to ingest more and more—often with quite some difficulty and disgust—contrary to their volition."

Loss of control also suggests that addictive drugs can start a biochemical chain reaction experienced by an addict as an uncontrollable physical demand for more drugs. Drug addicts are people who have allegedly lost their ability to control their ingestion of drugs.

In a speech in San Diego [in 1989, former] National Drug Policy Director William Bennett explained that a drug "addict is a man or woman whose power to exercise . . . rational volition has . . . been seriously eroded by drugs, and whose life is instead organized largely—even exclusively—around the pursuit and satisfaction of his addiction."

Yet, there is a contradiction in Bennett's point of view. If an addict's power to exercise rational volition is seriously eroded, on what basis does the addict organize life "largely even exclusively around the pursuit and satisfaction of his addiction"? An act of organizing is clearly a volitional act, an act of will.

THREE MODELS OF DRUG USE

Etiological paradigms for understanding drug use can be distilled into three models. Aside from the disease model, there are two other ways of looking at drug addiction: the free-will model and the moralistic model. In the free-will model drug use is envisioned as a means of coping with environmental experience, a behavioral choice and a function of psychological and environmental factors combined. The nervous system of the body is conceived of as a lens, modulating experience as self and environment interact. The self is like the film in a camera, where experience is organized and meaning is created. The self is not the brain.

Individual physiological differences affect the experience of self. They do not create it. The quality of a camera lens affects the image of the environment transposed to the film. When the image is unpleasant, drugs are used to modify the lens.

The self is the executor of experience in this model, not the nervous system. Drug use may or may not be an effective means of lens modification. The assessment of drug effectiveness and the price of drug use are viewed as moral, not medical, judgments.

The recommended therapy for the drug user is: (1) a matter of choice; (2) concerned with awareness and responsibility; (3) a process of values clarification; (4) a means of support to achieve specific behavior goals; and (5) an educational process that involves the learning of coping strategies.

The moralistic model harkens back to the days of the temperance movement and is often erroneously equated with the free-will model. Here, addiction is considered to be the result of low moral standards, bad character, and weak will. Treatment consists of punishment for drug-using behavior. The punitive nature of America's current war on drugs with its call for "user accountability" is typical of the moralistic perspective.

Addicts are viewed as bad people who need to be rehabilitated in "boot camps." They are said to be lacking in values. President Bush gave a clear example of this during the televised debates of the 1988 presidential campaign. When asked how to solve the drug problem, he answered, "by instilling values."

The drug user's loss of values is often attributed to the presence of a disease. A "plague" and "epidemic" of drug use are said to be spreading across the land. Since users are sick and supposedly unaware of their disease, many people feel justified in coercing them into treatment, treatment that is primarily religious in nature. Thus, the moralistic model is paternalistic.

In the disease or medical model, addicts are considered to have physiological differences from normal people, differences based in a genetic source or created through the chemical effects of drugs. Instead of focusing on the interaction between the self and the environment, advocates of the disease model view the interaction between physiology and the chemicals in drugs as both the disease and the executor of behavior and experience. In this sense the model is mechanistic. The person is viewed as a machine, a highly complex machine, but a machine nevertheless. The disease of addiction is considered to be incurable. People in treatment can only reach a state of perpetual recovery. Treatment of symptoms involves admitting that one is ill by breaking through denial of the disease and turning over one's life to a "higher power" in a spiritual sense and psychological support to achieve sobriety. Addicts are not bad but sick people. Intervention is required because the machine has broken. Thus, the disease model is both paternalistic and mechanistic.

ADDICTION REDEFINED

Proponents of the will and the disease models disagree with the moralistic perspective, but for different reasons. The former believe addicts should not be punished for having unconventional values. They believe treatment should focus on changing the psychological and environmental conditions conducive to drug use. Coping skills should be taught along with the building of self-esteem and self-efficacy. The latter believe that addicts should not be punished for being sick and that treatment should focus on the biological factors that cause and reinforce drug use.

James R. Milam and Katherine Ketcham, authors of *Under the Influence* (1983), are popular spokespersons for the disease-model camp. They argue that alcoholics should not be held accountable for their actions because these are the "outpourings of a sick brain. . . . They are sick, unable to think rationally, and incapable of giving up alcohol by themselves."

Similarly, physician Mark S. Gold, an expert on cocaine use and treatment, says in his book *800-COCAINE* (1985) that cocaine should not be regarded as a benign recreational drug because it can cause addiction. As with alcoholism, says Gold, there is no cure for cocaine addiction except permanent and total abstention from its use. Cocaine produces "an irresistible compulsion to use the drug at increasing doses and frequency in the face of serious physical and/or psychological side effects and the extreme disruption of the user's personal relationships and system of values." According to Gold "if you feel addicted, you are addicted." Addiction, be it to alcohol or cocaine, is, as far as Milam, Ketcham, and Gold are concerned, identical to loss of control. The drug itself and physiological changes in the addict's body are said to control further ingestion of drugs in what is viewed as an involuntary process.

It may be helpful to look at how the term "addiction" has developed. Its use in conjunction with drugs, disease, loss of control, withdrawal, and tolerance developed out of the moralistic rhetoric of the temperance and anti-opium movements of the nineteenth century, not through scientific inquiry. Such a restrictive use of the word served multiple purposes according to psychologist Bruce Alexander of Simon Fraser University in British Columbia, lead author of an article on the subject. Linking addiction to drugs and illness suggested it was a medical problem. It also helped to scare people away from drug use, a tactic that became increasingly important with anti-opium reformers. Etymologically, the word "addiction" comes from the Latin "*dicere*" (infinitive form) and, combined with the preposition "*ad*," means "to say yes to," "consent." Consent implies voluntary acceptance.

The idea of choice, volition, or voluntariness inherent in the meaning of the word "addiction" is significant to will-model proponents because the concept of addiction as a disease depends so much on the loss-of-control theory. Most people think of addiction with the element of volition decidedly absent. Studies of alcoholics and cocaine and heroin addicts conducted over the past twenty-six years appear to refute this claim, however.

THE MYTH OF LOSS OF CONTROL

In 1962 British physician and alcohol researcher D. L. Davies rocked the alcoholism field by publishing the results of a long-term followup study of patients treated for alcoholism at the Maudsley Hospital in London. Abstinence, long considered the only cure for alcoholism, was seriously questioned as the only form of treatment when seven out of ninety-three male alcoholics studied exhibited a pattern of normal drinking. Physiological differences purportedly present in alcoholics did not seem to affect their ability to control drinking.

Four years later, *The Lancet* published an important study by British psychiatrist Julius Merry that supported Davies's findings. Alcoholics who were unaware they were drinking alcohol did not develop an uncontrollable desire to drink more, undermining the assertion by supporters of the disease model that a small amount of alcohol triggers uncontrollable craving. If alcoholics truly experience loss of control, then the subjects of the study should have reported higher craving whether they believed their beverages contained alcohol or not.

According to the loss-of-control theory, those with the disease of alcoholism cannot plan their drinking especially when going through a period of excessive craving. Yet, psychologist Nancy Mello and physician Jack Mendelson, leading alcoholism researchers and editors of the *Journal of Studies on Alcohol,* reported in 1972 that [they] found alcoholics bought and stockpiled alcohol to be able to get as drunk as they wanted even while undergoing withdrawal from previous binges. In other words, they could control their drinking for psychological reasons; their drinking behavior was not determined by a physiologically uncontrollable force, sparked by use of alcohol.

As Mello and Mendelson wrote in summary of their study of twenty-three alcoholics published in *Psychosomatic Medicine*: "It is important to emphasize that even in the unrestricted alcohol-access situation, no subject drank all the alcohol available or tried to 'drink to oblivion.' These data are inconsistent with predictions from the craving hypothesis so often invoked to account for an alcoholic's perpetuation of drinking. No empirical support has been provided for the notion of craving by directly observing alcoholic subjects in a situation where they can choose to drink alcohol in any volume at any time by working at a simple task. There has been no confirmation of the notion that once drinking starts, it proceeds autonomously."

A significant experiment conducted by Alan Marlatt of the University of Washington in Seattle and his colleagues in 1973 supported these findings by showing that alcoholics' drinking is correlated with their beliefs about alcohol and drinking. Marlatt successfully disguised beverages containing and not containing alcohol among a randomly assigned group of sixty-four alcoholic and social drinkers (the control group) asked to participate in a "taste-rating task." One group of subjects was given a beverage with alcohol but was told that although it tasted like alcohol it actually contained none. Subjects in another group were given a beverage with no alcohol (tonic) but were told that it did contain alcohol.

As Marlatt and co-authors reported in the *Journal of Abnormal Psychology,* they found "the consumption rates were higher in those conditions in which subjects were led to believe that they would consume alcohol, regardless of the actual beverage administered." The finding was obtained among both alcoholic and social drinker subjects. Marlatt's experiment suggests that according to their findings the ability of alcoholics to stop drinking alcohol is not determined by a physiological reaction to alcohol. A psychological fact—the belief that they were drinking alcohol—was operationally significant, not alcohol itself.

Similar findings have been reported in studies of cocaine addiction. Patricia G. Erickson and her colleagues at the Addiction Research Foundation in Ontario concluded, in their book *The Steel Drug* (1987), after reviewing many studies on cocaine that most social-recreational users are able to maintain a low-to-moderate use pattern without escalating to dependency and that users can essentially "treat themselves." They state, "Many users particularly appreciated that they could benefit from the various appealing effects of cocaine without a feeling of loss of control."

Erickson and co-authors cite in support a study by Spotts and Shontz (1980) that provides "the most in-depth profile of intravenous cocaine users to date." They state: "Most users felt a powerful attachment to cocaine, but not to the extent of absolute necessity. [A]ll agreed that cocaine is not physically addicting . . . [and] many reported temporary tolerance."

In a study by Siegel (1984) of 118 users, 99 of whom were social-recreational users, described by Erickson et al. as the only longitudinal study of cocaine users in North America, "all users reported episodes of cocaine abstinence."

These results thus further support the hypothesis that drug use is a function of psychological, not physiological, variables. Even the use of heroin, long considered "the hardest drug," can be controlled for psychological and environmental reasons that are important to heroin addicts. A notable study of 943 randomly selected Vietnam veterans, 495 of whom "represented a 'drug-positive' sample whose urine samples had been positive for opiates at the time of departure" from Vietnam, was commissioned by the U.S. Department of Defense and led by epidemiologist Lee N. Robins. The study shows that only 14 percent of those who used heroin in Vietnam became readdicted after returning to the United States. Her findings, reported in 1975, support the theory that drug use is a function of environmental stress, which in this example ceased when the veterans left Vietnam. Veterans said they used heroin to cope with the harrowing experience of war. As Robins and coauthors wrote in *Archives of General Psychiatry*:

> . . . [I]t does seem clear that the opiates are not so addictive that use is necessarily followed by addiction nor that once addicted, an individual is necessarily addicted permanently. At least in certain circumstances, individuals can use narcotics regularly and even become addicted to them but yet be able to avoid use in other social circumstances. . . . How generalizable these results are is currently unknown. No previous study has had so large and so unbiased a sample of heroin users.

The cocaine and heroin studies are important for several reasons. They challenge the contention that drug addiction is primarily characterized by loss of control. Moreover, these and similar studies support the idea that what goes on outside of a person's body is more significant in understanding drug use, including alcoholism, than what goes on inside the body.

Consider for a moment how a person enters and exits drug use. While disease-model proponents such as Milam, Ketcham, and Gold claim that abstinence is the only cure for this "special disease," implying that strength of will is irrelevant, we must recognize drug use, and abstinence from it, for what they really are —volitional acts.

ADDICTION AND THE LAW

This is a markedly different process from that in real diseases. A person cannot will the onset of cancer, diabetes, or epilepsy. Nor can these diseases be willed away. While people may exercise responsibility in relation to their diseases, they cannot be held responsible for actually creating them. Research supports the idea that drug use does not automatically lead to loss of control—a drug-ingestion frenzy devoid of any volitional component. Unfortunately, viewing addiction as a disease has often led to attempts to absolve drug users of their responsibility for criminal actions.

The extent of an addict's responsibility for criminal behavior has been debated in the courts for more than twenty-five years. . . . In *Traynor* v. *Turnage* (1988), the Supreme Court upheld the right of the Veterans Administration (VA) to define alcoholism to be the result of willful misconduct. The petitioner in this case asserted he was unable to claim VA education benefits because he was an alcoholic; he further claimed that he suffered from a disease called alcoholism and that the law prohibits discrimination on the basis of a disease. The VA called his alcoholism "willful misconduct." Soon thereafter, however, Congress passed a law for veterans that expressly forbids considering the disabling effects of chronic alcoholism to be the result of willful misconduct. However, this law does not define alcoholism as a disease, nor does it prohibit drug addiction from being regarded as "willful misconduct."

According to Herbert Fingarette, a professor of philosophy at the University of California in Santa Barbara and an expert on addiction and criminal responsibility, much of the controversy arising from Traynor and similar cases—such as *Powell* v. *Texas* (1968), a case involving the disease-model defense of a man convicted for public intoxication—stemmed from a Supreme Court ruling in *Robinson* v. *California* (1962).

In this case the Court decided that narcotics addiction is a disease and held that criminal punishment of a person thus afflicted violates the Eighth Amendment's prohibition against cruel and unusual punishment. As Justice William O. Douglas concurred, "The addict is a sick person." But the Court ruled only insofar as Robinson's status as a drug addict was concerned. Its decision had nothing to do with any acts stemming from that status.

In *Powell* the Court held against the use of status as an alcoholic as exculpatory. Powell, an alcoholic, was held to be responsible for his criminal actions. In *Traynor,* the Court upheld the decision made in *Powell.* Traynor and Powell were not absolved of responsibility for their actions because of their alcoholism disease. Robinson, however, was absolved of criminal responsibility because of his status as a drug addict. In *Robinson,* the Court equated punishment for the status of narcotics addiction with punishment for disease affliction. From this viewpoint, an addict's acts are considered to be inseparable from his status as an addict because they are a symptom of the disease and thus an involuntary result of status.

The critical point here is the inseparability of status and act. Certain acts are considered to be part of disease status. Disease is involuntary. Therefore, acts stemming from the disease are exculpable. Are the acts that stem from status really involuntary? This belief is the legal corollary to Jellinek's notion of loss of control.

DISEASE VS. BEHAVIOR

According to professor of psychiatry Thomas Szasz at the State University of New York in Syracuse, a disease, as textbooks on pathology state, is a phenomenon limited to the body. It has no relationship to a behavior such as drug addiction, except as a metaphor. Szasz argues against the disease model of addiction on the basis of the following distinction between disease and behavior. In *Insanity: The Idea and Its Consequences* (1987) he writes:

> [B]y behavior we mean the person's "mode of conducting himself" or his "deportment" . . . the name we attach to a living being's conduct in the daily pursuit of life. . . . [B]odily movements that are the products of neurophysiological discharges or reflexes are not behavior. . . . The point is that behavior implies action, and action implies conduct pursued by an agent seeking to attain a goal.

The products of neurophysiological discharges or reflexes become behavior when they are organized through intent, a willful act. Drug-taking behavior is not like epilepsy. The former involves intentional, goal-seeking behavior. An epileptic convulsion is an unconscious, unorganized neurophysiological discharge or reflex, not a behavior.

In another example, smoking cigarettes and drinking alcohol are behaviors that can lead to the diseases we call cancer of the lungs and cirrhosis of the liver. Smoking and drinking are behaviors. Cancer and cirrhosis are diseases. Smoking and drinking are not cancer and cirrhosis.

The alleged absence of voluntariness or willfulness forms the basis of legal rulings that extend beyond the minimalist interpretation of *Robinson,* exculpating criminal behavior on the basis of a person's supposed disease status. Yet because behavior such as drug use involves voluntariness it seems an individual who uses drugs should not be absolved of responsibility for criminal behavior on the grounds that his actions are involuntary symptoms of drug addiction disease.

Many advocates of the disease model cite as further evidence for their view the results of genetic studies involving the heritability of alcoholism. Recently, the dopamine D_2 receptor gene was found to be associated with alcoholism. A study by Kenneth Blum and co-authors, published in the *Journal of the American Medical Association,* suggests that this gene confers susceptibility to at least one form of alcoholism. The goal of this and similar studies is to identify the at-risk population in order to prevent people from becoming alcoholics and drug addicts.

What such studies do not tell us is why people who are not predisposed become alcoholics and why those who are predisposed do not. It seems more than reasonable to attribute this variance to psychological factors such as will, volition, and choice, as well as to environmental variables such as economic opportunity, racism, and family settings, to name just a few. Experimental controls accounting for genetic versus environmental influences on alcoholic behavior are sorely lacking in these studies.

The basis upon which people with alleged alcoholism disease are distinguished from mere heavy drinkers is arbitrary. No reliable explanation has yet been put forth of how the biological mechanisms theoretically associated with alcoholism and other forms of drug addiction translate into drug-taking behavior. Moreover, Annabel M. Bolos and co-authors, in a rigorous attempt to replicate the Blum findings, reported higher frequencies of the D_2 receptor gene found in their control population than in the alcoholic population in the same journal seven months later.

TREATMENT

Finally, the contribution of treatment to exposing the myth of addiction disease warrants mention. Since his arrest at the Vista Hotel in Washington, D.C., Marion Barry has undergone treatment for alcohol addiction and chemical dependency at the Hanley-Hazelden clinic in West Palm Beach, Florida, and at the Fenwick Hall facility near Charleston, South Carolina. Barry said he needs treatment because he has "not been spiritual enough." His plan is to turn his "entire will and life over to the care of God . . . using the twelve-step method and consulting with treatment specialists." He said he will then "become more balanced and a better person."

The twelve-step program Barry is attempting to follow is the one developed by Alcoholics Anonymous (AA), a spiritual self-help fellowship. AA is the major method dealing with alcoholism today. All good addiction treatment facilities and treatment programs aim at getting the patient into AA and similar programs such as Narcotics Anonymous. Yet several courts throughout the United States have determined that AA is a religion and not a form of medicine, in cases involving First Amendment violations, most recently in *Maryland* v. *Norfolk* (1989). Anthropologist Paul Antze at York University in Ontario has written extensively on AA and describes the "point-by-point homology between AA's dramatic model of the alcoholic's predicament and the venerable Protestant drama of sin and salvation."

Successful treatment from this perspective is dependent upon a religious conversion experience. In addition, patients are required to adopt a disease identity. If they do not, they are said to be in denial. But such an approach is a psychologically coercive remedy for a moral problem, not a medical one. And here—in their concepts of treatment—is where the disease model and moralistic model of addiction seem to merge.

With so much evidence to refute it, why is the view of drug addiction as a disease so prevalent? Incredible as it may seem, because doctors say so. One leading alcoholism researcher asserts that alcoholism is a disease simply because people go to doctors for it. Undoubtedly, addicts seek help from doctors for two reasons. Addicts have a significant psychological investment in maintaining this view, having learned that their sobriety depends on believing they have a disease. And treatment professionals have a significant economic investment at stake. The more behaviors are diagnosed as diseases, the more they will be paid by health insurance companies for treating these diseases.

Most people say we need more treatment for drug addiction. But few people realize how ineffective treatment programs really are. Treatment professionals know this all too well. In fact, the best predictor of treatment success, says Charles Schuster, director of the National Institute on Drug Abuse, is whether the addict has a job or not.

George Vaillant, professor of psychiatry at Dartmouth Medical School, describes his first experience, using the disease model and its effectiveness in diagnosing alcoholism, in *The Natural History of Alcoholism* (1983):

> ... I learned for the first time how to diagnose alcoholism as an illness ... Instead of pondering the sociological and psychodynamic complexities of alcoholism. ... [A]lcoholism became a fascinating disease. ... [B]y inexorably moving patients into the treatment system of AA, I was working for the most exciting alcohol program in the world. ... After initial discharge, only five patients in the Clinic sample never relapsed to alcoholic drinking, and there is compelling evidence that the results of our treatment were no better than the natural history of the disease.

This is important information because the definition of who an alcoholic or drug addict is and what constitutes treatment as well as treatment success can affect the lives of people who choose not to use drugs as well as those who choose to. For example, Stanton Peele has written extensively on how studies show that most people arrested for drinking and driving are directed into treatment for alcoholism disease, yet the majority are not alcoholics. Those receiving treatment demonstrate higher recidivism rates, including accidents, driving violations, and arrests, than those who are prosecuted and receive ordinary legal sanctions.

Furthermore, in a careful review of studies on treatment success and followup studies of heroin addicts at the United States Public Health Service hospital for narcotics addicts at Lexington, Kentucky, where "tens of thousands of addicts have been treated," the late Edward M. Brecher concluded in *Licit & Illicit Drugs* (1972) that "[a]lmost all [addicts] became readdicted and reimprisoned . . . for most the process is repeated over and over again . . . [and] no cure for narcotics addiction, and no effective deterrent, was found there—or anywhere else."

Brecher explained the failure of treatment in terms of the addictive property of heroin. Vaillant suggested that tuberculosis be considered as an analogy. Treatment, he said, rests entirely on recognition of the factors contributing to the "resistance" of the patient. And here is the "catch-22" of the disease model. Addiction is a disease beyond volitional control except when it comes to treatment failure, wherein "resistance" comes into play.

Neither Brecher nor Vaillant recognized that treatment does not work because there is nothing to treat. There is no medicine and there is no disease. The notions that heroin as an addictive drug causes addicts not to be treated successfully, or that "resistance" causes alcoholics to be incurable, are mythical notions that only serve to reinforce an avoidance of the facts: Addicts and alcoholics do not "get better" because they do not want to. Their self-destructive behaviors are not disturbed. They are disturbing.

All of this is not to suggest that the people we call addicts are bad, suffering from moral weakness and lack of willpower, character, or values. Drug addicts simply have different values from the norm and often refuse to take responsibility for their actions. Public policy based on the disease model of addiction enables this avoidance to continue by sanctioning it in the name of helping people. As a result, criminals are absolved of responsibility for their actions, drug prevention and treatment programs end up decreasing feelings of personal self-worth and power instead of increasing them, and people who choose not to use drugs pay higher taxes and health insurance premiums to deal with the consequences of those who do.

Drug use is a choice, not a disease. Still, our current drug policies give the drug user only two options: treatment or jail. But if the drug user is sick, that is, is not responsible for his behavior, why should he go to jail for his illness? And if the drug user is someone who chooses to use drugs because he finds meaning in doing so, why should he be forced into treatment for having unconventional values? "Unconventional values" is not a disease.

"Treatment" for drug addiction is a misnomer. Education is a more appropriate term. In this modality a drug addict is given psychological and environmental support to achieve goals based on an identification of values and behavior-value dissonance. Behavioral accountability is stressed insofar as people learn about the consequences of their actions.

The legal arguments set forth to exculpate criminals because of addiction disease do not seem to be supported by scientific findings. Quite to the contrary, research suggests that drug addiction is far from a real disease. And as long as drug addiction can be blamed on a mythical disease, the real reasons why people use drugs—those related to socioeconomic, existential, and psychological conditions including low self-esteem, self-worth, and self-efficacy—can be ignored.

REFERENCES

Alexander, B. K. (1990). *Peaceful Measures: Canada's Way Out of the "War on Drugs."* Toronto: University of Toronto Press.

Blum, K., E. P. Noble, P. J. Sherida et al. (1990). "Allelic Association of Human Dopamine D_2 Receptor Gene in Alcoholism." *Journal of the American Medical Association* 263: 2055–60.

Boles, A. M., M. Dean, S. Lucas-Derse, M. Ramsburg, G. L. Brown, and D. Goldman. (1990). "Population and Pedigree Studies Reveal a Lack of Association between the Dopamine D_2 Receptor Gene and Alcoholism." *Journal of the American Medical Association* 264: 3156–60.

Brecher, E. M., and the editors of *Consumer Reports*. (1983). *Licit and Illicit Drugs*. Boston: Little, Brown and Co.

Davies, D. L. (1985). "Normal Drinking in Recovered Alcohol Addicts." *Quarterly Journal of Studies on Alcohol* 23: 94–104.

Douglas, M. (ed.). (1987). *Constructive Drinking: Perspectives on Drink from Anthropology.* New York: Cambridge University Press.

Erickson, P. G., E. M. Adlaf, G. F. Murray, and R. G. Smart. (1987). *The Steel Drug: Cocaine in Perspective*. Lexinton, Mass.: Lexington Books.

Fingarette, H. (1988). *Heavy Drinking: The Myth of Alcoholism as a Disease*. Berkeley, Calif.: University of California Press.

———. (1989). "The Perils of Powell: In search of a Factual Foundation for the Disease Concept of Alcoholism." *Drugs & Society* 7: 1–27. (Originally published in *Harvard Law Review* 83 [1970]: 793–812.)

———. (1987). *Insanity: The Idea and Its Consequences*. New York: John Wiley & Sons.

Gold, M. S. (1985). *800-Cocaine*. New York: Bantam Books, Inc.

Institute of Medicine. (1990). *Broadening the Base of Treatment for Alcohol Problems*. Washington, D.C.: National Academy Press.

Jellineck, E. M. (1960). *The Disease Concept of Alcoholism*. New Haven, Conn.: Hillhouse Press.

Marlatt, G. A., B. Deming, and J. B. Reid. (1973). "Loss-of-Control Drinking in Alcoholics: An Experimental Analogue." *Journal of Abnormal Psychology* 81: 233–41.

Mello, N. K., and J. H. Mendelson. (1972). "Drinking Patterns during Work-Contingent and Noncontingent Alcohol Acquisition." *Psychosomatic Medicine* 34: 139–64.

Merry, J. (1962). "The 'Loss-of-Control' Myth." *Lancet* 1: 1257–58.

Milam, J. R., and K. Ketcham. (1983). *Under the Influence: A Guide to the Myths and Realities of Alcoholism*. New York: Bantam Books, Inc.

Peele, S. (1989). *Diseasing of America: Addiction Treatment Out of Control*. Lexington, Mass.: Lexington Books.

Peele, S., A. Brodsky, and M. Arnold. (1991). *The Truth about Addiction and Recovery*. New York Simon and Schuster.

Robins, L. N., J. E. Helzer, and D. H. Davis. (1975). "Narcotic Use in Southeast Asia and Afterward: An Interview Study of 898 Vietnam Returnees." *Archives of General Psychiatry* 32: 955–61.

Siegel, R. K. (1984). "Cocaine and the Privileged Class: A Review of Historical and Contemporary Images." *Advances in Alcohol and Substance Abuse* 4: 37–49.

Szasz, T. S. (1985). *Ceremonial Chemistry: The Ritual Persecution of Drugs, Addicts, and Pushers*. Holmes Beach, Fla.: Learning Publications.

Vaillant, G. (1983). *The National History of Alcoholism*. Cambridge, Mass.: Harvard University Press.

23

Vietnam Veterans Three Years after Vietnam: How Our Study Changed Our View of Heroin*

Lee N. Robins, John E. Helzer, Michi Hesselbrock, and Eric Wish

In May of 1971 two congressmen who went to Vietnam reported that there was extensive heroin use among American soldiers. Almost immediately thereafter, the Department of Defense, under Dr. Jerome Jaffe's urging, set up a urine screening program intended to detect all men using heroin at the time of their departure from Vietnam. They were then to be detoxified so that they would not arrive in the United States still addicted.

On his return from overseeing the establishment of the urine-screening program, Dr. Jaffe asked us to design and carry out a followup study of returning veterans to learn the consequences of heroin use in Vietnam. In response we interviewed about 900 of the 14,000 Army enlisted men who returned to the United States in September 1971, the first month in which this urine screening and detoxification system was operating uniformly throughout Vietnam.

The interviews took place between May and October of 1972, eight to twelve months after the men's return (Robins, 1974). The men interviewed had been randomly selected from a computer tape of returning veterans provided by the Department of Defense. We also had access to the Surgeon General's list of men who had been detected as drug users at departure. A random selection from this list allowed us to oversample men detected as drug users at departure. We did this to have a large number of men who would be at high

Reprinted with permission from *The Yearbook of Substance Use and Abuse* (New York: Plenum Publishing Corporation, 1980), 2: 213–30.

*We are grateful to Dr. Jerome Jaffe for suggesting this study, and for Dr. Robert Dupont's support of it through the Special Action Office and NIDA, and for their encouragement to pursue research in the natural history of heroin use, whether or not it conforms to popular and scientific stereotypes.

risk of using drugs after their return. In this report this high-risk group has been weighted appropriately so that our figures apply to the general population of returning veterans.

In 1974 we selected 617 men for reinterview. These men were interviewed between October and December of 1974, three years after their return from Vietnam, at the average age of 24. We had reduced the sample from 900 to 617 to have enough funds to interview a nonveteran comparison group. We interviewed 284 nonveterans, matched to the veterans for age, eligibility for military service, and education and place of residence as of the veterans' date of induction. The diligent interviewing team provided by the National Opinion Research Center secured a very high recovery rate of our target population for both interviews. On the first interview we reached 96 percent of the target population, and in the second interview 94 percent. Thus we have two interviews covering three years since return for 91 percent of a random sample of Army enlisted men who spent an average of a year in a country with cheap, potent heroin.

Having access to a random sample of men who had been heavily exposed to heroin in Vietnam provided a remarkable opportunity to learn something about the natural history of heroin use. Practically every man we interviewed had had an opportunity to use heroin in Vietnam. Eighty-five percent of the men told us that they had been offered heroin while they were there—often quite soon after their arrival. (One soldier was offered heroin as he descended from the plane on which he arrived in Vietnam by a soldier preparing to board that same plane to return home. He was offered the heroin in exchange for a clean urine sample so that the man due to leave would be able to get through the urine screen.) Thirty-five percent of Army enlisted men actually tried heroin while in Vietnam, and 19 percent became addicted to it.

This opportunity to study heroin use in a highly exposed normal population was unique because there is nowhere else in the world where heroin is commonly used. It has been possible to study cannabis use in India and Jamaica, and cocaine use in Bolivia, but there has been no equivalent opportunity to study heroin.

In the United States itself, heroin use is so rare that the National Commission survey (1973) of 2,400 adults turned up only about twelve people who had used heroin in the last year. Similarly, our nonveteran sample of 284 young men matched to veterans for age, location, education, and eligibility for service provided only seven and consequently will not be discussed in this report.

Because heroin users are scarce both worldwide and in the United States, most of our information about heroin before the Vietnam study came from treated and criminal samples. Yet only one in six of the veterans who used heroin in the last two years came to treatment. We must wonder whether the heroin histories of men who come to treatment are representative, or whether we may not have gotten a biased picture of heroin from them.

We investigated five common beliefs about heroin: First, does the use of heroin rapidly progress to daily use and addiction? Second, is heroin use so much more pleasurable than the use of other drugs that it supplants them? Third, is heroin addiction more or less permanent unless there is prolonged treatment? Fourth, does maintaining recovery from heroin addiction require abstention from heroin? Fifth, is heroin use a major social problem?

DOES THE USE OF HEROIN RAPIDLY PROGRESS TO REGULAR USE AND ADDICTION?

To determine whether a drug is especially likely to lead to regular use, daily use, or addiction, one must compare it with other drugs. In our interview we asked about use of twenty-one different drugs in the last two years. We also asked whether each drug had been used more than weekly for a month or more in the last two years, which we define as "regular" use. Ten drugs had been used by more men than used heroin, and ten had been used less. Thus, in terms of any use, heroin fell in the middle. There were more regular users of heroin, however, than of most other drugs, suggesting that heroin use is more likely to progress to frequent use.

Only three drugs had more *regular* users than heroin: marijuana, used regularly by 30 percent of the veterans; amphetamines, used regularly by 16 percent; and barbiturates, used regularly by 4 percent. Heroin itself had been used regularly by 3 percent of veterans for some period in the last two years. Those drugs used at least once by more persons than used heroin, but used less often regularly include LSD, cocaine, quaalude, Darvon, opium, mescaline, and Valium. We will confine our comparisons of heroin to amphetamines, marijuana, and barbiturates because these were the only drugs used regularly by enough men.

One reason why there are so many more regular users of marijuana and amphetamines than of heroin is that there are simply more users of all kinds. More than half the veterans (54 percent) used marijuana in the last two years, 30 percent used amphetamines, and 15 percent used barbiturates, while only 8 percent used heroin. However, when we looked only at users, we found that less than half the heroin users used it regularly, that is, more than once a week for a month or more (Figure 23.1). Users of amphetamines or marijuana were more likely than heroin users to become regular users, and barbiturate users were less likely. We find the same pattern for daily use. Only one-quarter of those who used heroin in the last two years used it daily at all, about the same proportion as amphetamine users, while about one-third of marijuana users were daily users of that drug.

How are we to understand the fact that heroin use progresses to daily or regular use no more often than use of amphetamines or marijuana, when lab-

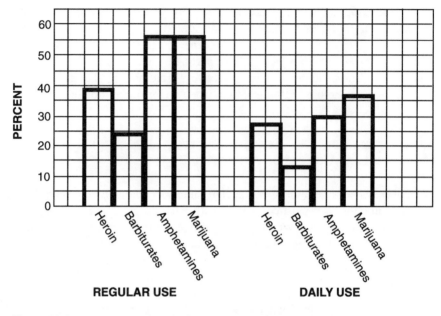

Figure 23.1   **Progression to Regular and Daily Use by Veteran Users of Four Drugs in the Last Two Years**

oratory experiments have shown it to be a highly addicting drug? We suspect that the quality of the heroin available in the United States may explain the fact that it can be used sporadically or even regularly by so many people without progressing to daily use. In Vietnam, where heroin was pure, 54 percent of all users became addicted to it and 73 percent of all who used it at least five times became addicted, a very substantial proportion indeed. (We cannot, unfortunately, look at progression to regular and daily use in Vietnam because in the first interview we asked those questions only about narcotics as a class, not about heroin specifically.)

To say that daily use among heroin users is no more common than among marijuana and amphetamine users does not necessarily mean that heroin is no more addicting. Daily use may not imply addiction equally for all drugs. It is difficult to compare addiction liability among drugs of different classes, since evidence for addiction differs: Users of all four of the drugs we are considering here, heroin, amphetamines, barbiturates, and marijuana, develop tolerance, but withdrawal symptoms are clear only for barbiturates and heroin.

Amphetamines are typically used in daily runs of ten to twelve days, followed by periods of fatigue and depression, but it is not clear to what extent those symptoms are withdrawal symptoms and to what extent they are the

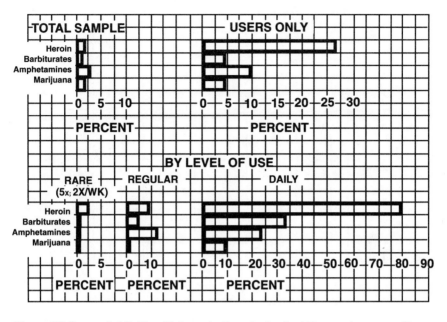

Figure 23.2   **Addiction Veteran's Psychological Dependence on Four Drugs**

result of prolonged sleep loss. Continuous, heavy use of marijuana in an experimental setting can produce withdrawal symptoms similar to those produced by narcotics (Jones, Benowitz, & Bachman, 1976), but as used generally, the major complaint is apathy, which may not be an indication of physiological dependence.

Because it is difficult to compare the addiction liability of heroin with that of nonnarcotic drugs, we limited our comparison to the one sign of dependence that all drugs share—psychological dependence. We asked, "Did you ever use _____ enough in the last two years so that you began to feel you needed it, that is, you would feel uncomfortable when you couldn't get it?" Figure 23.2 shows that in the total sample there were more men who felt dependent on amphetamines than on heroin, and about the same number felt dependent on marijuana. This result, however, depends entirely on the fact that heroin is used by fewer men than these other two drugs.

Among users, about one-quarter of the heroin users felt dependent at any time in the last two years, a distinct minority. Certainly heroin use and dependence were not synonymous. Nonetheless, heroin use was more associated with dependence than was the use of the other drugs. The bottom of Figure 23.2 shows that feeling dependent on all drugs almost required daily use, but many more daily users of heroin felt dependent—four out of five—than did

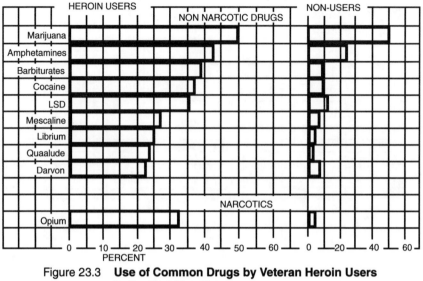

Figure 23.3   **Use of Common Drugs by Veteran Heroin Users
in the Last Two Years**

daily users of barbiturates (one out of three), amphetamines (one out of four), or marijuana (one out of ten). Users of drugs other than heroin rarely felt dependent, even when they were daily users.

In answer to our first question, then, use of the heroin purchased on the streets of the United States in 1974 did not lead rapidly to daily or compulsive use, no more so than did use of amphetamines or marijuana. On the other hand, most heroin users who used the drug daily did perceive themselves as dependent on heroin, while this was not true of daily users of the other commonly used drugs.

Does Heroin Use Supplant the Use of Other Drugs?

Heroin users are supposed to like the drug so well that they lay all other drugs aside in its favor. Our finding shows quite the contrary. In Figure 23.3 we note that veterans who used heroin in the last two years were more likely to use every common drug during that same period than were veterans who did not use heroin. Indeed, the use of other narcotics was almost exclusively restricted to heroin users.

There are a number of possibilities that might allow us to reconcile this finding with our idea that heroin is by far the most pleasurable of drugs. For instance, one might think that heroin users' use of other drugs is always casual,

TABLE 23.1: THE "MAIN" DRUG OF HEROIN USERS

Men using more than one drug (including heavy drinkers)

Heroin Users

"Main" drug during the last two years	Total (97) (%)	Addicts (31) (%)	Other Drugs Only (237) (%)
Heroin	10	41	—
Other narcotic	5	3	0
Marijuana	42	30	40
Alcohol	18	22	44
Any other drug	15	2	3
Barbiturates	9	1	0
Amphetamines	5	0	0
A combination or none	10	1	13
	100	100	100

and that it occurs only when they can't get heroin. However, we find that their use is not casual at all. While 99 percent of heroin users have used marijuana at all in the last two years, 92 percent have used it regularly (several times a week for at least a month), and a third have felt dependent on marijuana.

One might think that perhaps it is only the heroin "tasters" who use other drugs—that men seriously involved with heroin would not be interested in less satisfying drugs. Again, the finding is just the opposite. It is the addicts who are most likely to be deeply involved with other drugs. When we asked men who told us that they had been addicted to heroin in the last two years (in response to the question "Were you ever strung out or addicted in the last two years?") about the use of other drugs, we found that addicts had used 10.4 other drugs on the average out of the 20 we inquired about, as compared to 7.9 for less regular heroin users.

In keeping with popular views of heroin as the most exciting and pleasurable of drugs, we would certainly expect that regardless of their use of a multitude of other drugs, it is heroin that is really the drug that counts with the heroin user. We also found that this was not so. We asked everyone who had used more than one illicit drug or who had taken illicit drugs and had also drunk heavily in the last two years, what was the "main drug they had been into" in the last two years. All heroin users were asked because all had used other drugs. In Table 23.1 we note that heroin was considered to be the main drug of only 10 percent of heroin users. Less than half even of those who reported addiction to heroin, reported it as their main drug. Instead, the main drug for heroin addicts was often marijuana or alcohol.

In answer to our question, then, heroin does *not* seem to supplant the use of other drugs. Instead, the typical pattern of the heroin user seems to be to use a wide variety of drugs plus alcohol. The stereotype of the heroin addict as someone with a monomaniacal craving for a single drug seems hardly to exist in this sample. Heroin addicts use many other drugs, and not only casually or in desperation. Drug researchers have for a number of years divided drug users into heroin addicts versus polydrug users. Our data suggest that such a distinction is meaningless.

Is Addiction to Heroin More or Less Permanent without Prolonged Treatment?

One out of five in our sample reported themselves to have been addicted to heroin in Vietnam, and that self-description was substantiated by their report of prolonged heavy use and severe withdrawal symptoms lasting more than two days. Only 1 percent of our sample reported addiction to heroin during the first year back from Vietnam, and only 2 percent reported addiction in the second or third year after Vietnam. Any sample in which the addiction rate drops so dramatically obviously contains many people experiencing long-lasting remissions. Indeed, of all the men addicted in Vietnam, only 12 percent have elapsed to addiction at any time since their return, that is, at any time in the last three years. Can we attribute this recovery to treatment?

Half of the 281 men addicted in Vietnam received treatment while there. Of those treated, 4 percent were readdicted in their first year back. Of those not treated, again 4 percent were readdicted in their first year back. It may be thought that recovery without treatment was found in this sample only because of the enormous change in the availability of heroin and the circumstances of its use when men left Vietnam for the United States. To see whether this is a sufficient explanation, we have to look at their experience with addiction after the return to the United States. This is difficult because even without oversampling of men with positive urines on departure from Vietnam, we have only twenty men who were addicted in the first year after Vietnam. Nonetheless, we did look to see whether their addiction continued in the second period after Vietnam (the period between the first and second interviews).

Of those men who were addicted in the first year back, half were treated and half were not. In all, only 30 percent (six of the twenty men addicted in their first year back) were addicted at any time during the second period, that is, in the last two years. Of those treated, 47 percent were addicted in the second period; of those not treated, 17 percent were addicted. One should not conclude from these results, which show no better results for treated than untreated men whether treated in Vietnam or later, that treatment was useless. Treatment was often very brief (typically only two weeks during the first

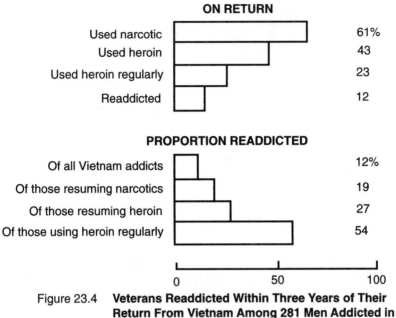

Figure 23.4   **Veterans Readdicted Within Three Years of Their Return From Vietnam Among 281 Men Addicted in Vietnam**

year back). Furthermore, those more seriously addicted were more likely to receive treatment. (In our sample of daily users in the last two years, all who used heroin daily for six months or more came to treatment, compared with only half of those who used heroin from one to six months, and only 6 percent of those who used it daily for less than a month.) What we can conclude, however, is that treatment is certainly not always necessary for remission.

We can also learn something about rates of remission in the last two years, a period during which there were thirty-one addicts. We asked them how many had used any heroin at all, even once in the last two weeks. Less than one-half had (47 percent). Thus at least half of those addicted within the last two years had not been addicted at any time in the last two weeks. We also asked how many had used any heroin at all in the last three or four days. Only one-quarter of the addicts had done so. Consequently, a minimum of three-quarters had recovered from their addiction before the interview. We collected urine samples at the end of the interview. Only one of the men who said they had been addicted in the last two years had a urine positive for morphine.

Heroin addicts are supposed to continue to be bothered by a persistent craving for the drug long after acute withdrawal symptoms subside. To see if this was true, we asked ex-heroin addicts who had not used any narcotic at all in the last two years if they felt like taking narcotics at any time and if so

TABLE 23.2: LOOKING FOR PREDICTORS OF READDICTION AMONG 171 VETERAN ADDICTS WHO RETURNED TO NARCOTIC USE

Factor tested		Results
Demographic characteristics		
Race	City size	
Age	Social class of upbringing	
Education	Religion	Negative
Own problems before service		
Dropout	Drugs, injection	
Arrest	Fighting	
Drinking	Truancy	
Drug-using friends	Psychiatric care	Negative
Parents' problems		
Broken home	Arrests	
Drinking	Psychiatric care	
Drugs		Negative
Drug use in Vietnam		
Long use of narcotics	Complications of use	
Which narcotics	Other users in unit	
Injection	Number of other drugs	
Treatment for drugs	Detected as user	Negative
Other military information		
Discipline problems	Psychiatric treatment	
Heavy drinking	IQ	
Combat	Draftee or volunteer	Negative

whether it was a real craving or just a thought that crossed their minds. Only one-quarter reported a craving. Thus craving can occur and can be extremely persistent—the four men reporting craving had not used any narcotic at all during the last three years—but it seems that prolonged craving is a rare residual effect of heroin addiction.

DOES RECOVERY FROM ADDICTION REQUIRE ABSTINENCE?

It is commonly believed that after recovery from addiction, one must avoid any further contact with heroin. It is thought that trying heroin even once will rapidly lead to readdiction. Perhaps an even more surprising finding than the high proportion of men who recovered from addiction after Vietnam was the number who went back to heroin without becoming readdicted. As figure 23.4 shows, half of the men who had been addicted in Vietnam used heroin on their return but only one-eighth became readdicted to heroin. Even when heroin was used frequently, that is, more than once a week for a considerable period of time, only one-half of those who used it frequently became readdicted.

Unfortunately, our finding that half of the men could go back to heroin use and not become readdicted is not very useful from a clinical point of view, because we have not been able to detect any characteristics predicting who can safely return to use and who cannot. We looked at thirty-five different variables including early drug history, demographic characteristics, discipline problems, Army intelligence test scores, psychiatric treatment, and whether men got off heroin through treatment or on their own, to search for predictors of readdiction. None of these was successful in predicting which users would be able to use heroin again safely (Table 23.2).

The factor that we could not investigate, which may be the most important variable of all, is the quality of the heroin used. Certainly the quality of heroin varies considerably from time to time and place to place in the United States. This may be the missing explanatory variable.

DOES THE USE OF HEROIN CONSTITUTE A MAJOR SOCIAL PROBLEM?

Veterans themselves believe that heroin use is very dangerous. When asked what one drug had done the most harm in Vietnam, 90 percent of veterans named heroin whether they themselves had used it or not. The antiheroin attitude of of veterans is surprisingly resistant to their own experience. When asked if drug laws should be changed, and if so how, half of both veterans and nonveterans favored legalizing marijuana, but only 4 percent of veterans and 1 percent of nonveterans favored reducing penalties for or legalizing narcotics. The veterans' attitudes closely resembled those of nonveterans, despite their considerably greater experience with heroin.

The veterans' view that heroin is more dangerous than other drugs is confirmed when they report on their own experience instead of more general opinions. Users of each drug were asked whether that drug had interfered with their lives (Figure 23.5). Although only one-quarter of heroin users thought that heroin had interfered with their lives, they more often believed this about heroin than users of other drugs believed it about their drugs. Thus the great majority of heroin users do not think that they have been harmed by it, even though they tend to think it is worse than any other drug.

But what about more objective measures? Heroin addicts are believed to account for much of our crime and welfare problems. To find out whether veterans' heroin use had contributed to crime, we considered what proportion

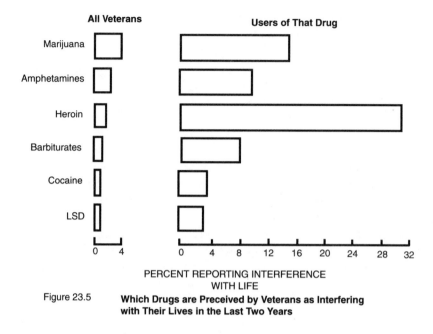

Figure 23.5   **Which Drugs are Preceived by Veterans as Interfering with Their Lives in the Last Two Years**

of those arrested were heroin addicts. In all, about one-quarter of veterans (22 percent) reported having a nontraffic arrest in the last two years. Nontraffic arrests are much more frequent among heroin addicts than in the general population of veterans. Among heroin addicts more than two-thirds (69 percent) reported an arrest. On the other hand, heroin addiction was so rare that heroin addicts accounted for only 5 percent of those who had been arrested.

Heroin addicts of course made their heaviest contribution to narcotics arrests. Sixty percent of all those arrested for a narcotics offense had been addicts. Heroin addicts also contributed disproportionately to property offenses. Twenty-four percent of those arrested for theft (stealing, armed robbery, or burglary) were heroin addicts, as were 8 percent of those arrested for bad checks. Heroin addicts contributed no more than their expected proportion (that is, 2 percent, since they constituted 2 percent of the population of veterans) to violent crime, vandalism, alcohol arrests, or arrests for nonnarcotic drugs.

Table 23.3 shows the proportion of addicts arrested for each offense and their employment status at the time of interview. Note that although heroin addicts accounted for more than their proportion of property offenders, only one-third of them had had a property offense in the preceding two years. Thus heroin addiction does not inevitably lead to theft to support the habit.

Table 23.3 also shows that heroin addicts had a great deal of difficulty holding jobs. At the time of the interview one-third of all those who had been

TABLE 23.3: JOB AND ARRESTS OF MEN ADDICTED TO HEROIN IN THE LAST TWO YEARS

	Heroin addicts (31) (%)	Other veterans (540) (%)
Job		
Employment status at interview		
Full-time job or school	44	87
Part-time job or school	23	5
Completely unemployed	33	8
	100	100
Months out of 24 unemployed and not in school		
None	21	63
1 to 5	13	25
6 to 11	33	9
12+	33	3
	100	100
Arrests		
Any nontraffic	69	21
Property	31	3
Conduct	28	5
Drugs	13	7
Alcohol	10	7
Violence	0	*
* < 0.5%.		

addicted at any time in the last two years were totally without work and not in school, and less than one-half were fully occupied in school or on a job. Their unemployment had been persistent: Two-thirds had been totally out of work and school for six months or more in the last two years. Their rate of current unemployment was much greater than that of other veterans, only 8 percent of whom were totally unemployed at followup; and their rate of total unemployment lasting six months or more was also much greater, only 12 percent of other veterans having been out of work that much.

To give an overall estimate of the social costs of heroin as compared to other drugs, we counted how many of eight problems each had experienced in the last two years: the use of hard drugs on a regular basis, alcohol problems, job problems including severe unemployment and many job changes, crime, divorce, credit difficulties, violence, and transiency. Heroin users in

TABLE 23.4: MEAN NUMBER OF RECENT ADJUSTMENT PROBLEMS (OUT OF EIGHT) FOR MEN USING VARIOUS DRUGS IN THE LAST TWO YEARS

| | Any use | Frequency of use | | |
		Occasional	Regular, but not daily	Daily
Marijuana	1.9	1.4	1.3	2.7
Amphetamines	2.5	1.9	3.0	3.1
Barbiturates	2.9	2.7	2.9	4.3
Heroin	3.2	2.8	2.4	4.5

the last two years had experienced more of these eight problems than the sample as a whole (they averaged 3.2 versus 1.3 for the sample as a whole), as well as more problems than users of any other drug (Table 23.4). For all drugs, problems increased as use became daily, but heroin led the other drugs both among occasional and daily users.

From the findings thus far presented one might conclude that even if heroin addiction does not always lead to property crimes, and even if it actually accounts for only a small proportion of the nation's crimes, still heroin addiction does have serious social consequences. However, heroin's bad reputation may limit its use to the kinds of people who are very likely to have social problems in any case. In addition, as we showed above, the use of heroin is associated with the use of many other drugs. It could well be the variety and quantity of drugs in general rather than heroin specifically that accounts for the high level of social problems among heroin users. Thus before deciding that heroin has an important role in creating social problems, we must take these two possibilities into account.

To take into account the fact that people who use heroin may have differed from nonusers long before they began taking heroin, we developed what we call a Youthful Liability Scale. This scale was made up of the best predictors of heroin use in Vietnam. It is composed of demographic factors (race, living in the inner city, being young at induction) and the individual's behavior before he was inducted into the service (truancy, dropout or expulsion from school, fighting arrests, early drunkenness, and use of many types of illicit drugs). His social class of origin and parents' problems are omitted because social class was not found to predict heroin use either in Vietnam or later, and parents' problems did not add measurably to the predictive power of the remaining variables.

TABLE 23.5: MEAN YOUTHFUL LIABILITY SCORES OF VETERANS WITH DIFFERENT TYPES OF DEGREES OF DRUG USE IN THE LAST TWO YEARS

	No use	*Any use*	*Light*	*Degree of use* *Regular, but not daily*	*Daily*
Marijuana	3.7	6.5	5.5	6.4	7.6
Amphetamines	4.2	7.3	6.8	7.8	7.7
Barbiturates	4.7	7.9	7.8	6.9	9.2
Heroin	4.9	8.0	8.1	7.7	8.0

The Youthful Liability Scale, composed entirely of items ascertainable before the soldiers went to Vietnam (and thus before almost all of them were introduced to heroin) was well correlated with heroin use in Vietnam ($r = 0.47$). It was also well, if less strongly, correlated with heroin use in the last two years ($r = 0.28$). It is interesting, however, as one can see in Table 23.5, that the Youthful Liability Scale did not predict the *degree* of heroin use in the last two years. Daily users had no higher scores than did occasional users. Nonetheless, heroin users had higher Youthful Liability scores than did the users of any other drug.

The Youthful Liability Scale was also correlated with each of the eight problems used to assess recent adjustment. Indeed, its correlation with the number of adjustment problems in the last two years was even stronger ($r = 0.53$) than its correlation with heroin use. Our suspicions are thus confirmed. The men who used heroin were those who were especially disposed to adjustment problems even before they used the drug.

To answer the question of whether heroin use is still associated with social problems after we take into account the kinds of people who use it and the number of other drugs they use, we matched each man who had used heroin in the last two years with a veteran who had not used heroin—if we could find a nonuser who had an identical score on the Youthful Liability Scale, who had used the same number of other drugs, and who had used the identical other drugs regularly. By this matching procedure we hoped to compare individuals who differed only with respect to whether they had used heroin, but who were identical with respect to other predictors of social problems. We then compared the number of social problems other than drug abuse that they had had in the last two years. We went through the same matching procedures for marijuana users, amphetamine users, and barbiturate users.

Our findings are that the *occasional* use of any of these drugs *was not* associated with a significant increase in social adjustment problems. *Regular* use of each of these drugs except marijuana, again defined as use more than once a week for more than a month, was associated with an increase in social adjustment problems. The excess problems experienced by those who used heroin regularly (0.9 more problems on the average out of seven) was no greater than the excess problems experienced by those who used amphetamines regularly (1.3) or barbiturates (1.1), and the association of heroin with social problems was less statistically significant than was the effect of either amphetamines or barbiturates.

Thus the reason that we find higher levels of social disability among heroin users than among users of other drugs is probably attributable to the kinds of people who use heroin. Men disposed to social problems are likely to use drugs, and those with the very greatest predisposition to social problems are the ones likely to use heroin. Yet regular heroin use does seem to have an added effect—whether because of the drug itself or because of its legal status, we still don't know. But its effects are no greater than the effects of regular use of amphetamines and barbiturates. These latter drugs constitute a more serious social problem than heroin, since they add at least as much to the level of social problems of users, and because so many more people use these drugs than use heroin.

SUMMARY

Despite its reputation as a rapidly addicting drug, heroin in the forms available in the United States in late 1974 was no more likely to be used regularly or daily, if used at all, than were marijuana or amphetamines. It was more likely to be used regularly than other narcotics and other nonnarcotic drugs. Compared with marijuana and amphetamines, what is distinctive about heroin is not its liability for daily use, but the fact that daily users perceive themselves as dependent. Despite their dependence, they manage to quit using the drug much more often than anyone would have guessed and can often even return to use without becoming dependent again.

Heroin users are extreme polydrug users. And heroin addicts use an even greater variety of other drugs than do less regular heroin users. Other drugs, and particularly marijuana, have been described as stepping stones to heroin because they almost always precede heroin use. A better image than stepping stones might be the cornerstones on which the edifice of varied drug use is built. The process is one of accretion, not of succession.

People who use heroin are highly disposed to having serious social problems even before they touch heroin. Heroin probably accounts for some of the problems they have if it is used regularly, but heroin is "worse" than amphetamines or barbiturates only because "worse" people use it.

What are the policy implications of our findings? It would seem that our society has overemphasized the importance of treatment for heroin per se, failing to pay attention to the many other problems that heroin addicts have. Heroin addicts are deeply involved with a great variety of other drugs at the same time that they are involved with heroin, and they have all kinds of social adjustment difficulties that are not entirely attributable to heroin. It is small wonder that our treatment results have not been more impressive, when they have focused so narrowly on only one part of the problem.

The results that we have reported here have come from a survey of a general population of young men of an average age of about 24 who were heavily exposed to heroin in Vietnam. This sample has its limitations: The men in Vietnam had been selected for psychiatric health, insofar as the draft boards and the Army could do so. They were exposed to generous supplies of heroin for only one year and in an extraordinary situation—far from home and under fire. Our findings may have been influenced by these special circumstances, but we cannot be sure whether they have been because there is no equivalent study of heroin use in a general population that has provided enough regular heroin users for comparison.

Certainly our results are different from what we expected in a number of ways. It is uncomfortable presenting results that differ so much from clinical experience with addicts in treatment. But one should not too readily assume that differences are entirely due to our special sample. After all, when veterans used heroin in the United States two to three years after Vietnam, only one in six came to treatment.

REFERENCES

Drug Use in America: Problems in Perspective. Second report of the National Commission on Marihuana and drug abuse, 1973. Washington, D.C.: U.S. Government Printing Office, 1973, Table 11-27.

Jones, R. T., N. Benowitz, and J. Bachman. "Clinical Studies of Cannabis Tolerance and Dependence." *Annals of the New York Academy of Science* 282 (1976): 221–39.

Robins, L. N. *The Vietnam Drug User Returns.* Special action office monograph, series A, no. 2. Washington, D.C.: U.S. Government Printing Office, May 1974.

24

Rat Park Chronicle

Bruce Alexander, Patricia Hadaway, and Robert Coambs

The opiate drugs, especially heroin, have a demonic reputation. "Junkies" have been viewed as fools who toyed with irresistible pleasure and became enslaved, much as earlier unfortunates were thought to be possessed by demons for their sins. Fortunately Isidor Chein, Stanton Peele, Norman Zinberg, and others are dispelling the devil-drug imagery and advocating a more human understanding of opiate addicts as people who need the powerful analgesic and tranquilizing effects of narcotics to cope with the stress of life.[1] The new understanding makes it possible to respond to heroin addiction more productively and to view the larger problem of addiction to alcohol, pills, work, gambling, love, etc., more clearly.

Curiously, there is a *scientific* roadblock to this progress. We first encountered it [in 1976] during a university seminar on addiction. The class was organized around the "coping" concept of addiction, which was acceptable to almost all the students. One dissenter, however, insisted on the importance of the fact that rats and monkeys consume large amounts of opiate drugs, including heroin, in experimental settings. Does this not prove that coping problems are irrelevant? After all, how much coping is required of a laboratory animal living alone in a perfectly controlled environment? Isn't the craving for heroin, and other opiate drugs, more simply a natural affinity for the pleasure the drugs produce, a weakness of the flesh which *Homo sapiens* shares with its mammalian cousins?

It has to be admitted that many psychologists and psychiatrists (perhaps most) accept this interpretation of the biomedical research that it seems to justify the extreme measures which have been applied to the heroin addiction

Originally published in the *British Columbia Medical Journal* 22, no. 2 (February 1980). Reprinted by permission of the publisher.

problem. If opiate addiction is caused by a powerful natural affinity, then it cannot be cured or even prevented, any more than the sex or hunger drives can. It follows that the most reasonable defense against the threat of opiate addiction is effective prohibition—Drug Squads must be bolstered, borders guarded, and junkies kept out of circulation, lest they spread the habit.

Two of us protested this interpretation, but we were not able to carry the day. Our class rat expert had hard data, but we only had the suspicion that the animals' affinity for opiate drugs existed precisely because they were isolated in laboratory cages. Who wouldn't want to be stoned during a life of solitary confinement? The "natural affinity" interpretation of the animal data has been questioned by other psychologists, including Stanton Peele and Edward Khantzian, but they have not provided direct evidence which refutes it.[2]

Finding ourselves unable to convincingly win the argument in the seminar, we decided to bring the case to the laboratory. The crucial test, we decided, would be to compare the opiate consumption of rats in radically different environments. One environment would be the "normal" housing for laboratory animals in psychopharmacology experiments, i.e.: individual cages mounted on steel racks, constructed so that the animals could not see or touch each other. The second environment was the most natural habitat we would contrive in the laboratory, so we named it "Rat Park." Rat Park is open and spacious, with about 200 times the square footage of a standard cage. It is also scenic (with a peaceful, British Columbia forest painted on the plywood walls), comfortable (with empty tin cans and other *desiderata* strewn about the floor), and friendly (we ran coed groups of sixteen to twenty rats).

Would the opiate consumption in the two environments differ? in order to find out, we had to develop a means of measuring each individual's opiate consumption. This was accomplished by allowing the rats to drink solutions containing precisely measured amounts of opiate drugs. Oral consumption of opiate drugs has the same effect as injection except, of course, that the injection takes effect faster, producing the famous "rush," so renowned in junkie lore. Regardless of the romance of the "rush" and the needle, injection is not essential to addiction. Opiate addiction was widespread in North America before syringes were available and many present day opiate addicts never inject their opiates unless a drug shortage makes the more efficient injection technique necessary.[3] This was especially true in Vietnam during the war when heroin was, for a time, very cheap, and a majority of the soldier-addicts preferred to smoke, snort, or drink their heroin.

In the cages, opiate consumption was measured simply enough by fastening drinking bottles containing narcotic and inert solutions on each cage and weighing them daily. In Rat Park it was more difficult to measure individual consumption, especially since we didn't want to disrupt life in what we hoped would become an idyllic community. We built a short tunnel opening into Rat Park which was just large enough to accommodate one rat at a time. At the end of the tunnel, the rats could release a fluid from either of two drop dispensers and drink it. A video camera recorded how much each rat drank of each solution.

We obtained a small supply of morphine through the Health and Welfare Ministry of the federal government. Heroin is a form of morphine (diacetyl-morphine), and the psychoactive effects of the two drugs are very similar, provided the doses are equivalent. This is widely recognized both by professionals and by narcotics addicts.

Now we were ready for the experiments. It occurred to us that there are at least three ways of offering narcotics to rats, analogous to the ways they become available to people. The first, which we call the "Easy Access" procedure, is a situation where the drugs are freely available and very cheap. We made two solutions available around the clock both in the cages and in Rat Park. One solution contained morphine, dissolved in sugar water to mask its bitter taste. The alternative solution was also bittersweet (in fact we concocted it to taste *exactly* the same to us), but the bitterness came from a non-narcotic, quinine. Thus, as far as we could arrange it, the narcotic solution was just as available and palatable to the rats as the inert alternative and they had no other source of fluids. In hedonic cost, the drug was precisely as "cheap as water."

We called our second mode of presentation the "Seduction" procedure, based on the idea that people are sometimes lured into heroin use by an extraneous payoff, like group acceptance or a feeling of successful rebellion. In our rodent microcosms, the "seduction" involved, again, a constantly available choice of water and morphine solution. This time the water in both environments was pure tap water, but the morphine solution was sweetened. Every five days the sweetness was progressively (and diabolically) increased toward levels which should be irresistible even to the most straitlaced rat, since all rats have a powerful "sweet tooth."

Finally, we had a "kicking-the-habit" procedure, simulating the dilemma faced by a person who is physically dependent on heroin and then has to either maintain the habit or endure the effects of withdrawal. In our version, the rat junkies were given nothing but morphine solution to drink for fifty-seven days, long enough by far, according to current research findings, to produce tolerance and physical dependence. They were then given free choice between water and morphine solution under three different experimental regimes.

We first ran the "Easy Access" experiment. To our complete surprise, after the first day, rats in both environments drank the quinine solution almost exclusively, so the possibility of an environmental effect could not even be tested. Undaunted (almost), we proceeded to the "Seduction" and "Kicking-the-habit" experiments. In them, the environmental effects were crystal clear. No matter how much we induced, seduced, or tempted them, the

Rat Park rats resisted drinking the narcotic solution. The caged rats drank plenty, however, ranging up to *sixteen times* as much as the Rat Park residents in one experimental phase, and measuring ten times as much in some other phases. The females, curiously, drank more morphine in both environments, but the Rat Park rats always drank far less than the caged rats. These data were duly transformed and statistically analyzed and proved to be statistically significant, at an extremely high level of confidence.[4]

Obviously, we think these results are socially as well as statistically significant. If rats in a reasonably normal environment consistently resist opiate drugs, then the "natural affinity" idea is wrong, an overgeneralization of experiments on isolated animals.

These animal findings are compatible with the new "coping" interpretation of human opiate addiction if one keeps in mind that rats are by nature extremely gregarious, active, curious animals. Solitary confinement causes extraordinary psychic distress in human beings and it is likely to be just as stressful to other sociable species, and therefore to elicit extreme forms of coping behavior such as the use of powerful analgesics and tranquilizers, in this case, morphine.

It may also be that socially housed rats *resist* morphine because it is such a powerful anesthetic and tranquilizer. As such, it interferes with a rat's (or a person's) ability to play, eat, mate, and engage in all the other active behaviors which make life rewarding. We presently are guessing that this second possibility is the primary cause of the environmental effect because of the fact that neither group consumed much morphine in the "Easy Access" procedure, and because of some newer data which are not yet ready for publication.

The Rat Park results seem to fit with the most careful observations of opiate addiction in our own species. For example, Chein has shown that in the city neighborhoods where heroin is most freely available, most people simply ignore it, and those that don't suffer unusually severe family problems and have the most painful self-concepts.[5] Robins has shown that over 90 percent of heroin-addicted soldiers returning from Vietnam kicked that habit, stateside, with little problem.[6] Numerous observers have reported that more than 90 percent of those made physically dependent by hospital medication have no hint of a craving for opiates upon recovery from their illness and release from the hospital.

Rats in Rat Park, ghetto dwellers, soldiers home from Vietnam, patients released from the hospital all seem to be telling us the same story. Namely that, contrary to the "natural affinity" view, individuals are vulnerable to opiate drugs under some circumstances, but not others. Solitary confinement puts rats in a state of vulnerability. We are investigating whether it is the solitude, absence of sensory input, lack of activity, or some other aspect of the rats' housing which makes them vulnerable, but we believe that the more vital task is to determine the conditions in which people are vulnerable.

Alienation, loneliness, self-hate, and helplessness are terms which suggest themselves, but they are too vague, in current usage, to be a basis for action. The state of vulnerability must be described well enough so that we can identify its causes and reduce them, as we guide the evolution of our society.

We have now spent four years in the gloom of our rat laboratory and we believe our faithful rodents have graciously told us something new and important. Our problem now is to perceive the dimensions of our own cages as clearly as we see those which house the rats.

NOTES

1. I. Chein, D. L. Gerrard, R. S. Lee, and E. Rosenfeld, *The Road to H: Narcotics, Delinquency, and Social Policy* (New York: Basic Books, 1964); N. E. Zinberg, W. M. Harding, S. M. Stelmack, and R. A. Marblestone, "Patterns of Heroin Use," *Annals of the New York Academy of Science* 3 (11) (1978): 10–24.

2. E. J. Khantzian, "Opiate Addiction: A Critique of Theory and Some Implications for Treatment," *American Journal of Psychotherapy* 28 (1974): 59–70.

3. E. M. Brecher, *Licit and Illicit Drugs* (Boston: Little, Brown, 1972).

4. B. K. Alexander, R. B. Coambs, and P. F. Hadaway, "The Effect of Housing and Gender on Morphine Self-Administration in Rats," *Psychopharmacology* 58 (1978): 175–79; P. F. Hadaway, B. K. Alexander, R. B. Coambs, and B. Beyerstein, "The Effect of Housing and Gender on Preference for Morphine-Sucrose Solutions in Rats," *Psychopharmacology* 66 (1979): 87–91.

5. Chein et al., *The Road to H.*

6. L. N. Robins, D. H. Davis, and D. N. Nurco, "How Permanent Was Vietnam Drug Addiction?" in M. H. Greene and R. L. Dupont, eds., *The Epidemiology of Drug Abuse*, NIDA Journal Supplement, Part 2, Vol. 64, Stock number 041-010-000 19. (Washington, D.C.: U.S. Government Printing Office, 1974).

25

Cocaine and Addictive Liability*

Patricia G. Erickson and Bruce K. Alexander

INTRODUCTION

The drug literature often singles out cocaine as a powerfully addictive drug (e.g., Kalant, 1987; Jaffe, 1985; Cohen, 1985; Allen, 1987) and points with alarm to the growing number of treatment admissions for cocaine dependence (Kozel and Adams, 1985; CEWG, 1987). The prevalent "disease model" of cocaine addiction usually asserts that exposure to cocaine causes addiction, that claims of moderate cocaine use entail "denial" of addiction by the user, and that apparently nonaddicted users will eventually become addicted (Gold, 1984; Du Pont, 1984).

In spite of an apparent consensus concerning cocaine's great "addictive potential" and "addictive liability," there is no consistent definition of these and similar terms in the scholarly literature. More important, there are indications that the consensus may not have a substantial basis (e.g., Clayton, 1985; Anthony, 1987).

This chapter critically examines the meaning of "addictive liability" and the sometimes conflicting evidence concerning the addictive liability of cocaine. These issues require review because an inaccurate estimate of cocaine's addictive potential may seriously compromise public policy. Underestimation of cocaine's addictiveness may lead to public negligence, whereas overestimation may lead to panic and wasteful diversion of re-

Originally published in *Social Pharmacology* 3, no. 3 (1989). Reprinted by permission.

*The views expressed in this paper are those of the authors and do not necessarily reflect those of the Addiction Research Foundation or of Simon Fraser University.

We wish to thank Kevin Fehr, Mary Ann Linseman, and Reg Smart for their incisive comments on an earlier draft of this paper.

sources from more serious hazards. We believe that a cross-disciplinary and cross-cultural review of contemporary research literature can provide an improved assessment of cocaine's addictiveness.

This chapter concerns the addictiveness of cocaine hydrochloride. Whereas the consequences of cocaine use on health, safety, and performance are also important issues, we shall not address them here (for reviews see Adams and Durrell, 1984; Anglin, 1985; Grinspoon and Bakalar, 1985; Alexander, 1990). We shall also not attempt to discuss "crack" in this review, because objective evidence is still scanty (see review by Reinarman and Levine, 1995).

DEFINING ADDICTIVE LIABILITY

The meaning of the term "addiction" has become uncertain in the face of recent debates on its definition. There are at least two negative consequences of this uncertainty. One is that claims about addiction and addictiveness can be made too freely, since there is no simple way to check them. The other is that addiction has come to have mysterious connotations, as an ill-defined disease rather than an ordinary human problem (Alexander, 1987).

The issue of definition cannot be fully addressed in this chapter (see review by Alexander and Schweighofer, 1988), but we will try to achieve a degree of precision by consistently following convention. In contemporary drug literature, addiction is usually defined with reference to compulsive drug-seeking behavior, whereas "dependence" is usually associated with withdrawal symptoms and tolerance (Kozel and Adams, 1985, p. 222). Dependence on cocaine has not been clearly established, because of the lack of distinct physical withdrawal symptoms after cessation of regular use (Jacobs and Fehr, 1987). Therefore, the term "dependence" will be avoided here.

There are a number of acceptable definitions of addiction based on the behavioral concept. Cocaine addiction has been defined as "compulsion to use the drug, loss of control over the amount used, and continued use in spite of adverse consequences" (Wesson and Smith, 1985, p. 200). Gawin and Kleber (1985; 1986) have proposed that cocaine addiction is most accurately described by a recurrent pattern of cyclic binges, rather than continuous daily use and withdrawal symptoms modeled on alcohol and heroin abuse. The World Health Organization has also produced a definition of "drug dependence" that will here be applied to cocaine addiction. The definition is as follows: "a syndrome manifested by a behavioral pattern in which the use of a given psychoactive drug, or class of drugs, is given a much higher priority than other behaviors that once had higher values" (Edwards, Arif, and Hodgson, 1982, p. 10).

We shall use the term "addictive liability" throughout this chapter to mean the likelihood that use of cocaine will be followed by addiction in the sense of a behavioral disorder as described above. Thus, addictive liability becomes a measurable aspect of an individual's drug use in a particular social context (see also Zinberg, 1984; Krivanek, 1988). The term "controlled use" will here refer to noncompulsive, nonexcessive, nondestructive use (Zinberg, Harding, and Apsler, 1978). With these terms of reference, we shall assess evidence regarding the addictive liability of cocaine from animal research, clinical studies, population surveys, and community samples of cocaine users.

ANIMAL RESEARCH

Claims that cocaine has an extraordinarily high addictive liability are often based on studies of self-administration of cocaine by laboratory animals. These studies can be divided into two types, those providing animals with periodic access to cocaine and those providing continuous access. Given periodic access to cocaine, members of many mammalian species press levers that deliver injections of cocaine into their bloodstream. If the concentration of the injected solution is raised, the animals respond proportionately less and if it is lowered they respond proportionately more. There are signs of stimulation from the drug, but convulsions are rare (review by Johanson, 1984).

When animals are given *continuous* access to cocaine, however, much more cocaine is self-administered. In one experiment, two rhesus monkeys given continuous access to cocaine were in a situation where each lever-press produced infusions of cocaine. Both monkeys died in convulsions following massive self-administered doses after three to five days. In another experiment, three monkeys were put in cages where they were allowed to press only one of two levers every fifteen minutes. One lever produced an infusion of cocaine and the other produced five food pellets. Over an eight-day experiment, all three monkeys chose cocaine almost exclusively. Even on trials where they did not choose cocaine they did not press the food lever. The animals averaged 6-10 percent weight loss and produced strange stereotyped behaviors (see Johanson, 1984). In an experiment at Concordia University, twelve rats were given continuous opportunity to self-inject cocaine. Ten injected significant amounts. The cocaine-using rats lost an average of 29 percent of their body weight and several experienced convulsions. By the end of the thirty-day experiment, nine out of the ten who administered cocaine had died (Bozarth and Wise, 1985).

The preference displayed by animals in continuous access conditions for cocaine over other drugs, food, water, or sex led to its identification as the most "efficacious reinforcer" known (Brady and Lukas, 1984, p. 66). Such research is often interpreted as reflecting the fate of human beings if cocaine were as freely available. S. Cohen (1985, p. 152) has stated:

> Under conditions of access to large amounts of cocaine the human response remarkably resembles that of the laboratory animal. Cocaine-dependent humans prefer it to all other activities. They will continue using until they are exhausted or the cocaine is depleted. . . . All laboratory animals can become compulsive cocaine users. The same might be said of humans.

However, the generalizability of these animal findings to the "real world" of animals (see Greenberg, 1983) as well as human beings is questionable, for many reasons.

Thoughtful observers have long noted that drug self-administration by animals may not be equivalent to human addiction (Thor, 1972). Monkeys, for example, are intensely gregarious, highly active, and curious animals, with a great resistance to being handled or restrained. The same is true of wild rats (Lore and Flannelly, 1977), and, to a lesser extent, of their laboratory-bred descendants. Animal studies isolate such creatures in small cages, tethered twenty-four hours a day to an injection apparatus, and surgically implanted with a canula. There is little for them to do but to press a lever on the wall that produces a temporary euphoric stimulation. Recent data indicate that rats housed in isolation self-inject much more cocaine in daily self-administration tests than rats housed in groups between self-administration tests (Schank, Lacelle, Gorman, and Amit, 1987). An earlier study of oral self-administration of cocaine found greater cocaine consumption in rats that had been housed in groups. However, the results of this experiment are equivocal because the socially housed rats were permanently removed from the social housing condition five days before the drug self-administration tests began and were housed in isolation throughout the sixteen days of testing (Hill and Powell, 1976).

The failure of animals to eat in some experiments may be because cocaine is a potent appetite suppressant in animals as well as human beings (Papasava and Singer, 1985). When, under conditions of continuous availability, experimental animals ignore their food, the appetite-suppressing effects of cocaine provide a more parsimonious explanation than addiction.

There is another line of animal research that is sometimes cited in support of the claim that cocaine has a high addictive liability. This concerns the effect of cocaine on the "reward centers" of the brain (Frawley, 1987; Wise, 1984). Experimental animals repetitively activate circuits that stimulate such areas with small doses of electricity. Reward centers can also be stimulated by neural stimuli generated by eating and drinking, and by cocaine and opiates in the bloodstream.

Because drugs research the reward center directly, it is currently hypothesized that they affect it more powerfully than sensations transmitted through a series of neurons to the reward center. Therefore, cocaine and opiate drugs are thought to be extraordinarily powerful reinforcers (Frawley, 1987; Wise, 1984).

Other researchers dispute this hypothesis, citing the diversity of response to drugs even in animals, and the lack of a unifying theory of addiction (Science, 1988). In spite of eloquent argumentation (Wise, 1988), this research provides no proof that cocaine is more reinforcing under normal circumstances than other reinforcers, or that use of cocaine necessarily leads to intense craving. Human motivation is multiply determined. It seems simplistic to try to explain complex life choices on the basis of the activity of any single brain center.

There are more general reasons to be cautious in applying the results of animal studies of cocaine self-administration to human beings. Experimental models of addiction to alcohol, minor tranquilizers, cannabis, nicotine, and caffeine are very difficult to engender in laboratory animals (Clarke, 1987; Collins, Weeks, Cooper, Good, and Russell, 1984; Griffiths, Bigelow, and Henningfield, 1980; Grupp, 1981; Numan, Naparzewska, and Adler, 1984). Yet human beings have the potential to become profoundly addicted to many substances besides cocaine and morphine (Jacobs and Fehr, 1987; Orford, 1985). Thus it is not appropriate to uncritically extend a drug hierarchy of addictive liability based on animal studies to human drug-taking behavior. One can recognize the importance of the biological component of addiction without resorting to rigid biological determinism. The next section examines the major evidence for assertions of cocaine's high addictive liability in human beings, i.e., studies of cocaine users in treatment.

CLINICAL STUDIES

There has been a substantial increase in clients seeking help for cocaine problems in the United States (Kozel and Adams, 1985; Schnoll, Karrigan, Kitchen, Daghestani, and Hansen, 1985; CEWG, 1987). Canadian data (Firth, 1988) have also shown an increasing proportion of cocaine-related treatment registrations in the 1980s. When patients with a new type of problem begin to present at treatment facilities, it is difficult initially to assess the significance of the situation. We will consider the size of the new group of cocaine patients and whether they can be considered the tip of an iceberg of users in need of treatment.

Clayton (1985) attempted to place American clinical data on cocaine in perspective by relating them to other drug problems. The Drug Abuse Warning Network (DAWN) reported that cocaine accounted for only 3.1 percent of all emergency room, drug-related events in 1982. Tranquilizers, narcotics, and sedatives were much more highly represented. Moreover, of the 3.1 percent only 29 percent of these emergency room episodes involved cocaine alone; in the remainder at least one additional drug was involved.

Similarly, in the Treatment Outcome Prospective Study (TOPS), only 3.7

percent of the clients listed cocaine as their primary drug problem. Moreover, about 70 percent of this group reported at least weekly use of alcohol and cannabis, and 21 percent to 27 percent used tranquilizers, amphetamines, and heroin at least weekly. Clayton (1985, p. 17) concludes that clients who identify cocaine as their primary problem are "likely to be abusing a number of other drugs at the same time" and are "essentially multiple drug users." Although some "cocaine only" patients have been identified, they are relatively uncommon (Schnoll et al., 1985; Spotts and Shontz, 1985). Therefore, those in treatment for cocaine addiction comprise neither a substantial fraction of those who require treatment for drug problems, nor are they an unidimensional group whose only drug problem is likely to be cocaine.

It must be understood that patients in treatment for cocaine addiction are not simply the tip of the iceberg of all cocaine users. Clinical samples contain only those individuals who have developed a serious enough problem with cocaine that they have decided to seek help. Naturally, their experiences with cocaine have been destructive.

Clinical research, however, does provide important guidance about events that are associated with progression from experimental to addictive use. There is a consistent association between entering treatment for cocaine problems and being male, being a multiple drug user, administering cocaine intravenously or by smoking, and using cocaine for several years (reviews by Clayton, 1985; Kozel and Adams, 1985). Cocaine users in treatment, compared to untreated users, are also more deviant in other lifestyle areas such as unemployment, social isolation, and criminal records (Chitwood and Morningstar, 1985). Clearly clinical subgroups are not representative of the entire population of users.

Users who call the "800-COCAINE" hotline (Gold, 1984) are similarly atypical. These callers are a self-selected sample of cocaine users who call to report their problems with cocaine. Therefore the data they provide cannot represent cocaine users in general. The characteristics of a random sample of 500 callers were similar to clinical samples in that most were nearly daily users, with about 40 percent reporting a preference for intravenous use or smoking and over 90 percent displaying a wide variety of adverse physical, social/financial and psychological effects (Gold, Washton, and Dackis, 1985). With respect to addiction, 66 percent of this group of callers felt addicted, 75 percent felt they had lost control, and 83 percent said they were unable to refuse cocaine when it was available (Gold et al., 1985). Clearly these data present a picture of acute distress and addiction to cocaine, but there is no basis to generalize these findings to cocaine users in general.

SURVEY RESEARCH

Random surveys provide the best available information on the proportion of cocaine users, and their levels of cocaine use, in the general population. These survey sources, while likely to underrepresent the heaviest users who appear in the treatment settings, span the whole range of involvement with cocaine. Of all countries, the United States has conducted the most systematic surveys of drug use in the population.

The National Survey on Drug Abuse, which began in 1971 and continued every two or three years to 1985, randomly sampled members of the household population aged twelve and over. The number of Americans who had ever tried cocaine nearly quadrupled between 1974 and 1982 (from 5.4 million to 21.6 million) and the number of current users who had used cocaine in the past year rose from 1.6 million in 1974 to 4.2 million in 1982 (Adams and Durrell, 1984). In retrospect, 1979 appears to represent a peak year for cocaine use in the general population, with indications of a leveling-off trend in the 1980s (Jaffe, 1985; Clayton, 1985). Those aged eighteen to twenty-five show the highest rate of having used any cocaine during the past month, namely 7 percent in 1982, compared to 2 percent of those aged twelve to seventeen, 3 percent of those aged twenty-six to thirty-four, and 0.5 percent of those thirty-five years or more (Abelson and Miller, 1985). Those who use cocaine more frequently are also likely to be multiple drug users, often concurrently using marijuana and/or alcohol in combination with cocaine (Abelson and Miller, 1985).

A second major national survey, conducted annually since 1975, involves random sampling of high school seniors in the United States. From 1976 to 1979, those reporting any use of cocaine in the past twelve months doubled in this population, from 6 percent to 12 percent. There were only minor fluctuations in subsequent years up to 1983 when the rate was 11.4 percent (O'Malley, Johnston, and Bachman, 1985). Monthly prevalence rates (any use in past 30 days) have also stayed quite constant between 1980 and 1983 at about 5 percent of high school seniors (O'Malley et al., 1985).

Data on addictive liability were provided by asking recent cocaine users among high school seniors whether they had ever tried to stop using cocaine and found they could not stop. Relatively few, 3.8 percent in 1983, responded affirmatively (in comparison to 18 percent of cigarette smokers). Also, only 4 percent of cocaine-using high school seniors in 1983 reported ever injecting cocaine, although 24 percent reported having smoked it (O'Malley et al., 1985). A followup study of a subset of this sample reached the following conclusion:

> Most of those who used [cocaine] in high school do not show a cross-time progression to heavier use in the three to four years following graduation, which suggests that dependence either develops rather slowly or develops with rela-

tively low frequency among moderate and light users. (Johnston, O'Malley, and Bachman, 1986, p. 221).

In conjunction with the National Survey, these findings show that most of those who try cocaine are found in the infrequent categories of use, and even use in the past year or past month is neither indicative of current compulsive use patterns nor predictive of future ones.

Other surveys in the United States have produced similar results. White (1988) reported that while both quantity and frequency of cocaine use increased significantly over a three-year period in a sample of New Jersey adolescents, "the average user . . . is still using only about twice a month and using an average quantity of six lines per occasion" (White, 1988: 130). Kandel, Murphy and Karus (1985) randomly selected a cohort of approximately twenty-five years of age in New York State. These authors found that of those who had ever tried cocaine, about 60 percent had used it no more than ten times in their entire lives and about 3 percent had used it as often as 1,000 times. Moreover, a large proportion of the people who had been frequent users fluctuated to lower levels or ceased using in a relatively short period of time. Of those who had ever used cocaine daily (about two percent of the cohort), about one-fifth continued to do so in the year of the study (Kandel et al., 1985, pp. 80–81). Newcomb and Bentler (1986) found similar low levels of frequent use in a study of young adults from Los Angeles, aged nineteen to twenty-four, of which 5 percent of the men and 4 percent of the women reported using cocaine one or more times per week in the past six months. When these more frequent users were compared to nonusers, they reported significantly more problems with their health and lifestyle—similar to those of users in treatment. An unanswered question in such studies is whether anxiety, depression, and other serious problems in heavy cocaine users are causes of cocaine use, effects of cocaine use, or both.

Various indirect indicators in Canada, such as arrests, convictions, seizures of drugs, admissions for treatment, and case reports, all pointed to some increase in the use of cocaine between 1970 and 1980 (Smart, 1983). In Ontario, high school survey data have shown that the annual prevalence (i.e., any use in the past twelve months) of cocaine use among students has remained quite stable, around 4 percent or 5 percent, between 1977 and 1985 (Erickson, Adlaf, Murray, and Smart, 1987, p. 51). The 1987 "Ontario Household Survey" provided the only trend data available for Canadian adults eighteen and over (Smart and Adlaf, 1987). The proportion of respondents reporting ever using cocaine nearly doubled, from 3.3 percent to 6.1 percent between 1984 and 1987. The increase in the proportion who reported using cocaine *in the past twelve months,* however, was insignificant: 1.7 percent in 1984 and 1.8 percent in 1987 (Smart and Adlaf, 1987, p. 34). Thus, while more people experimented with cocaine in the three-year interval between the surveys, most did not continue the practice. About 95 percent of those who had ever used cocaine reported using it less than once a month in 1987.

The highest-reported cocaine use in any Canadian subpopulation not in treatment was reported among university students. Of 107 students interviewed at Simon Fraser University, 40.2 percent had used cocaine at some time in their life. When the behavior of this group is examined fully, however, there is little indication of addiction. Whereas 3.7 percent of these university students had used cocaine in the previous thirty days, none used it daily during that period. One student reported having been dependent on cocaine in the past, but was no longer (Alexander, 1984).

Thus, the evidence of American and Canadian survey statistics runs counter to the claim that cocaine has a high addictive liability. In both countries, most of the population never tries cocaine; of those who do, most use it only a few times; very few become compulsive users. These studies confirm that people who use cocaine frequently are generally multiple drug users.

Survey statistics do not provide much information on any special characteristics of users who develop compulsive patterns nor on whether addicted-users may revert to controlled use. These issues are essential to assessing cocaine's addictive liability. Fortunately, four recent community studies provide relevant data from the United States, Canada, and the Netherlands.

COMMUNITY STUDIES

These four studies involve cocaine users who were neither in treatment nor in prison, and who were contacted through advertising and/or a personal network. Such samples are largely self-selected and hence not representative of all cocaine users. They are, however, likely to be more typical of cocaine users in the community than are clinical samples, and they provide more in-depth information than surveys.

Siegal (1980; 1985) recruited 99 frequent cocaine users (average three times per week) in 1974 in the Los Angeles area and followed them up for several years. Subjects were contacted every six months. All were initially classified as social-recreational users of one to four grams of cocaine per month for at least one year. Three-quarters were students aged twenty-one to thirty-eight years and 84 percent were male. After four years of followup, all subjects remained social-recreational users, with occasional "binges" of intensified use.

The fifty subjects still in the study from 1978 to 1982 showed less consistency. Whereas half were still social-recreational users, frequency of use had increased in the other half. Four were classified as intensified daily users and five as compulsive users; the latter five were all freebase users. Thus nine of fifty subjects, or 18 percent could be regarded as addicted. Since half of the sample had been lost to attrition by this point, the 18 percent can only be an approximation.

Siegal (1985) suggests that the changing patterns in later years were related to a decline in purity of street cocaine, purchase of larger amounts, diversification of the paraphernalia industry, growing preference for smoking cocaine, perception that intranasal ingestion was a safer route, and increased multiple drug use.

Another longitudinal study of relatively frequent cocaine users was conducted in the San Francisco area. Twenty-seven cocaine users who were initially interviewed in 1974–75 (Waldorf, Murphy, Reinarman, and Joyce, 1977) were followed up after eleven years. Murphy, Reinarman, and Waldorf (1989) reinterviewed twenty-one of the original twenty-seven respondents. There had been no formal contact with the respondents in the eleven-year hiatus. The original sample was characterized as a "naturally occurring friendship network" in which the age range was sixteen to fifty-one, the sex ratio was about equal and the majority were middle-class college graduates or attending university. In 1977, the investigators did not consider any of the twenty-seven respondents to be addicted, most were described as "casual" users, and four were daily users. After the second wave of interviews, Murphy et al. (1989) concluded that a sizable number of the group had subsequently had severe physical and psychological problems with the drug when they began to use it more heavily and for a longer period.

What is revealing from their intensive, retrospective, year-by-year probing of each user, is the striking fluctuation between periods of compulsive and controlled use. After eleven years, only one of the 21 respondents, who was described as heavy user in 1974, was currently a compulsive cocaine user. Eleven other users reported having used daily at some point, but were no longer doing so. Seven of these subjects had reduced their consumption (from as much as three grams a week to one-quarter gram or less) but continued to use in a controlled way. Four had adopted abstinence after periods of heavy, uncontrolled use; this group had experienced the most cocaine-related problems. All but one of this group, an injector, favored the intranasal route. Seven other respondents were characterized as "continuous controlled users" who had maintained moderate use patterns throughout the eleven-year period. Two other past users of this continuous, controlled type had stopped using entirely for two and five years, respectively, prior to the followup period. Their reasons for quitting included nervousness, increased alcohol use as a counterbalance to this effect of cocaine, and expense.

Since this research is reported primarily in the case study format, it does not provide much detail about quantities and frequencies related to compulsive use periods. It does, however, provide important insights into the users' own mechanisms for restraining their intake of cocaine in a context of ready availability. Factors mentioned included the responsibilities of parenting, an avoidance of injecting or freebasing, health concerns, and a norm that "small amounts on special occasions is the best way to enjoy cocaine" (Murphy et al., 1989). In addition, all respondents were gainfully employed at followup, many of them in professional or managerial careers. What is especially relevant to our effort to arrive at some reasonable estimate of cocaine's addictive liability is the figure of 5 percent (one in twenty-one respondents) who had developed a pattern of addiction and remained a compulsive user after eleven years. For the rest of their sample, Murphy et al. (1989) conclude that respondents managed to regain, or retain, rational control over the use of cocaine. For four of them, this had meant abstinence; therefore, if they are included in the calculation of addicted users *at some time in their cocaine-using career,* the estimate of addictive liability would be closer to 25 percent (five of twenty-one respondents).

Two other studies examined community samples at one point in time. A recent study of 160 "nondeviant" cocaine users and former users in Holland (Cohen, 1987) was directed at establishing a reliable estimate of the dependency-producing properties of cocaine. The sample was 60 percent male and the mean age was thirty years. All respondents had used cocaine at least twenty-five times and favored the intranasal route. Of the 160 people interviewed, about a third never exceeded a low (< 0.5 g/wk) level of use, despite an average duration of use of five years. At the other extreme, the maximal level of use for 21 percent of the sample had exceeded 2.5 g/wk at some point. While one-fifth of the sample had stopped using, the current heavier users showed a great deal of fluctuation over time in levels of use. This study provides further evidence of prolonged periods of controlled cocaine use and also for reversals of progression, from heavier to lower levels of use. Cohen (1987, p. 13) concludes that the "dependency-producing characteristics of cocaine may have been overstated."

In Canada, Erickson et al. (1987) interviewed 111 cocaine users who had at least one experience with cocaine in the past three years. A sample of typical users was sought. Two-thirds of the respondents were male, age range twenty-one to forty-four, and all had been employed in the year prior to the interview. Nearly all respondents favored the intranasal route, and the average duration of time since first exposure to cocaine was seven years. While 58 percent had used less than ten times in the past year, 9 percent reported 100 or more occasions of use in that period. Less than half of the total group (45 percent) had used cocaine in the previous month and, of these, only one-quarter had used cocaine six or more times in the month. Quantities consumed on any given occasion were generally small (six lines or less) over several hours although many of the respondents had experienced occasional "binges" of intensive use and "runs" lasting two days or more. Respondents reported considerable fluctuation in their consumption of cocaine since first trying it: 51 percent reported more intensive periods of use in the past, usually of short duration and mainly in response to greater availability. Over half (61 percent) reported cutting back their cocaine use at some time and provided a variety of reasons including less availability, concern with physical risks and overuse, loss of interest, and lifestyle changes.

All users were asked about any feelings of an uncontrollable desire or craving to use the drug. Of these 111 respondents, half reported never experiencing this feeling, nearly one-third said they rarely or sometimes did, and one-fifth acknowledged that craving occurred most times or always when using cocaine. Usually this was expressed as using up all that was there. This "craving to use" reaction was strongly related to past high frequency of use, to reported weight loss, and to physical/mental exhaustion. Similarly, while the risk of addiction was identified by very few of the less frequent cocaine users in this sample, nearly one-quarter of the "heavier" users did consider the possibility of addiction as the least appealing aspect of cocaine use.

Most of those interviewed by Erickson et al. (1987) were relatively infrequent users who clearly were able to limit their use of cocaine. Restricting use to party situations or special occasions, buying little or not at all, having a stable employment and/or domestic situation, and appreciating the risks of cocaine were some of the factors that were said to reinforce the controlled use of cocaine. The majority of those who had engaged in more intensive periods of cocaine use said they cut back on their own initiative. Seven individuals had sought treatment related to cocaine use, mainly for medical complications. Although a study conducted at one point in time cannot provide a figure for the proportion who might later develop addiction, the seven-year average duration of use is a fairly lengthy one. It is similar to the five-year average duration noted in the Netherlands by Cohen (1987). Again, between 5 percent and 10 percent of a sample of those who have tried cocaine developed very heavy or compulsive use patterns at some time.

Taken together, these community studies suggest that most social-recreational users can maintain a fairly low use pattern over lengthy periods without escalation to addiction.[1] Users appear to recognize the need to limit their use of cocaine, and most seem to be able to accomplish this without professional intervention. The longitudinal designs of Siegal (1985) and Murphy et al. (1989) demonstrate, however, that there can be no completely "safe" period of controlled use—escalation and even compulsive use emerged for some people after several years of using at social-recreational levels. Whereas those who got into the most problems with cocaine tended to impose abstinence on themselves, other heavy users drew back to lower levels of use and maintained them. In all these studies, social norms about appropriate ways to use cocaine and concerns for health were identified as restraints on cocaine use.

CONCLUSION

Patterns of cocaine use vary widely, from occasional experimentation to regular, compulsive use that dominates the life of the user. The latter pattern—cocaine addiction—is an incontestable reality. However, the evidence reviewed here indicates that the likelihood that cocaine users will become addicted has been greatly overstated.

Unlike laboratory animals under conditions of continuous intravenous access, most human cocaine users never use it immoderately, and most choose the intranasal route over smoking or injecting cocaine. Careful estimates of the proportion of those who try cocaine that progress to more intensive use converge around 5 percent to 10 percent. Of individuals in the more frequent use category, a reasonable estimate of those who progress to compulsive use, at some time, is between 10 percent and 25 percent. Those who use weekly or more often are at greatest risk of becoming compulsive users, as are those who begin to inject or smoke cocaine. Other risk factors include a history of multiple drug use and other socially deviant activities. Of those who become addicted, most seem able to regain control, some with, but most without, therapeutic intervention.

Thus, cocaine is not unlike other substances and activities that are used to excess by a minority of people, but not by the majority of users. Cocaine's addictive liability does not appear to be extraordinarily high. If this claim is borne out, it will have major social implications. The current focus on cocaine as a uniquely addictive drug may prove to be counterproductive for both treatment and prevention. The notion of cocaine's high addictive liability provides a scenario of "epidemic levels of destructive use" (Kozel and Adams, 1985, p. 224) in which many more, if not the majority, of cocaine users will eventually be casualties of the drug (Gottheil, 1986). A realistic appraisal of treatment needs might, however, place these estimates at much lower levels, thus avoiding the diversion of resources from more serious problems.

When attention is focused on the addictive qualities of a particular drug, cocaine, and individual vulnerability to it, as is the case now, this may even discourage people from seeking treatment. The fear of cocaine's great addictive liability may also divert addicts' attention from the need to explore their own behavior in relation to their addiction. This extreme view of cocaine's power may entice people on the fringes of society or risk seeking adolescents who are drawn to uniquely dangerous practices. An effective prevention program must convey the real risks of cocaine addiction in a way that is credible to current and potential users. Moreover, unwarranted preoccupation with the addictive liability of any particular drug may cause society to collectively overlook the deeper structural problems which cause so many people to compulsively embrace diversions from reality.

* * *

At this point, our estimate of cocaine's addictive liability must remain tentative, for three reasons. First, there is no single way to assess the way cocaine is used in a large population at any given time. Triangulation of data from different sources—clinical samples, surveys, and community user studies—offers the most accurate way of assessing the current situation, but more data must be assembled before conclusions can be secure. Second, investigators have not yet systematically compared the likelihood of addiction among cocaine users with practitioners of other habits. Third, the meanings of a drug, and consequently, the patterns of use, change over time in society. Cocaine's social meaning has been highly volatile and patterns of use will likely change in the future. Ultimately, we believe that judicious analysis of research can defuse some of the current overstatements, and even hysteria, surrounding the cocaine issue and contribute to a more rational debate on appropriate social responses and policies.

NOTE

1. A fifth community study, recently reported from Australia, offers further support for this general conclusion (Mugford, 1989).

REFERENCES

Abelson, H. I., and J. D. Miller. (1985). "A Decade of Trends in Cocaine Use in the Household Population." In N. J. Kozel and E. H. Adams, eds., *Cocaine Use in America: Epidemiologic and Clinical Perspectives.* (Research Monograph No. 61, pp. 35–49). Rockville, Md.: National Institute on Drug Abuse.

Adams, E. H., and J. Durrell. (1984). "Cocaine: A Growing Public Health Problem." In J. Grabowski, ed., *Cocaine: Pharmacology, Effects and Treatment of Abuse.* (Research Monograph No. 50, pp. 9–14). Rockville, Md.: National Institute on Drug Abuse.

Alexander, B. K. (1984). "Drug use, Dependence and Addiction at a British Columbia University: Good News and Bad News." *Canadian Journal of Higher Education* 15:13–29.

———. (1987). "The Disease and Adaptive Models of Addiction: A Framework Evaluation." *Journal of Drug Issues* 17:47–66.

———. (1990). *Peaceful Measures: Canada's Alternatives to the War on Drugs.* Toronto: University of Toronto Press.

Alexander, B. K., and A.R.F. Schweighofer. (1988). "Defining 'Addiction.' " *Canadian Psychology* 29:151–62.

Allen, D., ed. (1987). *The Cocaine Crisis.* New York: Plenum.

Anglin, L. (1985). *Cocaine. A Selection of Annotated Papers from 1880 to 1984 Concerning Health Effects.* Toronto: ARF Books.

Anthony, J. (1987). "The Epidemiology of Adult Cocaine Use." *DIS Newsletter* 4(1):4–5.

Bozarth, M. A., and R. A. Wise. (1985). "Toxicity Associated with Long-Term Intravenous

Heroin and Cocaine Self-Administration in the Rat." *Journal of the American Medical Association* 254:81–83.

Brady, J. V., and S. E. Lukas. (1984). *Testing Drugs for Physical Dependence Potential and Abuse Liability.* (Research Monograph No. 52). Rockville, Md.: National Institute on Drug Abuse.

Chitwood, D. D., and P. C. Morningstar. (1985). "Factors which Differentiate Cocaine Users in Treatment from Nontreatment Users." *International Journal of the Addictions* 20:449–59.

Clarke, P. B. S. (1987). "Nicotine and Smoking: A Perspective from Animal Studies." *Psychopharmacology* 92:135–43.

Clayton, R. R. (1985). "Cocaine Use in the United States: In a Blizzard or Just Being Snowed?" In Kozel and Adams, *Cocaine Use in America: Epidemiologic and Clinical Perspectives,* pp. 8–34.

Cohen, P. A. (1987). "Cocaine Use in Amsterdam in Nondeviant Subcultures." Paper presented at the International Council of Alcohol and Addictions Congress, Lausanne, Switzerland, May/June.

Cohen, S. (1985). "Reinforcement and Rapid Delivery Systems: Understanding Adverse Consequences of Cocaine." In Kozel and Adams, *Cocaine Use in America: Epidemiologic and Clinical Perspectives,* pp. 151–57.

Collins, R. J., J. R. Weeks, M. M. Cooper, P. I. Good, and R. R. Russell. (1984). "Prediction of Abuse Liability of Drugs Using IV Self-Administration by Rats." *Psychopharmacology* 82:6–13.

Community Epidemiology Work Group (CEWG) (1987). *Patterns and Trends of Drug Abuse in the United States and Europe.* Proceedings of the Community Epidemiology Work Group, June 1987. Rockville, Md.: National Institute on Drug Abuse.

Du Pont, R. L. (1984). *Getting Tough on Gateway Drugs.* Washington, D.C.: American Psychoactive Press, Inc.

Edwards, G., A. Arif, and R. Hodgson. (1982). "Nomenclature and Classification of Drug- and Alcohol-Related Problems: A Shortened Version of a WHO Memorandum." *British Journal of Addiction* 77:3–20.

Erickson, P. G., E. M. Adlai, G. F. Murray, and R. G. Smart. (1987). *The Steel Drug: Cocaine in Perspective.* Lexington, Mass.: D.C. Heath & Co.

Firth, J. (1988). "Registrations with Cocaine as the Major Problem Substance, July 1983/December 1987." Unpublished data. Toronto: Clinical Institute, Addiction Research Foundation.

Frawley, P. J. (1987). "Neurobehavioral Model of Addiction." *Journal of Drug Issues* 17:29–46.

Gawin, F. H., and H. D. Kleber. (1985). "Cocaine Use in a Treatment Population: Patterns and Diagnostic Distinctions." In Kozel and Adams, *Cocaine Use in America: Epidemiologic and Clinical Perspectives,* pp. 182–92.

———. (1986). "Abstinence Symptomology and Psychiatric Diagnosis in Cocaine Abusers." *Archives of General Psychiatry* 43:107–13.

Gold, M. (1984). *800-Cocaine.* New York: Bantam Books.

Gold, M. S., A. M. Washton, and C. A. Dackis. (1985). "Cocaine Abuse: Neurochemistry, Phenomenology and Treatment." In Kozel and Adams, *Cocaine Use in America: Epidemiologic and Clinical Perspectives,* pp. 130–50.

Gottheil, E. (1986). "Cocaine Abuse and Dependence: The Scope of the Problem." *Advances in Alcohol and Substance Abuse* 6:23–30.

Greenberg, J. (1983). "Natural Highs in Natural Habitats." *Science News* 124:300–301.

Griffiths, R. R., G. E. Bigelow, and J. E. Henningfield. (1980). "Similarities in Animal and Human Drug-Taking Behavior." *Advances in Substance Abuse* 1:1–90.

Grinspoon, L., and J. B. Bakalar. (1985). *Cocaine: A Drug and Its Social Evolution.* 2d ed. New York: Basic Books.

Grupp, L. A. (1981). "An Investigation of Intravenous Ethanol Self-Administration in Rats Using a Fixed Ratio Schedule of Reinforcement." *Physiological Psychology* 9:359–63.

Hill, S. Y., and B. J. Powell. (1976). "Cocaine and Morphine Self-Administration: Effects of Differential Rearing." *Pharmacology, Biochemistry & Behavior* 5:701–704.

Jacobs, M. R., and K. O'B. Fehr, (1987). *Drugs and Drug Abuse: A Reference Text.* 2d ed. Toronto: Addiction Research Foundation.

Jaffe, J. H. (1985). "Foreword." In Kozel and Adams, *Cocaine Use in America: Epidemiologic and Clinical Perspectives,* p. v.

Johnston, C. E. (1984). "Assessment of the Dependence Potential of Cocaine in Animals." In J. Grabowski, ed., *Cocaine: Pharmacology, Effects and Treatment of Abuse.* (Research Monograph No. 50, pp. 54–71). Rockville, Md.: National Institute on Drug Abuse.

Johnston, L. D., P. M. O'Malley, and J. G. Bachman. (1986). *Drug Use among American High School Students, College Students and Other Young Adults: National Trends Through 1985.* Rockville, Md.: National Institute on Drug Abuse.

Kalant, O. J. (1987). *Mater's Cocaine Addiction. [Der kokainismus,* 1926]. Toronto: Addiction Research Foundation.

Kandel, D. B., D. Murphy, and D. Karus. (1985). "Cocaine Use in Young Adulthood: Patterns of Use and Psychosocial Correlates." In Kozel and Adams, *Cocaine Use in America: Epidemiologic and Clinical Perspectives,* pp. 76–110.

Kozel, N. J., and E. H. Adams. (1985). "Cocaine Use in America: Summary of Discussions and Recommendations." In Kozel and Adams, *Cocaine Use in America: Epidemiologic and Clinical Perspectives,* pp. 221–26.

Krivanek, J. (1988). *Addictions.* Sydney: Allen & Unwin.

Lore, R., and K. Flannelly. (1977). "Rat Societies." *Scientific American* 236(5): 106–16.

Mugford, S. (1989). "Letter to the Editor." *The Journal* 18, June. Toronto: Addiction Research Foundation.

Murphy, S. B., C. Reinarman, and D. Waldorf. (1989). "An 11-Year Followup of a Network of Cocaine Users." *British Journal of Addiction* 84:427–36.

Newcomb, M. D., and P. M. Bentler. (1986). "Cocaine Use among Young Adults." *Advances in Alcohol and Substance Abuse* 6:73–96.

Numan, R., A. M. Naparzewska, and C. M. Adler, (1984). "Absence of Reinforcement with Low Dose Intravenous Ethanol Self-Administration in Rats." *Pharmacology, Biochemistry & Behavior* 21:609–15.

O'Malley, P. M., L. D. Johnston, and J. G. Bachman. (1985). "Cocaine Use among American Adolescents and Young Adults." In Kozel and Adams, *Cocaine Use in America: Epidemiologic and Clinical Perspectives,* pp. 50–75.

Orford, J. (1985). *Excessive Appetites: A Psychological View of Addictions.* Chichester: Wiley.

Papasava, M., and G. Singer. (1985). "Self-Administration of Low-Dose Cocaine by Rats at Reduced and Recovered Body Weight." *Psychopharmacology* 85:419–25.

Reinarman, C. and H. G. Levine. (1995). "The Crack Attack: Politics and Media in America's Latest Drug Scare." In Joel Best, ed., *Images and Issues: Typifying Contemporary Social Problems.* New York: Aldine de Gruyer, pp. 147–86.

Schnoll, S. H., J. Karrigan, S. B. Kitchen, A. Daghestani, and T. Hansen. (1985). "Characteristics of Cocaine Abusers Presenting for Treatment." In Kozel and Adams, *Cocaine Use in America: Epidemiologic and Clinical Perspectives,* pp. 171–81.

Science. (1988). "The Biological Tangle of Drug Addiction." In Research News, *Science,* 23 July, 415–17.

Schenk, S., G. Lacelle, K. Gorman, and Z. Amit. (1987). "Cocaine Self-Administration in Rats Influenced by Environmental Conditions: Implications for the Etiology of Drug Abuse." *Neuroscience Letters* 81:227–31.

Siegal, R. K. (1980). "Long-Term Effects of Recreational Cocaine Use: A Four-Year Study." In F. R. Jeri, ed., *Cocaine.* Lima: Pacific Press.

————. (1985). "New Patterns of Cocaine Use: Changing Doses and Routes." In Kozel and Adams, *Cocaine Use in America: Epidemiologic and Clinical Perspectives,* pp. 204–20.

Smart, R. G. (1983). *Forbidden Highs: The Nature, Treatment and Prevention of Illicit Drug Abuse.* Toronto Addiction Research Foundation.

Smart, R. G., and E. M. Adlaf. (1987). *Alcohol and Other Drug Use among Ontario Adults 1977–1987.* Toronto: Addiction Research Foundation.

Smith, D. (1986). "Cocaine-Alcohol Abuse: Epidemiological, Diagnostic and Treatment Considerations." *Journal of Psychoactive Drugs* 18:117–29

Spotts, J. V., and F. C. Shontz. (1985). "A New Perspective on Intervention in Heavy, Chronic Drug Use." *International Journal of the Addictions* 20:1545–65.

Thor, D. H. (1972). "Can Rats Be Addicted to Opiates?" *Psychological Record* 22:289–303

Waldorf, D., S. B. Murphy, C. Reinarman, and B. Joyce. (1977). *Doing Coke: An Ethnography of Cocaine Users and Sellers.* Washington, D.C.: Drug Abuse Council.

Wesson, D. R., and D. E. Smith. (1985). "Cocaine: Treatment perspectives." In Kozel and Adams, *Cocaine Use in America: Epidemiologic and Clinical Perspectives,* pp. 193–203.

White, H. R. (1988). "Longitudinal Patterns of Cocaine Use among Adolescents." *American Journal of Drug and Alcohol Abuse* 14:1–15.

Wise, R. (1984). "Neural Mechanisms of the Reinforcing Action of Cocaine." In J. Grabowski, ed., *Cocaine: Pharmacology, Effects and Treatment of Abuse.* (Research Monograph No. 50, pp. 15–33). Rockville, Md.: National Institute on Drug Abuse.

————. (1988). "The Neurobiology of Craving: Implications for the Understanding and Treatment of Addiction." *Journal of Psychology* 97:118–32.

Zinberg, N. E. (1984). *Drug, Set and Setting: The Pasts for Controlled Intoxicant Use.* New Haven: Yale University Press.

Zinberg, N. E., W. M. Harding, and R. Apsler. (1978). "What Is Drug Abuse?" *Journal of Drug Issues* 8:9–35.

Part Seven

Do Drugs Cause Crime?

26

Cocaine Careers, Control and Consequences: Results from a Canadian Study[*]

Patricia G. Erickson and Timothy R. Weber

INTRODUCTION

One of the first studies of recreational or "controlled" cocaine use was initiated in Canada in 1983 (Erickson, Adlaf, Murray, and Smart, 1987). The *Steel Drug* study did not set out to challenge popular notions of the addictive power of cocaine; rather, the aim was to examine the variation in patterns of cocaine use in a noncaptive sample of users who were neither in jail nor in treatment. Erickson and her colleagues at the Addiction Research Foundation (ARF) had no preconceived idea of what patterns would predominate; they wanted to tap into as wide a range of experiences with this emerging drug of concern as possible. A major conclusion of their study, that most of their sample of 111 users were not addicted and used cocaine infrequently and with little ill effect, was echoed simultaneously or subsequently by the other contributors to this special issue (e.g., Cohen, 1987). Despite the consistency of these findings, in a variety of studies in different countries, they remain controversial. They call into question many of the prevailing assumptions about cocaine's inevitably destructive power over lives, careers, and health, and provide empirical evidence about a different reality (see Table 26.1). Thus it is valuable and timely to have this research on cocaine use careers brought together in one volume.

Originally published in *Addiction Research* 2, no. 1 (1994). © 1994 Harwood Academic Publishers GmbH. Reprinted by permission.

*The authors are grateful to Valerie Watson, Tammy Landau, and Joan Moreau for their important contributions to the data collection and analysis for this study. We also greatly appreciate the comments from Reg Smart, Ed Adlaf, Lana Harrison, and anonymous reviewers.

This research was supported by the National Health Research and Development Program, Ottawa, Canada.

TABLE 26.1: ASSUMPTIONS ABOUT COCAINE AND RESEARCH EVIDENCE FROM COMMUNITY STUDIES

Assumptions	Implications from Research
1) Addiction is inevitable	1) Compulsive, destructive use is rare
2) Escalation always occurs	2) Escalation is only one pattern and often the reverse occurs
3) Abstinence is the only sure way to prevent harm	3) Moderate use without harmful effects is possible
4) Controlled use is impossible	4) Controlled use is the norm
5) Cocaine is one of the most harmful drugs	5) Little or no harm results to most users
6) Users are disturbed or anti-social individuals	6) Most users are not different from non-users
7) Users turn to crime to obtain cocaine	7) Most users are law-abiding, apart from their drug-related behavior
8) Complete repression is the only viable possibility to prevent harm of cocaine	8) There are public-health based alternatives to abstinence and repression

A second, prospective study was designed by the ARF group to explore more fully the patterns and consequences of cocaine use among current users who had moved beyond the experimental stages. Recruitment of a new sample began in early 1989. The results from these interviews provide the basis for the present chapter. Compared to the community sample in the first study, which required only one use of cocaine in the past three years, the second study recruited those who had used at least ten times in the past twelve months. The first study contained predominantly social-recreational, intranasal users, with only seven respondents who had injected cocaine and no freebase users (Erickson et al., 1987, p. 70). (Crack was not identified in Canada until 1986). In contrast, this second study of 100 current users, also in the community, consisted of many more users with multi-mode experience: twenty-two had injected cocaine at some time, seventy-nine had used crack, including two exclusive crack users, while the remainder were also intranasal users (Cheung, Erickson, and Landau, 1991). Thus, this more diverse and experienced group of cocaine users provides a somewhat different perspective on the extent and persistence of patterns of controlled cocaine use. Since we reach essentially the same conclusions, the generality of the earlier findings is strengthened.

DESIGN

The sample was recruited from adult users, aged eighteen years or more, in the Metropolitan Toronto area. The major vehicle for publicizing the study was through advertisements in a wide variety of media. The wording invited those with recent experience with cocaine, aged eighteen years or older, to call a number at the ARF. Ads were placed in mainstream, arts and entertainment, and community newspapers. Cable television and radio public service announcements were repeated many times, and posters were put up in many public locations around the city. A phone number directly to our research office was provided, and an answering machine was activated for calls outside office hours. The phone line was answered personally on weekends after major ad campaigns. A screening interview was conducted to determine if callers met the entry criteria of age and recent experience with cocaine, i.e., at least ten times in the past twelve months. If the caller was eligible, an interview was arranged as soon as possible, either at our offices or at a restaurant or coffee shop of the caller's choosing. Assurance of confidentiality and protection of identities were established before the interview began. Interviews took from one to one and a half hours to complete. The ratio of calls to successfully completed interviews was 8:1, reflecting ineligibility much more than failure to show up. After one year, recruitment ceased when 100 cases were obtained. Although payment was not mentioned in the ad, respondents were paid $30.

Despite efforts to build snowball referral chains through those responding to the ads, this method produced very few additional contacts. (This was in contrast to the first study, in which researchers' personal networks of users produced nearly half the sample.) The great public and media attention paid to the perceived "crack menace" and the enhanced enforcement efforts during the period of our sample recruitment was, we suspect, a contributing factor in most respondents' reluctance to direct other users to us (Erickson, Watson, and Weber, 1992; Cheung and Erickson, 1997). Nevertheless, we believe that the "trustworthy" reputation of ARF, and the nonjudgmental approach and experience of the interviewers, promoted candor among respondents in describing sensitive and illegal behavior. Many professed a desire to share their experiences with cocaine in order to "help" others and some appeared genuinely interested in contributing to a research project. Some wished to provide their knowledge about cocaine's effects that was in marked contrast to what they read or heard in the media. While it is not possible to ascertain precisely how users who volunteer for such a study differ from those who do not, people engaged in illegal or socially disapproved activities will risk their anonymity and come forward if the topic is of interest to them and a secure research environment is available.

Who, then, does this sample of cocaine users represent? At the time of sample recruitment in 1989, a random household survey of Ontario adults eighteen years or over was also conducted (Adlaf and Smart, 1989). It reported that 2.1 percent had used cocaine in the previous year and less than 1 percent had used crack. Since only 5.5 percent of these current users report a frequency of once a month or more often, and the prevalence of use in the

Metropolitan Toronto area is about double that of the rest of the province, a minimum estimate of 10,000 monthly or more frequent users was derived (Adlaf and Smart, 1989). If underreporting of heavier use is likely, then the upper limit may be two or three times higher. This suggests that the sample of 100 community users is drawn from a population of between 10,000 to 30,000 current, more frequent users in Metro Toronto in 1989.

SAMPLE CHARACTERISTICS

Respondents were, for the most part, young (mean age = 27.2 years), male (70 percent) and single (71 percent). Racial composition was almost exclusively white and ethnic background was not solicited. Sample characteristics are summarized in Table 26.2. The highest level of education attained was high school for 41 percent, other postsecondary institution for 32 percent, and university for 26 percent. While 57 percent were employed full time, only 13 percent were actively jobhunting. Annual income was under $31,000 for nearly two-thirds (62 percent) of respondents; less than one in five (17 percent) was earning more than $40,000 annually (in Canadian dollars, worth almost 20 percent less than U.S. $). Most rented accommodation (62 percent) or lived with parents (17 percent).

Compared with cocaine users in the Ontario population survey, also shown in Table 26.2, the community sample displays similar characteristics with respect to sex, education, employment status, and living situation. Though none of the differences were statistically significant (applying a chi square test), the community sample is somewhat younger, with a greater proportion of single persons and those in lower income groups than cocaine users in the Ontario-wide random sample.

The majority of respondents had an extensive history of multiple drug use. Besides current alcohol, cannabis, and cocaine use by nearly all those interviewed, over 80 percent also reported lifetime experience with LSD, other hallucinogens, amphetamines, and other stimulants. One-third had tried PCP and one-fifth heroin at least once. Yet despite this considerable exposure, a relatively low proportion of respondents—10 percent or less—reported the use of any drug other than alcohol, cannabis, and cocaine in the past month. Aside from tobacco, also widely used by this group, these latter three appeared to be their drugs of choice. The age of onset or first use of this array of drugs began with tobacco, followed with alcohol then cannabis in the early teens, continued with prescription drugs and hallucinogens in the later teens, and was completed with heroin (where applicable), cocaine, and finally crack.

TABLE 26.2: DEMOGRAPHIC CHARACTERISTICS OF TWO SAMPLES OF COCAINE USERS

	Cocaine Users from the Community (N = 100) (%)	Cocaine Users from Ontario* (N = 62) (%)
Gender		
Male	70	66
Female	30	34
Age		
18-20	13	4
21-25	39	28
26-30	22	40
31-35	17	16
36-40	4	10
41+	5	1
Mean age 27.2 years		
Marital Status		
Single (never married)	71	45
Common-law	6	9
Married	9	38
Separated	9	} 8
Divorced	5	
Education		
Grade 9-11	16	16
Grade 12-13	25	24
Some postsecondary schooling	17	11
Postsecondary diploma/certificate	15	16
Some university	13	11
University degree	11	} 20
Graduate degree	2	
Gross Personal Annual Income		
$10,000 or less	18	4
$11,000 to $20,000	24	12
$21.000 to $30,000	20	32
$31,000 to $40,000	18	13
$41,000 +	17	31
No response	3	9
Employment Status		
Employed full-time	57	63
Looking for job	13	n/a
Employed part-time	8	16
Student	8	8
Social assistance	7	n/a
Illegal activities	2	n/a
Other	5	14
Living Situation		
Own house/condominium	7	n/a
Rent house/apartment	36	n/a
Rent shared accomodation	26	n/a
Live with parents	17	n/a
Live in hostel/residence/looking for place to live	13	n/a
No response	1	n/a

*Based on a sample of cocaine users (N = 62) drawn from a Gallup probability sample of Ontario adults aged 18 and over (Adlaf and Smart, 1989).

n/a = not available.

COCAINE EXPERIENCES

First Experience and Reasons for Trying

Most respondents were initiated to cocaine by a male friend in someone's home. The average age of onset was 22.7 years. While the intranasal route was by far the most common way to start (for 82 percent), smoking crack and injecting cocaine also occurred. When asked what influenced their decision to try cocaine, the most common responses were out of interest or curiosity (79 percent), simple availability (75 percent), the "adventure" (60 percent), and the positive reports from others (54 percent). The respondents were almost evenly divided as to whether cocaine had met their expectations or not. The most and least appealing aspects of their first experience were diverse. Some liked the euphoria, increased sociability, and energy boost. Dislikes included the financial costs, the weak effect, "coming down," and various physical and psychological effects. These perceived negative effects included nasal irritation and congestion, feeling "speedy," and not being able to sleep. Obviously, respondents were willing to persist in further experimentation despite some complaints and few "raves" about this first experience.

Cocaine Career

This sample contained an even split between those with relatively brief cocaine careers and those with more extensive ones. About half of respondents (52 percent) had used cocaine for less than three years; for a further 25 percent from three to less than six years had lapsed since first use, and 22 percent of subjects had used cocaine more than six years by the time they were interviewed. As already noted, this sample reflects multi-modes of administration. Less than a quarter of the sample had used cocaine only by "snorting" the powder. All of the twenty-two injection users had experience with both powder and crack, but two of the crack users had not used in any other way. Nevertheless, when asked their current preferences for mode of administration, most were not injecting, but rather were quite evenly split between smoking and snorting. This did not necessarily reflect two distinct groups of consumers. Many respondents with varied experience stated that the two modes elicited very different types of highs: Sometimes they preferred the intense rush from crack, other times the mellow, social high from snorting powdered cocaine. The powder-only users expressed satisfaction with this route and had little interest in trying what they perceived as the more dangerous and addictive modes.

Their past history of cocaine use was elicited by a number of questions about the frequency and amount of cocaine taken during the first twelve months of use, the period of heaviest use, and during the past three months

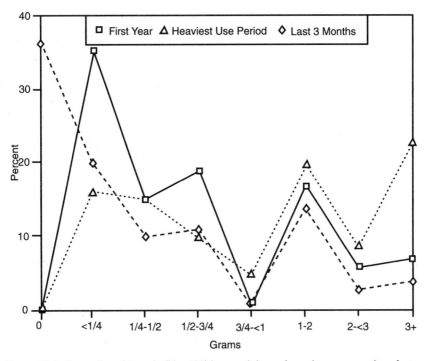

Figure 26.1   Proportion of sample (N = 100) by usual dose of cocaine per occasion of use during initial year, heaviest period, and last three months (prior to interview).

prior to the interview. As Figure 26.1 indicates, the overall pattern was for an increase in both amount and frequency, followed by a dropoff in recent use to less than the initial period. The average dose of cocaine consumed per occasion of use was less than one gram for over half of respondents when they started, whereas the proportion taking three or more grams tripled in the heaviest use period (from 7 percent to 23 percent). By the last three months, 36 percent reported no use, and of those still using the large majority were using less than one gram per occasion. The proportion of the sample using more than once per week rose from 41 percent in the first year to 85 percent during the heaviest use period, then dropped to 29 percent in the past three months. Followup data after one year further supported this pattern of diminishing and infrequent cocaine use for nearly all the respondents (Erickson, 1993).

Respondents were also asked a number of questions about their ongoing experiences with cocaine. The longest continuous interval of cocaine administration in a given episode of use, or "binge," was six or more days for 14 percent of the respondents. Only about a quarter had never extended a "run" for more than one day. About 90 percent of respondents also reported having voluntarily stopped using cocaine for one month or more. When asked how they would currently assess the most and least appealing aspects of cocaine use, the perceptions had changed little from those describing their first experiences. The positive aspects were still the euphoria, the "rush," and the increase in energy and sociability. Greater emphasis was placed on the negative aspects, that is the financial cost and the concern with addiction, than at initiation. A question about the importance of cocaine in their lives elicited an indifferent response from 90 percent of these users who answered not at all important or not very important. Only half of the group projected that they were very likely or quite likely to use cocaine in the next year. As mentioned above, this forecast was in fact borne out by the interviews conducted one year later (see Erickson, 1993).

A number of analyses were conducted (data not shown) in order to determine if there were typical patterns or subpatterns of use that could be related to variation in the demographic characteristics of the respondents. With only a couple of minor exceptions, we found no clear links between age, sex, education, or income, and frequency or type of cocaine experiences. Powder-only users were not different from crack-plus-powder users (Cheung et al., 1991). Those who had an injection history were somewhat more likely to be male (27 percent vs. 10 percent female), but otherwise male and female use patterns were very similar. The current more frequent users (i.e., more often than once a week) were older than the less frequent users: 75 percent aged twenty-six or more compared to 38 percent. The relatively homogeneous nature of the sample has likely obscured the potential relationship between individual characteristics and intensity of cocaine use. Next we shall consider the various impacts of cocaine use on health, social relation, and criminality, and how the more negative outcomes may be explained.

CONSEQUENCES

Health

In such a group of young adults, relatively few serious health problems would be expected. Data pertaining to respondents' personal satisfaction with their health and specific concerns have already been reported in detail elsewhere (Erickson et al., 1992) and will be summarized briefly here. In general, the large majority of respondents rated themselves as satisfied with a number of aspects of their lives involving general health and well-being (e.g., accomplishments, problem solving, decisions, attractiveness, self-confidence). Although the group with experience of all modes of cocaine administration showed somewhat less satisfaction than the powder-only or powder-plus-crack groups, differences were small.

When asked about more specific measures such as seeking medical attention, spending nights in [the] hospital or taking time off from school/work because of drug use, a poorer health profile emerged, especially for the multi-mode users. While only 5 percent of powder-only users had sought medical attention for any form of cocaine problem, about a quarter of the other respondents had done so. Crack users did so more often for a psychological reason while those with injection experience were more likely to seek help for a physical reason related to cocaine use. Nearly half of the respondents who had used crack and/or injected cocaine, but only a quarter of the powder-only group, felt that cocaine had changed their lives for the worse.

Reactions to cocaine may be divided into acute (short term) or chronic (long term). The most serious potential acute reaction is, of course, the fatal one. But other dramatic acute reactions such as hallucinations and convulsions may herald a possible overdose. Overall, 40 percent of respondents reported experiencing hallucinations at least once, and 22 percent identified having a convulsion, while using cocaine. It was not possible to ascertain if co-existing use of other substances or medical conditions contributed to these effects. When asked a direct question about whether they had ever experienced a cocaine overdose, 30 percent believed that they had.

Of the various chronic reactions that were specifically inquired about, the following proportion of respondents reported experiencing them most times or always: chronic insomnia (67 percent); inability to relax (54 percent); uncontrollable craving (48 percent); physical or mental exhaustion (44 percent); weight loss (42 percent); nasal congestion (39 percent); depression (37 percent); lack of sexual interest (26 percent); felt unable to think clearly (26 percent); sores or bleeding in nose (18 percent); abscesses (3 percent); hepatitis (1 percent). When these effects were related to frequency of cocaine use in the past three months, those who abstained during this period were more likely to have experienced all of these reactions than respondents who were currently either less or more frequent users. The one exception was weight loss, which was experienced by 50 percent of current nonusers and 62 percent of more frequent users (but only 17 percent of less frequent users). These results imply that current nonusers may have been prompted to cease use because of one or more of the adverse effects they had experienced during their periods of active cocaine use.

Addiction/Compulsive Use

One of the possible outcomes of cocaine use, loss of control, is of particular interest and will be examined in more detail. A number of questions were asked about cocaine users' perceptions and experiences relating to the possibility of addiction. As noted above, of the total sample, 48 percent reported experiencing an "uncontrollable craving or urge to use cocaine" most times or always; moreover, 33 percent had this feeling rarely or sometimes, and 19 percent said never. Given that three quarters of the respondents also acknowledged that they had *ever* been concerned about becoming addicted to cocaine, and this property was also identified as one of the least appealing aspects of cocaine use, it would appear that these experienced users have a healthy respect for cocaine's addictive potential. Findings reported earlier (Erickson et al., 1992) indicated that the vast majority (over 80 percent) of respondents, whatever their type of experience with modes of cocaine use, perceived a "great" risk in regular cocaine and crack use. The message of potential addiction seems an important one as a means of personal and informal control over escalating cocaine use.

This is not to ignore the evidence that a substantial number of these respondents did not indicate any difficulty in controlling their own cocaine use or concerns about possible loss of control. The importance of job, family, or other activities relegated cocaine to a minor leisure role. For other users, control did not present as a major issue. Some had learned to ignore or suppress cravings, while others imposed financial or temporal limits on the amount used.

For some users, as their personal accounts indicated, loss of control "snuck up" on them. One employed male in his thirties said that he was spending more and more money on cocaine, neglecting his work and his friends, but he did not recognize he had a problem until "some friends sat me down and made me see what was going on." For some, their recognition that cocaine use was having a negative impact on their lives, which could take the form of imminent job loss, a pregnancy, or a legal penalty, "brought them around" and they stopped abruptly. For others, recognition of a problem did not mean an immediate reversal, as one young man, employed as a bus driver revealed: "[T]he first time I was about to do some crack before going to work, I thought, 'I could have an accident, kill somebody.' I quit my job." What is clear is that, like other research on more heavily involved users (Waldorf, Reinarman, and Murphy, 1991; Cohen, 1989), many different routes and outcomes are possible besides sheer escalation. The conceptual model, shown in Figure 26.2, also reflects the empirical data of this study and others in this special issue (Erickson, 1993).

Social Relations

Respondents were asked whether their cocaine use had ever had an impact on various aspects of their work, finances, and relationships. Then they were asked whether the effect had been beneficial or harmful. About one-fifth to one-sixth of respondents thought that cocaine had improved, usually at an earlier stage of their use career, their quality of work in their jobs, their relations with their boss, helped their overall relationship with their spouse or other partner, and improved their sexual relations. Nevertheless, about three

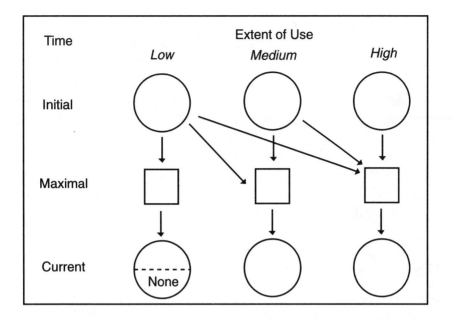

Figure 26.2   Conceptual model of cocaine use patterns during initial, maximal, and current periods of use.

times as many respondents also reported a negative impact on all these dimensions of social relations. The highest rating for a beneficial effect was on the amount of work, for which 44 percent of respondents reported improved output, but an even higher proportion, 69 percent, said that amount of work had ultimately been diminished by cocaine use. Three-quarters of respondents (74 percent) also said their financial situation had suffered from cocaine use.

These various social indicators were related to lifetime crack use. Those who had used crack forty or more times were compared to those who had used less than that. For all measures, the more frequent crack users reported a much higher degree of harmful effects. For example, comparing the more frequent crack users with the less frequent ones, 65 percent reported worsened reactions with bosses (vs. 38 percent less frequent use); 91 percent missed work because of cocaine use (vs. 52 percent); 74 percent of relations with partner suffered (vs. 45 percent); 57 percent had poorer sexual relations (vs. 32 percent). However, no other variable of cocaine use frequency or pattern of use was related to adverse social consequences in these realms.

TABLE 26.3: MEANS OF OBTAINING COCAINE OR MONEY TO BUY COCAINE FROM LEAST TO MOST COMMON

Means	Never	Seldom	3–9	10 or More
Stole a car	100	0	0	0
Stole from a car	98	0	2	0
Prostitution	96	2	2	0
Shoplifted	94	6	0	0
Broke in	94	2	4	0
Forged a check	89	4	6	2
Loan	87	7	4	2
Taken from family/friend	87	7	4	2
Stole money	85	6	6	4
Ran con games	80	7	9	4
Stole cocaine	76	11	9	4
Trade[d] sex for cocaine	72	13	9	4
Sold possessions	67	24	7	2
Sold other drugs	61	9	7	22
Borrow[ed] money from family/friends	48	17	17	19
Sold cocaine	46	20	6	28
Given	6	6	11	78
Bought with own money	2	4	9	85

Criminality

One possible consequence of becoming a cocaine user is arrest and prosecution for cocaine possession. Indeed, 5 percent had had such an experience. Realistically, most respondents did not anticipate a high risk of legal intervention. Only 7 percent thought it was likely or very likely that they would be caught by the police with cocaine in the next year. Presented with the hypothetical question as to what would be the most likely sentence they would receive in such an event, most selected a fine, probation, or other non-jail option. Prison was anticipated by 12 percent of respondents. The maximum penalty available in Canadian law (i.e., for possession of cocaine under the *Narcotic Control Act*) is, in fact, seven years, but the actual sentences awarded are much less severe. Nevertheless, since national sentencing data for 1989 show that 29 percent of all cocaine possession offenders were imprisoned, users may be overly optimistic about their risk of incarceration if caught (Erickson, 1992). On the other hand, if those imprisoned are more serious offenders than these respondents (e.g., prior record, trafficking suspects) the expectation of less severe sentences may be realistic.

Respondents were presented with a list of eighteen possible ways of obtaining cocaine, or money to buy cocaine, and asked if they had ever done any of them, and if so, how often. These results are shown in Table 26.3. The most common means of getting cocaine, by far, were to buy it with their own money or be given it. The next most frequent ways, for about half the respondents, were to borrow money from family or friends or to sell cocaine. About 40 percent had sold other drugs as well. Criminal activity, other than drug sales, was resorted to rarely. Fewer than 10 percent of respondents had ever shoplifted, broken into a building or car, or engaged in prostitution in order to obtain money to buy cocaine. These results belie the popular notion that cocaine use fuels various forms of predatory crime. They are consistent with the research of Waldorf et al. (1991) that people who are otherwise law-abiding, with stakes in conformity, are highly unlikely to embark on serious criminal activities as a result of even heavy cocaine use. Further analyses (data not shown) found little relationship between means of obtaining cocaine and other demographic or drug use history factors.

TME MEDIA PORTRAYAL OF COCAINE IN TORONTO

In 1988–89, we conducted a content analysis of the three major Toronto newspapers to examine and compare how two stimulant drugs, cocaine and tobacco (i.e., nicotine), were portrayed (Erickson and Moreau, 1990). Some of the key findings will be highlighted here. About half the cocaine articles were extracted during January and February 1989, just before the period of recruitment for the study of users, and the balance of articles during the remaining ten months. Thus the portrayal reflects what our community users were exposed to in Toronto papers. This media study corresponded to a period when heightened concern and coverage of cocaine, and especially crack, spilled over the border from the U.S. (Cheung and Erickson, 1997). "Devil drug has Metro in its grip" was not [an] atypical headline.

Over a twelve-month period, sixty-seven news stories about cocaine (including crack) were selected for analysis of themes and content. Half of the total sources of information cited in the stories were the police or other criminal justice officials. Scientific or health professionals were the sources only 6 percent of the time. Not surprisingly, the central theme and issues covered in the cocaine articles emphasized crime, smuggling, and enforcement in two-thirds of all stories. Details of raids and seizures were regular fare. Health aspects of cocaine use, the focus of about one-sixth of all stories, included addiction far more often (in half of these stories) than any other adverse physical or psychological effects. Thus users might sense that the official reaction was concerned more with criminalizing them than with concern for their health.

CONCLUSION

This chapter has examined the consequences of cocaine use and patterns of controlled use in a community sample of one hundred multimode users in Toronto, Canada. Some highlights of a media study during the period of recruitment were also reported. Although use at least ten times in the past year was a criterion for inclusion in the study, at the time of interview nearly one-third had not used cocaine in the past three months. The overall pattern was for a peak followed by a dropoff in both amount and frequency of use compared to initial periods of experimentation and heaviest use. Most had quit or reduced their use without professional help, suggesting that the natural history of cocaine use is a self-limiting phenomenon of relatively short duration (Cheung et al., 1991). Fear of adverse health, social, and financial consequences, rather than concern for legal consequences, was the most important influence on this deescalation.

One important question arising from these results is why so few relationships were found between patterns of cocaine use, adverse consequences, and individual characteristics of users. This is likely due in part to the fairly homogeneous nature of the sample. Most respondents were single, white males with no children and limited occupational and financial achievement. Most (79 percent) had already distinguished themselves by crack use, while as many had used powder only as had injected cocaine. Therefore, these are not patterns of just recreational snorters, though most used this mode in addition to smoking or injecting. From their multimode experience, most appeared to have undergone a learning experience about the benefits and risks of cocaine. Over time, the pleasurableness of cocaine waned and came to be overshadowed by the increasing costs and adverse effects of the drug. While it is tempting to conclude that the few who got into the most serious trouble with their cocaine use were distinguished by using too much, too often for too long, the personal factor clearly was vital in determining the "too." According to the "cocaine stories" of most respondents, it was rarely a specific event or intervention that led to marked change in cocaine use behavior, but rather a tipping of the balance between the perceived costs and benefits. In this sense, cocaine may be viewed as another, albeit risky, commodity, subject to consumer preferences and tradeoffs. Outcomes are highly individualized.

An important implication of this study for a health-directed social policy is that potential and early-stage cocaine consumers need accurate information about both the pleasures and pitfalls of this seductive drug. Users are concerned about and aware of many of the harmful effects of cocaine, but speak with hindsight rather than foresight. The criminal law, the dominant instrument of the current prohibitionist policy, neither is a major factor in decisions about initiating or persevering in illicit drug use activity, nor does it impede access (Bachman, Johnson and O'Malley, 1990; Erickson and Cheung, 1992). Despite the lack of a demonstrable deterrent effect, the criminal justice system continues to be mobilized to identify and punish severely the small proportion of users who are caught. This policy generates substantial personal, social, and economic costs to society. A more rational drug policy would focus on the risks and benefits of cocaine and other illicit drug use in all its forms, and aim to reduce the actual harm users do to themselves and the community.

REFERENCES

Adlaf, E. M., and R. G. Smart. (1989). *The Ontario Adult and Other Drug Use Survey, 1977–1989.* Toronto: Addiction Research Foundation.

Bachman, J. G., L. D. Johnson, and P. M. O'Malley. "Explaining the Recent Decline in Cocaine Use among Young Adults." *Journal of Health and Social Behaviour* 31 (June): 17–84.

Cheung, Y. W., and P. G. Erickson. (1997). "Crack in Canada A Distant American Cousin." In C. Reinarman and H. Levine, eds., *Crack in Context: Myths, Realities and Social Policies.* Berkeley and Los Angeles: University of California Press.

Cheung, Y. W., P. G. Erickson, and T. Landau. (1991). "Experience of Crack Use: Findings from a Community-Based Sample in Toronto." *Journal of Drug Issues* 21 (1): 121–40.

Cohen, P. (1987). "Cocaine Use in Amsterdam in Nondeviant Subcultures." Paper presented at the International Council on Alcohol and Addictions Congress, Lausanne, Switzerland, May 31–June 5.

Cohen, P. (1989). *Cocaine Use in Amsterdam.* University of Amsterdam: Institute of Social Geography.

Erickson, P. G. (1992). "Recent Trends in Canadian Drug Policy: The Decline and Resurgence of Prohibitionism." *Daedalus* 121 (Summer): 239–67.

———. (1993). "The Prospects of Harm Reduction for Psychostimulants." In N. Heather, A. Wodak, E. Nadelmann, and P. O'Hare, eds. *Psychoactive Drugs and Harm Reduction: From Faith to Science.* London: Whurr Publisher.

Erickson, P. G., and Y. W. Cheung. (1992). "Drug Crime and Legal Control: Lessons from the Canadian Experience." *Contemporary Drug Problems* 19, no. 2: 247–77.

Erickson, P. G. and J. A. E. Moreau. (1990). "A Tale of Two Stimulants: A Content Analysis of Cocaine and Tobacco in Toronto Newspapers." Addiction Research Foundation. Unpublished paper.

Erickson, P. G., E. M. Adlaf, G. Murray, and R. G. Smart. (1987). *The Steel Drug: Cocaine in Perspective.* Lexington: D.C. Heath.

Erickson, P. G., V. Watson, and T. Weber. (1992). "Cocaine Users' Perceptions of their Health Status and the Risks of Drug Use." In P. A. O'Hare, R. Newcombe, A. Matthews, E. C. Buning, and E. Drucker, eds., *The Reduction of Drug-Related Harm.* London: Routledge.

Waldorf, D., C. Reinarman, and S. Murphy. (1991). *Cocaine Changes: The Experience of Using and Quitting.* Philadelphia: Temple University Press.

27

Addiction and Criminal Responsibility[*]

Herbert Fingarette

For more than a decade courts have debated the scope of the addict's criminal responsibility; today the issue remains unsettled. These debates were triggered by the Supreme Court's decision in *Robinson* v. *California,*[1] which recognized that narcotic addiction is a "disease," and held that criminal punishment of a person thus "afflicted" violates the Eighth Amendment's prohibition of cruel and unusual punishment.[2] Subsequent cases discussed the possible conflicting interpretations of *Robinson.*[3] All agreed that *Robinson* held, at the very least, that the Constitution precludes criminal punishment of the addict simply for a condition of body and mind manifesting a "bare desire"[4] or "mere propensity"[5] to use the drug. It is over the tendencies to go beyond this "minimalist" interpretation of *Robinson,* however, that controversy flourishes. While the major trend in the courts has been to interpret *Robinson* in the minimalist way,[6] some courts have argued for extension of exculpation[7] to crimes related to addiction.

Arguments of this type appear in recent decisions in the District of

Reprinted by permission of The Yale Law Journal Company and Fred B. Rothman & Company from *The Yale Law Journal,* Vol. 84, pages 413–44.

*This project was supported in part by Grant No. I R03 MH 25193-01, awarded by the Center for Studies of Crime and Delinquency, NIMH, DHEW. I am greatly indebted to Ann Fingarette Hasse, whose collaboration in related studies and whose legal research in this area have been a significant contribution. She is not to be held responsible, however, for the specific theses or form of this article.

The present article is part of a comprehensive study in collaboration with Ann Fingarette Hasse, currently in progress; it covers all types of mental impairments that may affect criminal responsibility. See H. Fingarette, *The Meaning of Criminal Insanity* (1972); Fingarette, "The Diminished Mental Capacity Defence in [English] Criminal Law," *Modern Law Review* 37 (1974): 264; Fingarette, "The Perils of Powell: In Search of a Factual Foundation for the 'Disease Concept of Alcoholism,' " *Harvard Law Review* 83 (1970): 793.

Columbia, and in a number of powerfully argued dissents in cases decided by narrow majorities.[8] They claim either that the addict's use of the drug and some or all related offenses are inseparable from the addict's nonpunishable status or "disease,"[9] or that they are involuntary effects or symptoms of that status.[10] On the basis of such arguments some have urged that the *Robinson* immunity should be extended beyond the minimalist interpretation to include the addict's nontrafficking use, possession, and purchase of his drug; others would go farther and include offenses motivated by addiction, such as theft.[11]

In *Powell* v. *Texas,*[12] decided six years after *Robinson,* the Court again addressed these issues in four separate opinions. Four dissenting Justices argued that *Robinson* and common law principles rendered an alcoholic immune from criminal punishment for public drunkenness by virtue of his addiction.[13] Four Justices in the majority rejected this reasoning in affirming the appellant's conviction.[14] The fifth, Justice White, in his concurring opinion, seemed to support immunity from criminal punishment for the chronic alcoholic's drinking or being drunk, but he found that the factual record in the case could not support exculpation based on that principle.[15] In 1970 the Circuit Court of Appeals for the District of Columbia seemed close to a consensus that would clear up this confusion. In *Watson* v. *United States*[16] that court announced that a nontrafficking addict presenting a better factual record than appeared in the case before it ought to be able to invoke *Robinson* to win immunity from punishment for possession. But when the issue arose again in 1975 the same court rejected, in a five-to-four vote, immunity for possession by an addict.[17] Some of those opposing exculpation for the addict, however, rested their arguments more on the current state of legislation than on a square and self-sufficient rejection of the legal reasoning and factual assumptions of those favoring exculpation.[18]

The present study seeks to dispel the confusion that arises in the case law. The discussion begins with an analysis of the typical exculpatory arguments that are based on *Robinson.* It will be seen that, insofar as these arguments attempt to extend the immunity of the addict beyond the minimalist interpretation of *Robinson,* they ultimately rely on the assumption that behavior motivated by addiction is involuntary. The discussion then reviews the factual background of addiction[19] as it relates to the legal concept of involuntariness. It demonstrates that the assumption of involuntariness is plainly unsound. Finally, this study explores nonlegal theories of drug addiction in an attempt to show that these cannot function as exculpatory vehicles in the criminal law. All the exculpatory arguments, whether they originate within or without the legal arena, lead to oversimplified "solutions" to complex and ill-understood problems, thus injudiciously preempting the legislature's role. Though they are intended to be humane, they actually reflect a less humane, less realistic, and less helpful attitude toward the addict himself than would their rejection.

I. THE LEGAL ARGUMENTS

The principal lines of constitutional and common law argument designed to preclude criminal liability where addiction is at issue are often interwoven in the leading opinions. For clarity of analysis, however, the following sections of this chapter will distinguish them carefully and examine them successively. They resolve into three distinguishable lines of argument here labeled, for the sake of convenience, the "status argument," the "disease argument," and the "involuntariness argument."

A. The Status Argument:
A Minimalist Reading of *Robinson* v. *California*

The issue of "status" is central in *Robinson.* Referring to the statute under which the defendant had been found guilty, the majority wrote:

> This statute, therefore, is not one which punishes a person for the use of narcotics, for their purchase, sale, or possession, or for antisocial or disorderly behavior resulting from their administration. . . . Rather, we deal with a statute that makes the "status" of narcotic addiction a criminal offense. . . .[20]

The Court found that the statute violated the Eighth and Fourteenth Amendments: "We hold that a state law which imprisons a person *thus afflicted* as a criminal, even though he has *never touched* any narcotic drug within the State or been guilty of any irregular *behavior* there, inflicts a cruel and unusual punishment in violation of the Fourteenth Amendment."[21] In arriving at this holding the Court analogized punishment for the status of narcotic addiction to punishment for affliction with a disease.[22] The analogy suggests that the term "disease" carries an exculpatory force independent of that of "status"; alternatively, it suggests that disease is a species of status and is nonculpable simply because it can be so classified. This section of the discussion adopts the latter view; the former is discussed elsewhere.[23]

What, then, is the scope of exculpation for the status of addiction in *Robinson*? Certainly the case cannot be read to do away with all crimes of status. These have a long history in the common law and in statutory law; they have not been fundamentally challenged by the Court.[24] It is implausible to read *Robinson* to announce a new constitutional doctrine declaring crimes of status generally to be outside the scope of the criminal law.[25] The text and context of *Robinson* carry no such implication, nor has any court proposed such a reading of the case. It is therefore more accurate to read the case to bar punishment for status only insofar as, and just for the reason that, the status excludes any act at all. Indeed, a criminal offense, even though it may not itself be conduct, must generally be defined with some essential reference to conduct.[26] In *Robinson* the majority emphasizes the absence from the statute at issue of any requirement to prove that there was any drug use, purchase, possession, or sale, or any antisocial or disorderly behavior resulting from drug use.[27] In *Powell* v. *Texas* Justice Marshall reads *Robinson* to stand for the proposition that punishment may not be inflicted in the absence of proof of any *actus reus*.*[28] Many lower courts have focused on the distinction between status and act in making this, the minimalist argument.[29]

Does this concept of pure status as distinct from acts make sense in the context of addiction? Of course one may separate addiction status (some distinctive bodily state or mental desire) from the actual use of the drug by mere definition; the California trial court did so in *Robinson* in construing its statutory crime of "addiction."[30] But some would insist that the addict's purchase, possession, and use of the drug are "realistically inseparable from the status of addiction."[31] In this view California's definition of addiction is unduly arbitrary and unrealistic; regardless of our verbal freedom to define "addiction" only in terms of desire, the possession and use of the drug—and perhaps other acts—are seen as *factually* inseparable from the physiological and psychological status of addiction.

Two arguments have suggested the forms this alleged inseparability takes: (1) The addict's drug use is a symptom of disease. (2) The addict's use of drugs is an involuntary result of a status which is physiological or psychological, or perhaps both. If the status argument is pushed beyond the minimalist reading to exculpate other behavior associated with the status, it thus resolves into arguments based on disease or involuntariness. These arguments will lead us into complex factual issues about drug addiction that will be explored later in the chapter; we turn now to a closer examination of the arguments themselves.

B. The Disease Argument

Robinson opens the door to the argument that "disease" may preclude criminal liability. Justice Stewart's majority opinion acknowledges that persons addicted to narcotics are diseased or ill;[32] the emphasis on disease is central to his argument. Justice Douglas's concurring opinion asserts that the addict is sick, and that addiction is a disease.[33] Justice Clark's dissent speaks of "cure" and justifies confinement in a penal institution as "treatment."[34]

Although the theme of disease has remained pervasive in case law on the topic, its exculpatory force remains as ambiguous as it is in the *Robinson* opinions.[35] In applying that theme to the case of addiction, however, the skeleton of the argument is discernible in at least a generalized form. Its proponents would claim that it cannot be a crime to be afflicted with a disease,

---

*I.e., the criminal *act*, as compared to criminal *intent* (*mens rea*). (Ed.)

that addiction is a disease, and hence unpunishable. Others would argue further that some or all addictive conduct is either part of the disease,[36] "a compulsion symptomatic of the disease,"[37] or an "invariable"[38] symptom of the disease; as a result such conduct is unpunishable. Two questions must be explored in order to evaluate these arguments: Can the claim that addiction is a disease be usefully adapted to the context or a legal argument? Which, if any, of the phenomena associated with disease are inappropriate as grounds for punishment under the criminal law?

The first question is problematic because the term "disease" is vaguely defined within the medical profession.[39] The term suggests generally that a person manifests some distinguishable complex of abnormal conditions having, or surmised to have, a biological basis.[40] If one seeks to derive a relevant meaning of disease by analysis of the term "addiction," one confronts a plurality of concepts and definitions describing addiction.[41] Moreover, these are used in varying ways by various authorities within the health professions, sometimes overlapping and sometimes differing significantly in meaning.[42] Unresolved questions, problems, speculation, and controversy abound in this field.[43] Thus it is clear that any claim that drug addiction is a disease is not made on the basis of a consensus among researchers and health professionals about its manifestation. Obviously the claim that addiction is a disease has its suggestive, rhetorical, perhaps educational uses. But the controversy surrounding that claim makes it unsuitable as the premise for tightly reasoned argument leading to fundamental innovation in constitutional or common law doctrine.

Even if theories and definitions were clear and uniform, they would not in themselves make clear which aspects of the alleged disease should or should not be reached by the criminal law. In order to see how the lines of argument would be drawn, we list the specific kinds of phenomena associated with the rubric "addiction":[44]

1. *Autonomous somatic states*—specific neurological, physiological, or other bodily states that are effects of repeated past use of narcotics, barbiturates, alcohol, or other drugs, but which can exist even in the current absence of the drug.

2. *Autonomous mental phenomena*—the powerful desire for the drug, and the related subjective sensations, that can exist after repeated use but in the current absence of the drug.

3. *The autonomous and distinctive pattern of behavior*—the pattern of repeated, persistent, illegal use of the drug, and other behavior distinctively belonging to this pattern, even in the absence of the drug.

It is evident that a minimalist reading of *Robinson* forbids criminal punishment for the existence of the pure status phenomena included in the first category, mere somatic states per se. The phenomena in the second category, mere mental propensities or desires, are similarly protected. Thus insofar as a disease theory of addiction suggests the existence of autonomous bodily and mental states, criminal immunity is exactly coextensive with that arising from the minimalist reading of the status argument.

If the disease argument is to broaden the scope of criminal immunity for drug addiction, it must do so by immunizing the phenomena in the third category, addictive behavior.[45] Certainly it is inaccurate to claim that all disease-related behavior can escape the reach of the criminal law.[46] The state can require a nondiseased person to take steps to prevent his catching the disease;[47] it can require the diseased person to isolate or quarantine himself,[48] or to take measures to protect others.[49] But the criminal law may not reach involuntary conduct,[50] and it is this assumption that has formed the basis for arguments for criminal immunity for an addict's behavior.

Since the bodily condition associated with the disease is clearly protected by the status argument, the addict's conduct can be exculpated only insofar as it is involuntary. Thus arguments for immunity may describe the addict's behavior in terms that suggest involuntariness, such as "compulsion symptomatic of the disease."[51] Legal involuntariness, however, must be demonstrated as a matter of fact no matter how the conduct is related to the protected disease status.

The claim that addictive behavior is a "symptom" of the disease thus amounts to an attempt to gloss over the issue of involuntariness. There is no reason to assume that whatever is a medically recognized symptom must be legally involuntary. A symptom is simply an indicator or manifestation of disease.[52] There are some kinds of behavior that can be symptomatic movements of the body and that are not directly subject to the will in certain situations— e.g., fainting, tics, or squints. But there are also behaviors that can be symptomatic in medical terms and that can be directly subject to the will.[53] It is, then, a question of fact and not of definition whether symptomatic behavior is voluntary. Where a symptom is a voluntary act, there is no legal basis for declaring that merely because it indicates or manifests a disease, the person cannot be punished for it. Indeed, if such a voluntary act could cause serious social harm, is there any doubt that the state could invoke the criminal law to prohibit it?

One variant of the disease argument deserves particular mention at this point; it is the claim, explicit or implied, that addiction is a *mental* disease.[54] If this is meant to advance the argument by invoking the insanity defense, it only makes the addict's attempt to escape liability more burdensome: the defendant would have to prove both the existence of a mental disease and either a lack of understanding related to the offending act itself,[55] or a defect in volitional capacity.[56] Proof that addiction is a mental disease would be difficult; there is no consensus in the medical profession that addiction is a mental disease.[57] Although courts have shown sympathy for the doctrine that addiction is a disease, they have consistently refused to adopt the doctrine that addiction is a mental disease.[58] Moreover, the very concept of mental disease has been under severe scientific attack and is now plainly a controversial one.[59] But assume the defendant establishes that addiction is a mental disease. If he is being tried for use, possession, or addiction-related theft, for example, the issue of a lack of understanding is unlikely to arise. If an addict committed an act while under the influence of a drug, any resulting lack of understanding would not suffice to establish the insanity defense; such a lack of understanding would not result from the "disease" of addiction, but from the act of taking the drug. Thus, proof of defective volition would still be necessary; the addict would have to show that he was unable to exert the self-control necessary to refrain from drug use. Use of the insanity defense therefore does not avoid the necessity of showing involuntariness; that proof is only one part of the case such a defendant would have to make.

In summary, the disease argument relies on two assumptions in attempting to exculpate the addict. First, it suggests that his psychological and physiological condition, a pure status, is not punishable; this suggestion is unnecessary because it merely argues the minimalist holding in *Robinson*. Second, it implies that addictive behavior is involuntary. The latter suggestion has been made even more directly in the case law and is explored below.

C. The Involuntariness Argument

While *Robinson* contains only a brief and cryptic allusion to the involuntariness issue,[60] other cases have extended its implications to introduce directly considerations of involuntariness in ways that would seem to exculpate addictive behavior. Sometimes the argument is that the addictive behavior in question is involuntary;[61] sometimes it takes the more complex form that the addictive behavior is the involuntary result of a nonpunishable status.[62] Some forms of the argument use the word "involuntary,"[63] some the term "compulsion,"[64] and some the term "pharmacological duress."[65] Usually the involuntariness is said to extend to nontrafficking use, possession, and purchase; sometimes it is said to extend to behavior such as theft, if motivated by the need for money for a personal supply of the drug.[66] The theme of involuntariness has also been pressed vigorously in connection with addiction to alcohol. The premise proposed in the *Powell* dissent, and in the decisions in similarly inclined cases, is that alcoholism is a disease that is involuntarily and nonculpably caused and maintained.[67] Yet even where courts have doggedly resisted the exculpatory legal implications of these arguments, they often seem to do so without a firm logical basis. This is because, paradoxically, these courts often seem to acquiesce in the fundamental assumption of involuntariness, or at least fail to challenge it.[68]

On its face the involuntariness argument seems to raise a simple question: Does the addict have any control over the behavior motivated by his desire for the drug? To answer this question we must confront a set of deeply rooted myths about drug addiction. The legal issues can be clarified only if they are reviewed against a carefully redrawn picture of the factual background, one that reassesses these myths and stereotypes. In the face of such an analysis the simple picture of the narcotic addict as a slave to the drug disappears. We are left with deeper substantive insight, but also with greater humility, appreciating the extent of our ignorance, the complexity of the problems, and the hopeless inappropriateness of trying to deal with those problems in terms of a blanket concept of involuntariness.

II. THE FACTUAL BACKGROUND

A typical layman's view of drug addiction is dominated by the myth of the addict's slavery: In this view drugs typically associated with drug-dependency have powers such that their repeated use even for a short period will "hook" the user. Once hooked, he will be unable voluntarily to abstain from use thereafter; he will make any sacrifice to get his daily supply. If he fails to obtain a supply of the drug he will undergo excruciating withdrawal suffering. If he is forced to abstain for a period of time—as a result of imprisonment or compulsory hospitalization, for example—he will inevitably relapse into addictive use upon his release.

Greater sophistication will no doubt suggest that such an extreme view needs qualification. But the main substance of the portrait is widely accepted even in more sophisticated circles: indeed, the involuntariness argument presupposes acceptance of the myth for all practical purposes. This acceptance accounts for the widespread failure of the courts to challenge the fundamental assumptions of the argument. This section of the chapter offers such a challenge. It reports a number of basic factual considerations that cast doubt on the accuracy of this portrait of addiction. The discussion focuses on four aspects of drug use that belie this myth: the existence of a population of drug users who do not become addicts, the successful elimination of addictive patterns among formerly addicted groups, the relative rarity of a heavy physiological addiction in addicts in this country, and the correspondingly widespread influence of social and psychological inducements to addictive behavior.

The community's deep concern with the serious social problems associated with addiction undoubtedly focuses attention on those relative few who do take up an addictive pattern of use, thus distracting attention from the larger numbers who use drugs for medical or nonmedical purposes, but who do not take up such a pattern. Narcotics constitute the most effective analgesics (pain relievers) known to medicine, and their use is a widespread and conventional procedure for medical relief of substantial pain.[69] Yet only a small fraction of the many millions of patients who receive morphine ever attempt to take the drug again,[70] and only an exceedingly small proportion of addicts owe their dependence to medically initiated narcotic use.[71] These data alone prove that repeated use of narcotics does not automatically hook users to continued use of the drug.[72] One can make similar comments about the sedatives and tranquilizers; these can and do come to be used addictively, but only by a relative few of the many millions who use such drugs.[73]

Among the minority of drug users who do develop addiction, many give it up.[74] Contrary to widespread skepticism about drug rehabilitation, there has been substantial success in measures to control and eliminate addiction in the United States. Skeptics probably assume that anything less than 100 percent success in achieving total, permanent abstention from narcotics as the result of exposure to any one program is a failure and proof of the hopelessness of the task. This conclusion is unreasonable and misleading. More important than such total successes are the days spent free of drug use and the direction of the trend for a population even though specific individuals may relapse on occasion. Impressive achievement in these latter aspects[75] is often overlooked because attention is focused on the relapse incidents.

A . . . study of Vietnam veterans[76] confirms the notion both that addiction does not always follow drug use and that addiction can be eliminated voluntarily. The Vietnam experience was "a natural experiment in the exposure of masses of young men to narcotic drugs,"[77] barbiturates, amphetamines, and marijuana. Pure forms of heroin and other drugs were easily available, and at low cost. In Vietnam in 1971, "almost every soldier had the opportunity to experiment with heroin and almost all personally knew other soldiers who used heroin with some regularity."[78] In September 1971, the study examined the entire group of 13,240 young Army enlisted men who were then returning from Vietnam. Eight to twelve months later they reexamined this group with regard to drug use during the period following their return. Widespread use was not followed by comparable rates of addiction: Almost half had tried heroin or opium while in Vietnam, but only about 20 percent developed signs of physical or psychological dependence.[79] Where addictive patterns had developed, voluntary nonaddiction upon return home had almost always followed. Although about 20 percent of the total group of 13,240 had shown actual signs of addiction while in Vietnam, only 1 percent of the total experienced such signs at any time after their return to the United States.[80] A number of the ex-addicts among these veterans did use narcotics after their return, but without readdiction. The study concluded:

> These results are surprising not only in that men who report having been addicted in Vietnam so seldom report any addiction in the United States during the 8 to 12 months since their return, but that many of them avoided readdiction *without* completely abstaining from narcotics. The ability of men formerly

dependent on narcotics to use them occasionally without readdiction challenges the common view of narcotic addiction as a chronic and intractable condition.[81]

The phenomenon is not unique to Vietnam veterans.[82] The nature of drug dependency in this country further belies the myth of addict slavery to drugs. It is highly unlikely that much physiological addiction exists in the United States. Drugs sold illegally are usually highly adulterated. In one survey of street drugs in New York, 10 percent of the purchases contained no active ingredient whatever, and it has been estimated that illegally purchased bags of heroin typically range from 1 percent to 5 percent active material.[83] Thus, if we look solely at the chemical factors involved in drug addiction in this country, we find that the addict's strictly physiological dependence is at most moderate and very often quite mild in degree.[84]

On the other hand, the social inducements to adopt addictive patterns of behavior are often maximal. A very large proportion of new addicts in the United States today are young, psychologically immature, occupationally unskilled, socially uprooted, poor, and disadvantaged. Many engaged in crime before they were addicted.[85] The myth of the addict as a helpless slave to his habit only lends further strength to the inducements for addicts to continue addictive patterns. It provides such persons with a rationale for ignoring alternatives to crime and the drug culture. Young people who are disadvantaged, and alienated, may find the foundation of a socially authenticated identity in addiction. For such persons, drug use provides at last a "constructive" focal activity in life, generating its own occupational responsibilities, opportunities for success and achievement, social status, and ideological, philosophical, or religious meaning.[86] The "hustling" required by drug addiction is not always a burden[87] or a separation from a socially productive life; for certain groups it may be one natural outgrowth of the values of an alienated subculture, values that are by definition inconsistent with those of the dominant society.[88] When some writers characterize the addict as one who will seek the drug at "great risk"[89] or "at the cost of unbelievable sacrifices,"[90] the sacrifice in question may be one of values important only to the writer and not to the addict.[91] A person who has developed roots in conventional society and skills for leading a productive life is substantially less likely to find a meaningful social identity in the drug culture, and such a person can more readily abandon addiction once it develops.[92]

Because addiction in this country has far deeper social roots than physiological ones, judicious use of sanctions and threats of sanctions, especially if coupled with suitable constructive aid, can be an effective tool in deterring addicts from continuing drug use. Such sanctions may be rooted in the powers of the criminal law; they often are under present policies (e.g., revocation of parole, use of prison sentences).[93] Sanctions and aid may also be rooted in other values and institutions—for example, in personal freedom, work, or family.[94] What is essential, however, is that the addict perceive both the sanctions and the aid in terms of his own values.[95]

III. THEORIES OF DRUG ADDICTION

In light of the preceding factual discussion, we now turn to a discussion of the main types of hypotheses used to explain addictive drug use and to prove its involuntary nature. There are basically two types: one explains addiction in terms of physiology, the other in terms of psychology. It might be sufficient response simply to point out that there is no generally accepted scientific explanation of addiction,[96] and perforce no scientific basis for establishing that addictive behavior is generally involuntary. But if we are to dissolve the myths that dominate this field, we must go beyond this generalization and examine specific types of explanations that promote them.

The first type of hypothesis is a qualified version of the simple theory that mere use of a narcotic drug inevitably causes addiction in all persons. According to this hypothesis, the physiological effects of the drug interact with a biological, possibly genetically determined, sensitivity found only in a certain subgroup of all users; for this special subgroup the physiological impact of the drug suffices to produce an addictive pattern of conduct.[97]

As a scientific or empirical claim, this type of hypothesis is speculative, neither substantiated by medical evidence nor supported by medical consensus;[98] it hardly warrants reshaping constitutional or common law doctrine. But even if these hypotheses were substantiated to some extent, it is unlikely that such a biological predisposition could account for a significant portion of drug-related conduct. Biological signs indicate that many of those who demonstrate full-blown, extreme drug-addict patterns of conduct are, at most, only moderately physically dependent. Common addictive patterns of conduct exist in which the known biological after-effects of the particular drug used are minimal or nil.[99] It is empirically implausible, in the absence of strong independent evidence, that a physiological influence so slight, even if related to unique bodily predisposition, should absolutely and irresistibly transform a whole way of life. A conceptual incongruity also pervades this type of hypothesis, an incongruity in kind between the supposed biological cause and its supposed behavioral effects. There are, of course, instances where a particular physiological process or directly associated feeling may seem to produce an automatic behavior-response. It seems plausible, for example, that intractable and overwhelming pain, or the last extreme of exhaustion or of hunger, may lead to a kind of immediate, instinctive reflex, an uncontrollable sound or gesture. Yet even in such cases, the notion that this reaction is a direct behavioral effect of a physiological cause, that the mind can play no significant role in mediating the behavior, may be factually incorrect. The biological drive of hunger can be influenced by cultural and psychological factors. Indeed, eating can be suspended altogether to the point of death by the mediation of mind, either by a voluntary hunger strike or by neurotic loss of appetite. Recent medical research has dramatically revealed how much even our extreme pain-distress reactions are psychological rather than direct physical response.[100]

Yet even if one accepts the image of an automatic and involuntary behavioral response to a specific physiological drive, this very limited range of behavior does not constitute the kind of response that could account intelligibly and fully for the typically elaborate addictive lifestyle. A pattern of conduct must be distinguished from a mere sequence of reflex-like reactions. A reflex knee jerk is not conduct. If we regard something as a pattern of conduct, whether criminal or not, we assume that it is mediated by the mind, that it reflects consideration of reasons and preferences, the election of a preferred means to the end, and the election of the end itself from among alternatives. The complex, purposeful, and often ingenious projects with which many an addict may be occupied in his daily hustling to maintain his drug supply are examples of conduct, not automatic reflex reactions to a single biological cause.[101]

Nothing in the preceding is intended to deny that chemical predisposition or other biological causes may be some among a number of factors significantly influencing addictive patterns of conduct. But even if such causal factors were shown to exist, it would be implausible to expect that they would be sufficient to resolve the question of the legal voluntariness of the various kinds of conduct in which addicts engage. One must conclude that there is no substantiated biological explanation of drug addiction nor is there a reasonable hope that further research in this area could settle the questions of law concerning the voluntariness of addictive conduct and ways of life.

It is therefore necessary to turn to theories that would explain addictive conduct by introducing psychological considerations: theories of motivation, learning, or conditioning, or of personality structure and mental pathology. We turn first to theories based on motivation. These explanations of addictive conduct assume that either the drug-induced euphoria or the addict's withdrawal stress or both provide mentally overpowering motives for addictive behavior.[102]

Some would emphasize that either the experience of withdrawal stress or the fear of it can serve as an absolutely overriding motive[103] for continuing addictive patterns of conduct. Immediate total abstention from drugs, especially in heavy narcotic users, can be associated with a temporary but intensely distressing reaction that includes chills, muscle twitching, vomiting, diarrhea, and general debility. But "cold turkey" withdrawal from narcotics, in and of itself, is apparently never fatal; it is temporary, continuing at its worst for no more than several days.[104] Moreover, since most addicts are not heavily addicted physiologically, the reaction is not nearly so severe.[105] For the moderately addicted, it is comparable to a bad case of flu.[106] It is not uncommon for young people who think themselves heavily addicted to find that they can withdraw, "cold turkey," with only minimal discomfort.[107] And drugs associated with addictive conduct do not always produce withdrawal stress.[108] Most important, there is no need for "cold turkey" withdrawal. The standard, gradual withdrawal procedures used under professional care keep narcotic withdrawal discomfort to a quite moderate and readily bearable level.[109]

Furthermore, it is well established that withdrawal symptoms (as well as the effects of drug use) are mediated to a great degree by mental attitudes.[110] Not only can the intensity and stress of symptoms vary greatly with changes in the addict's state of mind and the social-psychological setting, they can even be made to appear and disappear with changes in setting or circumstance.[111] Drug dependence facilities take advantage of this fact: Increasing numbers of lay groups, therapeutic communities, and medical and social welfare agencies provide a variety of withdrawal and post-care settings in which the medical, social, and moral support is maximal.[112]

This discussion suggests that the experience or fear of drug withdrawal cannot render addictive conduct legally involuntary. The criminal law demands that citizens refrain from criminal conduct even at the cost of temporary moderate personal discomfort; fear of such discomfort alone could neither establish a criminal law defense nor an absence of *mens rea* on the ground of involuntariness. Thus arguments for defenses such as "pharmacological coercion"[113] due to drug addiction are fatally flawed. Such arguments implicitly reveal profound factual misapprehensions about the assumed horrors of withdrawal symptoms. The common law defense of coercion requires a showing of reasonable fear of imminent mortal or grave bodily injury;[114] only if one erroneously equates the narcotic addict's withdrawal stress with these dangers could a defense like pharmacological coercion have any legal force.

Moreover, if courts were to make this erroneous equation they would only encourage addictive conduct by validating the myth that withdrawal stress is an agony to be avoided at any cost; the myth often influences addicts themselves.[115] The belief in the myth of addict-slavery can encourage addicts to surrender to, and even to embrace, their "destiny" as hapless victims.[116] This attitude can provide a dimension of drama in a formerly drab or frustrating life. Such a belief and attitude, often reinforcing counterculture values, provide a rationale for pursuing a life of crime as a member of an addict culture.[117]

Euphoria is another important effect of drug use that many believe provides a principal motive for addiction.[118] It is obvious that in settings other than addiction prospective euphoria is not a motive that will normally serve to excuse criminal conduct. But one might argue that anticipation of euphoria in the case of drug addiction could be so intense that it could be shown to be overpowering to the point where it negates voluntariness in the criminal law. Even if one strains to entertain the logic of this argument, the facts are otherwise. The narcotic addict typically does not reach or anticipate reaching such an intense level of pleasure. Most addicts in this country cannot amass the money, even through a life of active crime, to buy the quantity of narcotics needed to achieve this kind of euphoria regularly. The "rush," which may be more common at stages of early use, becomes increasingly rare with the development of tolerance to the drug.[119] Thus a legal defense based on ecstatic drug euphoria would simply have no basis in fact. Nor could the prospect of the loss of tranquil euphoria associated with routine drug use preclude criminal liability for addictive conduct; presumably this motive would be even less overwhelming.[120]

Human beings respond to conditioning that influences complex forms of learning. Conditioning and habit-learning can operate without the necessity for (at times with hardly an opportunity for) conscious motivation or reflective choice or will. Could addiction be a form of conditioned or learned "automatic" response that overrides the conscious will? There is no empirical proof that simple pleasure conditioning or positive reinforcement in operant conditioning can of itself determine a whole way of life.[121] Of course a person may learn to alleviate certain discomforts by the use of a tranquilizing drug such as heroin that has short run, immediate effectiveness. That person may then develop a strong, habitual propensity to respond to subsequent discomfort this way. In the absence of strong countermotives, such as a commitment to law or to other cultural values reflected in it, a person who has been positively conditioned to desire and use a drug might indulge this desire persistently, in spite of the illegality of the conduct necessary to do so. But is it plausible that a person who has genuine, urgent contrary values and commitments would find it impossible either to inhibit such a conditioned or learned behavioral response, to substitute another, or at least to take steps that would indirectly bring about extinction of the learned or conditioned response? The availability of any of these measures[122] could establish the legal voluntariness of his drug use. The fact is that there is no independent empirical evidence or generally accepted scientific theory that warrants an assertion that human beings can be conditioned to the point where these options cease to exist. Theories along these lines remain highly speculative and controversial.[123]

Yet another group of psychological hypotheses are based on claims of psychiatric derivation. According to the arguments, whereas mentally healthy persons do not allow the pleasure, fears, or learning associated with drug use to become imperative or paramount in their lives, the addict is psychologically vulnerable. He suffers from "mental illness," "personality defect," "character disorder," or psychic "compulsion." In response to these arguments, one might point to the problems and inadequacies in invoking a generalized concept of disease (including mental illness) that were discussed in an earlier section; we deal here with more specific descriptions of mental illness and how they may relate to the criminal law.[124]

For example, one writer reports that a large portion of addicts suffer from "some form of personality disturbance, . . . [an illness often] manifested by a pattern of antisocial behavior, rather than by observable mental symptoms."[125] This concept of personality disturbance does little to distinguish the addict from other persons who have a tendency to get into difficulties with the law and with their neighbors and who often manifest no discernible mental abnormalities. Nor is it a helpful means of distinguishing addictive disorders to note that addicts manifest personal failings of the sort found in the general population: "The majority of addicts . . . do not fall into clear-cut nosological entities, but rather present mixtures of traits of the kind found in neuroses, character [personality] disorders, and inadequate personalities."[126]

The psychiatric concept of "compulsion" is perhaps the most widely accepted basis for an implicit argument that the addict's conduct is involuntary.[127] The term means something different in psychiatric usage than it does in criminal law. In criminal law "compulsion" designates what is conceptually and observationally quite simple in common sense terms: Either there is an exterior physical force greater than the person's physical strength to resist, or, if one considers coercion to be a form of compulsion, there is a plain and imminent threat by another person to do grave bodily injury or even mortal harm unless the victim acquiesces.[128] In psychiatric usage the term means neither of these things, but it does have several other meanings that cannot accurately be used to describe addictive behavior.

Being "compelled" is often regarded as the result of tensions among psychic energies or psychic forces within the individual.[129] In the latter usage, the psychic forces behind the addict's propensity to use the drug are presumed to be quantitatively stronger than any contrary forces. However, they are presumed stronger not because they have been independently measured, but because the theory, post facto, merely interprets in those terms the fact that the person engages in the repetitive conduct rather than inhibits it. In this usage, compulsion is a speculative theoretical construct about human behavior generally rather than a scientifically discovered, distinctive feature of the individual defendant's behavior.[130]

"Compulsion" may also be used in a more specific, descriptive sense in psychiatry to refer to "an insistent, repetitive, intrusive, and unwanted urge to perform an act which is contrary to the person's ordinary conscious wishes or standards."[131] This characteristic definition cannot apply generally to addictive conduct, however, since the drug and the life are often consciously and wholeheartedly "wanted."[132] Sometimes, however, psychiatrists define "compulsion" as an urge that *cannot* be inhibited.[133] But on what grounds and in what sense can one say that the addict cannot inhibit the impulse? Only two grounds are ever offered: (a) the observation that the addict does continue to use the drug in spite of attempts to threaten and persuade;[134] and (b) the theory of the balance of conflicting psychic forces; as noted above, it hypothesizes that the urge that wins out must therefore have been the strongest. But the latter explanation is only a restatement, in the terms of the theory, of the observed fact that the individual does persist.[135] Neither formulation is an independent scientific determination that the individual does so because he *must*.

Moreover, the question of legal voluntariness cannot be resolved until we know, at least, whether the addict had the option of taking some preventive measure that would have either eliminated the compulsive urge or restrained him from satisfying it. These and other legally essential questions are lost when courts employ too readily the psychiatric term; such questions are simply irrelevant in the psychiatric use of "compulsive."[136] Indeed, psychiatrists themselves recognize that the logical relation between the concepts of "psychic forces" in psychiatry and "will" and "choice" in the law remains unclear.[137] How, then, can the psychiatric formulations of "compulsion" warrant the creation of legal doctrine that labels addictive conduct involuntary?

In the scientifically perplexing context of addiction, all these concepts of mental disorder are mere vague rubrics. They obscure our vast ignorance in this area by imparting an aura of scientific knowledge because of their technical appearance. At most they merely obfuscate familiar facts: When we talk about "addicts," we often have in mind persons with an intense commitment, one that seems unreasonable and excessive, to a pattern of life centering on drug use.

CONCLUSION

In spite of a vast literature, professionals in the field of drug addiction acknowledge that no satisfactory scientific understanding of drug addiction has been reached. Thus there is no medical foundation for adopting the general proposition at the crux of the exculpatory legal arguments, the proposition that addictive conduct is involuntary. On the other hand, massive descriptive evidence indicates that individuals often make choices to abandon addictive conduct or abstain from drug use permanently or temporarily. Moreover, authorities observe that narcotic addiction often involves little in the way of chemical or biological influences. Yet it may provide an important individual or group identity for many who lack socially approved skills or are socially alienated. Popular beliefs about the chemically induced hell of withdrawal agony or the insatiable craving for ecstatic pleasures are profoundly at odds with the facts, though they have deeply colored the thinking of the courts. All this information forces abandonment of the argument that drug addiction—and acts associated with it—be regarded as legally involuntary.

Once we conclude that addictive conduct is legally voluntary, however, we do not express a basic substantive insight into addiction, but merely free ourselves from a false idea. Courtroom cliche has obscured the fact that the problems at issue concern intricate and poorly understood relationships that link character, personality, and mind to upbringing, social setting, and cultural values, and in turn to biochemical and neuropsychological processes. Indeed, courts have been ill-served by those psychiatrists who have promoted the notion that addiction is involuntary and who have seen this notion as a legal formula that will permit medical models to supersede the use of criminal sanctions.[138] The very complexity of the problem calls for legislative determinations concerning rehabilitation; regulation of drug trafficking,[139] and the general administration of criminal law in this area.[140]

Undoubtedly there are those who regard possible legal approaches to addiction in polar terms: Either we inflict harsh, punitive, and degrading measures on the addict, or we declare the person sick and therefore not responsible for his conduct. What is needed here is the abandonment of such extreme and fixed positions.[141] In the present antipunitive atmosphere in many enlightened circles, it is appropriate to recall that the lawful and proper threat of sanctions may be not only a pragmatically effective approach,[142] but also a morally humane approach. It regards the addict as an autonomous person, responsible for guiding his own life, and subject to law.[143] The medical approach can also reflect a humane concern, a concern for the weak and ailing and for those who cannot, in some respects, handle their own lives. By now it is no news that both of these approaches, however inspired, can in practice disregard human dignity when ignorance, social prejudice, well-intentioned dogma, lack of funding, or routinization take over. We need to rethink the implications of both approaches against the background of the limited knowledge that we have. Coordinating the attack on the complex problem of drug abuse is preeminently a legislative responsibility. For the courts to assume that addictive drug use or addiction-related conduct is involuntary and to build such an unworthy assumption into constitutional and common law doctrine would be a grave error.

NOTES

1. 370 U.S. 660 (1962).
2. Ibid., pp. 666–67.
3. *Powell* v. *Texas,* 392 U.S. 514 (1968): *People* v. *Zapata,* 220 Cal. App. 2d 903, 34 Cal. Rptr. 171 (1963), *appeal dismissed for lack of juris.,* 377 U.S. 406 (1964) *State* v. *Margo,* 40 N.J. 188, 191 A.2d 43 (1963).
4. 370 U.S. p. 679 (Harlan, J., concurring).
5. *Powell* v. *Texas,* 392 U.S. 514, 543 (1968) (Black, J., concurring).
6. *United States* v. *Rundle,* 429 F.2d 1316 (3d Cir. 1970) (per curiam) (conviction for unlawful use of drugs is not punishment for addiction): *Bailey* v. *United States,* 386 F.2d 1 (5th Cir. 1967) (no error in refusal to charge that addiction is disease creating compulsion under which defendant is not criminally responsible): *United States ex rel. Swanson* v. *Reincke,* 344 F.2d 260 2d Cir.), *cert. denied,* 582 U.S. 869 (1965) (statute prohibiting self-administration of narcotic drugs held constitutional); *People* v. *Zapata,* 200 Cal. App. 2d 903 34 Cal. Rptr. 171

(1963), *appeal dismissed for lack of juris.*, 377 U.S. 406 (1964) (imprisonment for possession of heroin for personal use not cruel and unusual punishment); *Nutter v. State*, 8 Md. App. 635, 262 A.2d 80 (1970) (addicts may be criminals because responsible for acts such as possession and control of a narcotic drug which are crimes even though they stem from the addiction); *People v. Borrero*, 19 N.Y.2d 332, 227 N.E.2d 18, 280 N.Y.S.2d 109 (1967) (penal sanction applied to addicts who committed crimes solely to procure money to purchase drugs not cruel and unusual punishment); *State v. Margo*, 40 N.J. 188, 191 A.2d 43 (1963) (punishment for being "under the influence" of narcotic, as distinguished from act of using drug, not cruel and unusual punishment); *Rengel v. State*, 444 S.W.2d 924 (Tex. Crim. App. 1989) (no error to refuse to instruct jury to render verdict of not guilty of possession of narcotics merely because appellant was admitted and known addict). See *Powell v. Texas*, 392 U.S. 514 (1968); *United States v. Moore*, 486 F.2d 1139 (D.C. Cir.), *cert. denied*, 414 U.S. 980 (1973).

7. The term is used here to mean immunity from criminal liability either on the ground that *mens rea** is absent or on the ground that addiction functions as a defense. Whether exculpation takes the former or the latter form is undoubtedly significant both in terms of litigation strategy and in terms of the consequences of a finding of "not guilty." See Goldstein and Katz, "Abolish the "Insanity Defense—Why Not?" 72 *Yale Law Journal* 853 (1963). Such discussion, however, is beyond the scope of this article.

8. *Powell v. Texas*, 392 U.S. 514, 554 (1968) (Fortas, J., dissenting) *United States v. Moore*, 486 F.2d 1139, 1236 (D.C. Cir.), *cert. denied*, 414 U.S. 980 (1973) (vacation of sentence, but not exculpation, for narcotic addict convicted under federal statute for possession of narcotics) (Wright, J., dissenting); *United States v. Carter*, 436 F.2d 200 (D.C. Cir. 1970) (conviction upheld where substantial testimony that defendant's alleged mental illness and narcotic addiction not causally connected with commission of robbery and assault) (Bazelon, C.J., concurring); *Watson v. United States*, 439 F.2d 442 (D.C. Cir. 1970) (insanity plea issue properly submitted to jury where plea made by narcotics addict); *Easter v. District of Columbia*, 361 F.2d 50 (D.C. Cir. 1966) (chronic alcoholism resulting in public intoxication not a crime; holding severely limited by *Powell v. Texas*, above); *Driver v. Hinnant*, 356 F.2d 761 (4th Cir. 1966) (statute punishing public drunkenness could not be applied to chronic alcoholic; holding severely limited by *Powell v. Texas*, above); *Hutcherson v. United States*, 345 F.2d 964, 971 (D.C. Cir.), *cert. denied*, 382 U.S. 894 (1965) (ten-year sentence for heroin addict convicted of narcotic trafficking not cruel and unusual punishment) (Bazelon, C.J., concurring in part and dissenting in part); *Lloyd v. United States*, 343 F.2d 242, 243 (D.C. Cir.), *cert. denied*, 381 U.S. 952 (1964) (denial of petition for rehearing for addict convicted for sale of narcotics) (Bazelon, C.J., dissenting); *United States v. Lindsey*, 524 F. Supp. 55, 59–60 (D.D.C. 1971) (defendant unable to show inability to abstain from narcotic drugs which would eliminate *mens rea* for nontrafficking possession of narcotic drug); *United States v. Ashton*, 317 F. Supp. 860 (D.D.C. 1970) (no liability for addict's nontrafficking possession of drugs); *People v. Malloy*, 58 Misc. 2d 538, 296 N.Y.S.2d 259 (Crim. Ct. 1968) (cruel and unusual punishment to charge certified addict with felony of escape when he is voluntarily incarcerated under valid civil commitment order for treatment).

9. See *Watson v. United States*, 459 F.2d 442, 475 (D.C. Cir. 1970) (McGowan, J.).

10. See *Powell v. Texas*, 392 U.S. 514, 567 (1965) (Fortas, J., dissenting); *Easter v. District of Columbia*, 361 F.2d 50 (D.C. Cir. 1966) (holding severely limited by *Powell v. Texas*, above); *Driver v. Hinnant*, 356 F.2d 761, 764-65 (4th Cir. 1966) (holding severely limited by *Powell v. Texas*, above).

11. Most of the debate has focused on nontrafficking use, purchase, and possession. At one end of the spectrum a state court held that *Robinson v. California*, 370 U.S. 660 (1962), did not even cover an addict's "being under the influence" of the drug. *State v. Margo*, 40 N.J. 188, 191 A.2d 431 (1963). At the other end, Judge Bazelon has argued for immunity on the

---

*That is, a guilty mind, referring here to criminal intent. (Ed.)

broadest grounds. *United States* v. *Carter,* 430 F.2d 200, 202 (D.C. Cir. 1970) (Bazelon, C.J., concurring). For a direct expression of disagreement among those who would extend the scope of *Robinson* v. *California,* above, compare *United States* v. *Moore,* 486 F.2d 1159, 1260 (D.C. Cir. 1973) (Bazelon, C.J., concurring in part and dissenting in part), with 486 F.2d at 1236 (Wright, J., dissenting).

The extensive case law debates over *Robinson* are paralleled by extensive discussion in journal literature. Amsterdam, "Federal Constitutional Restrictions on the Punishment of Crimes of Status, Crimes of General Obnoxiousness, Crimes of Displeasing Police Officers, and the Like," *Criminal Law Bulletin* 3 (1967): 205; Cuomo, "*Mens Rea* and States Criminality," *Southern California Law Review* 40 (1967): 463; Dubin, "*Mens Rea* Reconsidered: A Plea for a Due Process Concept of Criminal Responsibility," *Stanford Law Review* 18 (1966): 322; McKevitt, "The 'Untouchable' Acts of Addiction," *A.B.A. Journal* 55 (1969): 454; McMorris, "Can We Punish for the Acts of Addiction?" *A.B.A. Journal* 54 (1968): 1081, Note, "Criminal Law: Demise of 'Status'—'Act' Distinction in Symptomatic Crimes of Narcotic Addiction," *Duke Law Journal* (1970): 1053; Note, "The Cruel and Unusual Punishment Clause and the Substantive Criminal Law," *Harvard Law Review* 79 (1966): 635; Note, "Punishment of Narcotics Addicts for Possession: A Cruel but Usual Punishment," *Iowa Law Review* 56 (1971): 578. Legal commentators generally approve extension beyond the minimalist reading of *Robinson* to provide immunity from criminal punishment at least for the addict's nontrafficking use, possession, and purchase of the drug.

12. 392 U.S. 514 (1968).

13. Ibid., p. 584 (Fortes, J., dissenting, joined by Douglas, Brennan, and Stewart, JJ.).

14. Ibid., p. 514 (Marshall, J., joined by Warren, C.J., and Black and Harlan, JJ.).

15. Ibid., pp. 552–54 (White, J., concurring).

See *In re Foss,* 10 Cal. 3d 910, 519 P.2d 1073, 112 Cal. Rptr. 649 (1974) (cruel and unusual punishment to prohibit consideration of parole for a minimum period of ten years where addict convicted of furnishing heroin had a record of a prior heroin possession conviction). The court noted that, although statutes providing for increased penalties for habitual offenders are generally justified, in the case of the addict one must take into account the fact that the *repetition* of drug offenses may be "attributable solely to a psychological and/or physiological compulsion arising from an addiction." Ibid., p. 916, 519 P.2d at 1079, 112 Cal. Rptr. p. 656. The court notes that the penalty it strikes down falls somewhere between sanctions for status prohibited under *Robinson,* and the sanctions for overt acts that result from addiction, permissible under *Powell* v. *Texas,* 392 U.S. 514 (1968). Foss, apparently, can be punished for his second offense, since it was an "overt act," but not for the fact that it is a *second* offense, since *that* was a result of a "compulsion" due to nonpunishable addict status! The distinctions generated by *Robinson* and *Powell* are thus so strained as to substitute metaphysics for matter in order to reach exculpatory ends.

16. 439 F.2d 442, 452-53 (D.C. Cir. 1970).

17. *United States* v. *Moore,* 486 F.2d 1139 (D.C. Cir.), *cert. denied,* 414 U.S. 980 (1973).

18. Ibid., p. 1159 (Leventhal, J., concurring, joined by McGowan, J.).

19. Unless otherwise indicated, I will be discussing narcotic addiction as an example of the most acute addiction problem from the standpoint of the power of the craving and the consequent intensity and persistence of the quest to obtain and use the drug. For a discussion with similar conclusions in relation to alcohol, see Fingarette, "The Perils of Powell: In Search of a Factual Foundation for the 'Disease Concept of Alcoholism,' " *Harvard Law Review* 83 (1970): 793. I shall only occasionally comment specifically on other forms of addiction (e.g., those involving barbiturates, amphetamines, tobacco, and tranquilizers), although I maintain that, so far as the criminal law is concerned, the principal theses of this article and of the 1970 article, apply to all forms of conduct generally collected under the rubric "addiction." For concise and authoritative standard descriptions of the various types of addictions, see Eddy, Hal-

bach, Isbell, and Seevers, "Drug Dependence: Its Significance and Characteristics," *Bulletin of the World Health Organization* 32 (1965): 721; DeLong, "The Drugs and Their Effects," in *Dealing with Drug Abuse: A Report to the Ford Foundation* 62 (Staff Paper No. 1) (1972) [hereinafter cited as *Dealing*].

20. 370 U.S. 660, 666 (1972). The trial judge made a similar distinction in instructing the jury: He noted that addiction which the statute made a criminal offense, was a "condition" or "status" while the "use" of the narcotic was an "act." Unlike the act of using a narcotic, said the judge, the status of being an addict is a "chronic" offense that "continue[s] after it is complete." Ibid., p. 662.

21. Ibid., p. 667.

22. Ibid., pp. 666–67.

23. See pp. 309–12 below.

24. See generally Amsterdam, "Federal Constitutional Restructions on the Punishment of Crimes of Status," Cuomo, "*Mens Rea* and Status Criminality"; Lacey, "Vagrancy and Other Crimes of Personal Condition," *Harvard Law Review* 66 (1953): 1203.

Vagrancy, for example, is often characterized as a crime of status although a number of vagrancy statutes have been struck down for vagueness in defining the status, nowhere has the claim been accepted that vagrancy is immune simply because it is a status. See *Papachristou* v. *City of Jacksonville,* 405 U.S. 156 (1972); *Edelman* v. *California,* 344 U.S. 357 (1953).

25. Amsterdam's exhaustive 1967 survey notes that the questions as to how to construe *Robinson* with regard to status crimes have not even yet been structured. Amsterdam, "Federal Constitutional Restrictions on the Punishment of Crimes of Status," p. 240.

26. *Powell* v. *Texas,* 592 U.S. 514, 543 (1973) (Black, J., concurring). Justice Black notes that this requirement applies even for "offenses most heavily based on propensity, such as attempt, conspiracy, and recidivist crimes." See G. Williams, *Criminal Law: The General Part 1* (1961). In *Papachristou* v. *City of Jacksonville,* 405 U.S. 156, 170 (1972), Justice Douglas's majority opinion quotes with approval an English opinion, Frederick Dean, 18 Crim. App. 133, 134 (1924), that disapproves prosecution and conviction under the Vagrancy Act where there would not be enough evidence to charge the prisoner with an attempt to commit a crime. Lacey, "Vacrancy and Other Crimes of Personal Condition," p. 1204, finds that many statutes defining status crimes contain no reference to acts. But he acknowledges that in cases such as "common thief" status, one can argue that "evidence of past conduct is necessary." In analyzing these statutes it would seem clearer to distinguish between the *status* (admittedly not itself conduct) and an *implicit reference* to conduct necessarily made because proof of conduct is essential to prove the existence of the status.

27. 370 U.S. at 666.

28. 392 U.S. at 533.

29. In these cases "status" includes no more than the mere physical and mental state associated with desire. *United States* v. *Rundle,* 425 F.2d 1316 (3d Cir. 1970), *Bailey* v. *United States,* 386 F.2d 1 (5th Cir. 1967), *United States ex rel. Swanson* v. *Reincke,* 344 F.2d 260 (2d Cir.), *cert. denied,* 382 U.S. 869 (1965), *People* v. *Zapata,* 220 Cal. App. 2d 903, 34 Cal. Rptr. 171 (1963), *appeal dismissed for lack of juris.,* 377 U.S. 406 (1964) *Nutter* v. *State,* 8 Md. App. 635, 262 A.2d 80 (1970), *State* v. *Margo,* 40 N.J. 188, 191 A.2d 43 (1963); *People* v. *Borrero,* 19 N.Y.2d 332, 227 N.E.2d 18, 280 N.Y.S.2d 109 (1967): *Rengel* v. *State,* 444 S.W.2d 924 (Tex. Crim. App. 1969). But see the following cases and opinions which challenge this use of "status" by arguing either that certain addictive conduct inevitably and involuntarily flows from this immune addictive status or is indeed a part of the status itself: *Powell* v. *Texas,* 392 U.S. 514, 554 (1968) (Fortas, J., dissenting; *Watson* v. *United States,* 439 F.2d 442 (D.C. Cir. 1970); *United States* v. *Carter,* 436 F.2d 200, 243 (D.C. Cir. 1970) (Bazelon, C.J., concurring). *Easter* v. *District of Columbia* 361 F.2d 50 (D.C. Cir. 1966); *Driver* v. *Hinnant,* 356 F.2d 761 (4th Cir. 1966); *Hutcherson* v. *United States,* 345 F.2d 964, 971 (D.C. Cir.) (Bazelon, C.J., concurring

in part, dissenting in part), *cert. denied,* 382 U.S. 894 (1965), *Lloyd* v. *United States* 343 F.2d 242 243 (D.C. Cir.) (Bazelon, C.J., dissenting), *cert. denied,* 381 U.S. 952 (1964), *United States* v. *Lindsey,* 324 F. Supp. 55 (D.D.C. 1971); *United States* v. *Ashton,* 317 F. Supp. 860 (D.D.C 1970); *People* v. *Malloy,* 58 Misc. 2d 538, 296 N.Y.S.2d 259 (Crim. Ct. 1968).

    30. *Robinson* v. *California,* 370 U.S. 660, 662 (1962).

    31. *Watson* v. *United States,* 439 F.2d 442, 475 (D.C Cir. 1970) (McGowan, J.). See *Robinson* v. *California,* 370 U.S. 660, 686 (1962) (White, J., dissenting).

    32. 370 U.S. 650, 667 & n.8, citing *Linder* v. *United States,* 268 U.S. 5, 18 (1925).

    33. 370 U.S. at 674, 676.

    34. Ibid., pp. 681, 683, 680. However, Justice Clark insists that the issue which ought to be central is the voluntary quality of the addiction.

    35. But see *United States* v. *Brawner,* 471 F.2d 969, 1010 (D.C Cir. 1972) (Bazelon, C.J., dissenting).

    36. *Watson* v. *United States,* 439 F.2d 442, 470 (D.C. Cir. 1970) (Bazelon, C.J.) (appendix to rehearing en banc).

    37. *Powell* v. *Texas,* 392 U.S. 514, 569 (1968) (Fortas, J., dissenting) (quoting findings of the trial judge with approval). Compare *Marshall* v. *United States,* 414 U.S. 417, 433 (1974) (Marshall, J.) with *Powell* v. *Texas,* 392 U.S. 514, 526 (1968) (Marshall, J.).

    38. *Watson* v. *United States,* 459 F.2d 442, 470 (D.C. Cir. 1970) (Bazelon, C.J.) (appendix to rehearing en banc).

    39. Although Jellinek, one of the greatest authorities on alcoholism, defends the claim that "alcoholism is a disease," he admits that the proposition reflects a labeling decision rather than a discovery of fact: "[A] disease is what the medical profession recognizes as such." The term "disease" is a highly general, handy rubric, not itself the direct subject of any scientific demonstration. E. Jellinek, *The Disease Concept of Alcoholism* (New Haven: Hillhouse Press, 1960), p. 12. For a discussion of "disease" as it has been used in relation to alcohol addiction, see Fingarette, "The Perils of Powell."

    Meehl stresses that even in neurology and internal medicine, "there is actually no clearly formulable disease-entity model." Meehl, "Specific Genetic Etiology: Psychodynamic and Therapeutic Nihilism," *International Journal of Mental Health* (Spring–Summer 1972): 10, 20. Typical of innumerable medical texts as well as lists of nomenclature is E. Thompson and A. Hayden, *Standard Nomenclature of Disease and Operations,* 5th ed. (New York: Published for the American Medical Association [by] Blakiston Division, McGraw Hill, 1961), which uses the word "disease" as a general rubric but nowhere defines or explains it. The terminological difficulty is not overcome by shifting to the phrase "mental disease." Challenges to the use of this term are widespread both within and without the medical profession. See generally H. Fingarette, *The Meaning of Criminal Insanity* (1972), pp. 19–52.

    40. Stedman's *Medical Dictionary,* 22d ed. (Baltimore: Wiliams and Wilkins, 1972) defines "disease" as: "illness, sickness, an interruption, cessation or disorder of body functions, systems, or organs," or "[a] disease entity, characterized usually by at least two of these criteria: a recognized etiologic agent (or agents); an identifiable group of signs and symptoms; consistent anatomical alterations; caused by specific micro-organismic alterations" McHugh, "Psychologic Illness in Medical Practice," in *Textbook of Medicine* 3d ed. (P. Beeson and W. McDermott eds., 1971), p. 107, states: "The term 'disease' is difficult to define. . . . It is intended to convey the idea that among all the morbid changes in physical and mental health it is possible to recognize groups of abnormalities as distinct entities or syndromes separable from one another and from the normal and that these separations *will prove to have* some biologic explanation when the entities have been thoroughly investigated" (emphasis added). *Taber's Cyclopedic Medical Dictionary,* 12th ed. (Chicago: C. W. Tabor, 1973), p. D47, defines "disease" as: "a pathological condition of the body that presents a group of symptoms peculiar to it and which sets the condition apart as an abnormal entity differing from other normal or pathological body states." Those in the medical

profession tend to use the word "disease" even where they do not yet know the biological basis (if any) of the "disease entity"; they will do so because they assume that one exists. Similar use of the term in relation to addiction avoids some crucial legal questions. See pp. 316–19.

41. Jaffe, "Drug Addiction and Drug Abuse," in *Pharmacological Basis of Therapeutics,* eds. L. Goodman and A. Gilman, 3d ed. (New York: Macmillan, 1965), pp. 285, 286.

42. Experts in the field now avoid the term "'addiction." DeLong, "Drugs and Their Effects," p. 82. For a brief review of these definitional inadequacies, see Lewis, "Introduction: Definitions and Perspectives, in *Scientific Basis of Drug Dependence,* ed. H. Steinberg (New York: Grune and Stratton, 1969) [hereinafter cited as *Basis of Drug Dependence*]. For a fuller review, see National Commission Marijuana and Drug-Abuse, *Drug Use in America: Problem in Perspective* 120–40 (2d Rep. 1975) [hereinafter cited as *Drug America*]. See generally Eddy, Halbach, Isbell, and Seevers, "Drug Dependence," p. 721.

In 1964 the World Health Organization (WHO) formally abandoned the term "addiction" and began to develop a more complex terminology. WHO Expert Committee on Addiction-Producing Drugs, *Report No. 13* [(Tech. Rep. Ser. No. 273, 1964) hereinafter cited as *Report No. 13*]. Central to the new terminology was replacement of the term "addiction" with the word "dependence." (The proposed terminology is now widely but by no means universally used in the professional literature.) The Committee distinguished "psychic dependence" and "physical dependence" and classified drugs accordingly. The opiates and alcohol produce both kinds of dependence, and the study provides a set of categories that characterize the degree of dependence, e.g., "overpowering desire" (opiates) and "strong desire" (alcohol-barbiturate types). In a 1969 report, the concept "drug dependence" is itself defined: "A state, psychic and sometimes also physical, resulting from the interaction between a living organism and a drug, characterized by behavioral and other responses that always include a compulsion to take the drug on a continuous or periodic basis in order to experience its psychic effects, and sometimes to avoid the discomfort of its absence. Tolerance may or may not be present. A person may be dependent on more than one drug." WHO Expert Committee on Addiction-Producing Drugs, *Report No. 16* (Tech. Rep. Ser. No. 407, 1969). The definition is reaffirmed in a 1973 report. WHO Expert Committee on Drug Dependence, *Report No. 19* (Tech. Rep. Ser. No. 526, 1973).

The crucial concepts in the definitions of "dependence" (as distinguished from mere use) are those of "overpowering desire" (the early formulations) and of "compulsion" (1969 formulation and after). But no specific analysis or explanation of these concepts appears in any of the official texts (nor in any other treatises I have seen on the topic). The closest approach to such analysis is remote at best: In the 1973 report, a section entitled "Quantification of Drug-Dependence" lists five very general categories of questions whose responses "*may* help to define the problems associated with drug taking and provide a basis for quantifying the presence and intensity of drug dependence." Ibid., p. 20.

Some authorities have tried to replace the subjective and vague notions of "overpowering desire" or "compulsion" with more objective language. Isbell defines dependence in terms of "persistent seeking and undergoing great risks to obtain the drug," use of the drug as the chief means of adaptation to life, and a "strong tendency to relapse after treatment." Isbell, "Pharmacological Factors in Drug Dependence," in *Drug Abuse: Nonmedical Use of Dependence Producing Drugs* 36, 35–42 (S. Btesh ed. 1972) (vol. 20 of *Advances in Experimental Medicine and Biology*) [hereinafter cited as *Nonmedical Use*]. Lewis, *Scientific Basis of Drug Dependence,* p. 8, suggests defining dependence in terms of observable withdrawal symptoms and behavior.

In this chapter the word "addict" generally refers, as indicated in context, to any one or combination of the following: a person who shows distinctive *physical symptoms* upon abstinence from a drug he has been using, a person who experiences a powerful desire to continue using a drug as a result of frequent prior use; a person who shows through *behavior* a persistent and intense commitment to seeking and using a certain drug, even though lawfulness and analogous socially approved values must be sacrificed.

43. Authorities in the field agree on this point. With respect to the physical aspects, see A. Goldstein, L. Aranow, and S. Kalman, *The Principles of Drug Action* 605 (1969) [hereinafter cited as *Principles*]; Chruscial, "Perspectives in Pharmacological Research on Drug Dependence," in *Nonmedical Use,* p. 79; Jaffe, "Drug Addiction and Drug Abuse," p. 283. With respect to addictive life patterns, see DeLong, *Pharmacological Basis of Therapeutics,* pp. 79–81, Jaffe, "The Implementation and Evaluation of New Treatments for Compulsive Drug Users," in *Drug Dependence* 230–32 (R. Harris, W. McIsaac, and C. Shuster eds. 1970), *Drug America,* pp. 369–70. See generally note 96 below.

Preble and Casey's summary of the various historic phases of heroin use from World War I to the present notes how different they were. Preble and Casey, "Taking Care of Business: The Heroin User's Life on the Street," in *It's So Good, Don't Even Try It Once,* ed. D. Smith and G. Gay (Englewood Cliffs, N.J.: Prentice-Hall, 1972), 100–104 [hereinafter cited as *Don't Try It*].

44. This categorization is not intended as a definitive one but is formulated for the purposes essential to the argument that follows. It includes each of the main types of phenomena that authorities typically speak of as constituting addiction. See, e.g., *Report No. 13,* above, note 42. The factual questions that arise in connection with these phenomena are discussed below.

45. See *United States* v. *Moore,* 486 F.2d 1139, 1236 (D.C Cir.) (Wright, J., dissenting cert. denied, 414 U.S. 980 (1973).

46. *Robinson* v. *California,* 370 U.S. 660 (1962); *Holden* v. *Hardy,* 169 U.S. 366 (1897); Slaughter-House Cases 83 U.S. 36 (1873), *Dowell* v. *City of Tulsa,* 273 P.2d 859, 861 (Okla. Sup. Ct.), *cert. denied,* 348 U.S. 912 (1954). See note 27, above.

47. *Jacobson* v. *Massachusetts,* 197 U.S. 11, 23–24 (1905) (vaccination).

48. See ibid., p. 25, *Holden* v. *Hardy,* 169 U.S. 366, 398 (1897). *Compagnie Française* v. *Board of Health,* 186 U.S. 380, 387 (1901).

49. The classic situation involves a driving prohibition for those who know they may lose control because of their disease. Failure to observe reasonable precautions to protect others from such dangers can warrant criminal conviction if, for example, another person's death results. *People* v. *Freeman,* 61 Cal. App. 110, 142 P.2d 435 (1943); *People* v. *Decina,* 2 N.Y.2d 133, 133 N.E.2d 799, 157 N.Y.S.2d 558 (1956).

50. M. LaFave and A. Scott, *Handbooks on Criminal Law* §25, p. 130 (1972).

51. *Powell* v. *Texas,* 392 U.S. 514, 569 (1968) (Fortas, J., dissenting (quoting trial judge with approval), *Watson* v. *United States,* 439 F.2d 442, 470 (D.C. Cir. 1970) (Bazelon, C.J.) (appendix to rehearing en banc) ("Even if an addict retains some minimal 'free will' not to indulge at a particular moment in time, no one would deny that his use of narcotics is largely involuntary—indeed is the essence of his disease"). See *In re Foss,* 10 Cal. 3d 910, 922, 519 P.2d 1073, 1080, 112 Cal. Rptr. 649, 656 (1974) ("psychological and/or physiological compulsion arising from an addiction").

52. *Stedman's Medical Dictionary,* p. 1231 defines "symptom" as: "Any morbid phenomenon or departure from the normal in function, appearance, or sensation experienced by the patient and indicative of disease." E. De Gowin and R. De Gowin, *Diagnostic Examination,* 2d ed. (New York: Macmillan, 1969), says: "Symptoms are those variations from normal sensations or behavior that enter the patient's consciousness. They are *subjective.* . . . Physical examination discloses *physical signs*; these are *objective* manifestations of disease. . . ." *Tabor's Cyclopedic Medical Dictionary,* p. 5-140 says: "Any perceptible change in the body or its functions that indicates disease or the kind or phases of disease."

53. One large category of symptomatic behaviors subject to voluntary control includes partial paralyses or failures of bodily coordination symptomatic of various kind of neurological or other organic disease or defect. The behavioral malfunction is commonly both evident and symptomatic, but sufficiently limited in degree to be subject to a positive effort of will. For example, in cases where diverging eyes have resulted from partial paralysis of a muscle of one of the eyes, a partial closing of one eye is a typical symptomatic behavior; it can be reversed

with some attention and moderate effort of will. The double vision that is distinctively symptomatic of this condition can also be elicited or prevented at will by those who have sufficient use of the muscle to relax it or to activate it sufficiently. S. Duke-Elder, *System of Ophthalmology* (St. Louis: Mosby, 1958), p. 617. For other examples of partial paralyses influenceable by effort of will and of voluntary exercises recommended to help in therapy, see the medical treatment discussion of Bell's palsy, and of paralyses due to cerebrovascular accidents in Harvard, *Current Medical Treatment* (3d ed. 1970), pp. 454, 460.

54. Fifty years ago, when people spoke of "dope fiends," it was possible for a court to accept the notion that a morphine addict was per se insane. *Prather* v. *Commonwealth,* 215 Ky. 714, 287 S.W. 559 (1926). More recently the claim that addiction is a mental disease had been put forth by defendant addicts either as a generalized claim, *Robinson* v. *California,* 370 U.S. 660, 667 n.8, or with respect to the particular case at issue. *Gaskins* v. *United States,* 410 F.2d 987 (D.C. Cir. 1967): *Rivers* v. *United States,* 330 F.2d 841 (D.C. Cir. 1964). See *Hutcherson* v. *United States,* 345 F.2d 964, 970 (D.C. Cir. 1965), *cert. denied,* 382 U.S. 894 (1965) (Burger, J., concurring): *Horton* v. *United States,* 317 F.2d 595, 597 (D.C. Cir. 1963); note 58, below.

55. In M'Naghten's Case, 8 Eng. Rep. 718 (H.L. 1843) this lack of understanding is formulated as a defect of reason from disease of the mind, such that "[the accused did not] know the nature and quality of the act he was doing, or if he did know it, that he did not know he was doing what was wrong." This requirement appears as one option for proof of insanity in the *Model Penal Code* §4.01 (Proposed Official Draft 1962), and is described as a defect resulting from mental disease wherein the person "lacks substantial capacity . . . to appreciate the criminality of his conduct."

56. In *Davis* v. *United States,* 165 U.S. 373, 378 (1897) the Court described this defect as a condition in which "[the] will, . . . the governing power of his mind has been otherwise than voluntarily so completed; destroyed that his actions are not subject to it, but are beyond his control." The *Model Penal Code* § 4.01 (Proposed Official Draft 1962) describes this aspect of the insanity defense as an optional alternative to the ground described in note 55. Here the defendant "lacks substantial capacity . . . to conform his conduct to the requirements of law." Any trend toward allowing a mere showing that the offending act resulted from mental disease, without a specific showing of lack of knowledge or lack of free will, collapsed with the abandonment of the rule of *Durham* v. *United States,* 312 F.2d 847 (D.C. Cir. 1962) (act must be product of mental disease or defect) in *United States* v. *Brawner,* 471 F.2d 969 (D.C. Cir. 1972) (adoption of *Model Penal Code* test). See generally Fingarette, *The Meaning of Criminal Insanity*; A. Goldstein, *The Insanity Defense* (1967).

57. See notes 41–43 above; Fingarette, *The Meaning of Criminal Insanity,* pp. 19–52. Such a consensus would not in any event control the legal concept of "disease" or "defect" as applied in the insanity defense. See *MacDonald* v. *United States,* 312 F.2d 847, 851 (D.C. Cir. 1962), superseded by *United States* v. *Brawner,* 471 F.2d 969 (1972). See also *Powell* v. *Texas,* 392 U.S. 514, 541 (1968) (Black, J., concurring).

58. *Castle* v. *United States,* 347 F.2d 492, 495 (D.C. Cir. 1965) (Burger, J., concurring), *cert. denied,* 388 U.S. 915 (1967). *Robinson* does not assert more than that addiction is a disease, though there is a footnote quoting "without direct comment or clear contextual indication of attitude) the appellee's brief which claimed that heroin addiction is a state of mental and physical illness." 370 U.S. at 666 n.8. Courts have also stated that "a mere showing of narcotic addiction, without more does not constitute 'some evidence' of mental disease. . . ." *Bailey* v. *United States,* 386 F.2d 1, 4 (5th Cir. 1967), citing *Heard* v. *United States* 348 F.2d 43, 44 (D.C. Cir. 1965). See also *United States* v. *Collins,* 443 F.2d 550 (D.C. Cir 1970): *United States* v. *Freeman,* 357 F.2d 606 (2d Cir. 1966): *Hutcherson* v. *United States,* 345 F.2d 964 (D.C. Cir.), *cert. denied,* 382 U.S. 894 (1965), *Lloyd* v. *United States,* 343 F.2d 242 (D.C. Cir.), *cert. denied,* 381 U.S. 952 (1964); *People* v. *Bonero,* 19 N.Y.2d 332, 227 N.E.2d 18 (1967). Of course, an addict may make an insanity plea and a showing of mental disease independent of a claim of addiction. This strategy

may succeed in a case where addiction exists but the addiction per se is not in itself sufficient even to raise the insanity issue. *Castle* v. *United States,* above, at 494 (Wright, J.); ibid., pp. 496–97 (Burger, J., concurring). This approach was used successfully In *People* v. *Kelly* 10 Cal. 3d 565, 516 P.2d 875, 111 Cal. Rptr. 171 (1973). But see *Prather* v. *Commonwealth* 215 Ky. 714, 287 S.W. 559 (1926) (morphine addict held insane because of addictive status).

59. See generally Fingarette, *The Meaning of Criminal Insanity,* pp. 19–52.

60. 370 U.S. at 667. The Court offers two examples in which addiction may result involuntarily. One is the addiction resulting from medically prescribed narcotics; the other is the newborn infant's addiction resulting from the mother's addiction. Both are not only examples of rare types of addiction relative to the total addict population, but are also examples of innocent development of addiction rather than innocent subsequent, self-initiated use of the drug once addiction exists. It is the ability to refrain from use subsequent to addiction that is most commonly at issue when the assumption of the involuntariness of addict behavior is discussed. The *Robinson* majority opinion says nothing at all on that score, as Judge Wilkey notes in *United States* v. *Moore,* 486 F.2d 1139 (D.C. Cir.), *cert. denied,* 414 U.S. 980 (1973).

61. See *United States* v. *Moore,* 486 F.2d 1139, 1209-10 (D.C. Cir.), *cert. denied,* 414 U.S. 980 (1973) (Wright, J., dissenting).

62. See *Watson* v. *United Sates,* 439 F.2d 442, 475 (D.C. Cir. 1970) (McGowan, J.).

63. *Watson* v. *United States,* 439 F.2d. 442, 470 (D.C. Cir. 1970) (Bazelon, C.J.) (appendix to rehearing en banc).

64. See pp. 309–10 above; *United States* v. *Lindsey,* 324 F. Supp. 55, 59 (D.D.C. 1971).

65. *Watson* v. *United States,* 459 F.2d 442, 467 n.18 (D.C. Cir. 1970) (Bazelon, C.J.) (appendix to hearing en banc); *Castle* v. *United States,* 347 F.2d 492, 494 (D.C. Cir. 1965), *cert. denied,* 388 U.S. 915 (1967). See *United States* v. *McKnight,* 427 F.2d 75 (7th Cir.), *cert. denied,* 400 U.S. 880 (1970); *United States* v. *Henry,* 417 F.2d 267, 269 (2d Cir. 1969) ("pharmacological coercion").

66. *United States* v. *Moore,* 486 F.2d 1139, 1210 (D.C Cir.) *cert. denied,* 414 U.S. 980 (1973) (nontrafficking possession) (Wright, J., dissenting); ibid., p. 1260 (trafficking and robbery to obtain funds for purchase of drug) (Bazelon, C.J.); *Watson* v. *United States* 439 F.2d 442, 470 (D.C. Cir. 1970) (Bazelon, C.J.) (appendix to rehearing en banc); *Lloyd* v. *United States,* 343 F.2d 242. 245 (D.C. Cir. 1 64), *cert. denied,* 382 U.S. 894 (1965) (purchase and possession) (Bazelon, C.J., dissenting); *United States* v. *Lindsey,* 324 F. Supp. 55 (D.C. Cir. 1971) (nontrafficking possession). See *Easter* v. *District of Columbia,* 361 F.2d 50, 52–53 (D.C. Cir. 1966) (being drunk in public; holding severely limited by *Powell* v. *Texas,* 392 U.S. 514 [1968]); *Driver* v. *Hinnant,* 356 F.2d 761, 764 (4th Cir. 1966) (alcohol addiction, being drunk in public; holding severely limited by *Powell* v. *Texas,* above).

67. *Powell* v. *Texas,* 392 U.S. 514, 560–61, 567–68 (1968) (Fortas, J., dissenting; *Easter* v. *District of Columbia,* 361 F.2d 50 (D.C Cir. 1966) (holding severely limited by *Powell* v. *Texas,* above); *Driver* v. *Hinnant,* 356 F.2d 761 (4th Cir. 1966) (holding severely limited by *Powell* v. *Texas,* above). See generally Fingarette, *The Meaning of Criminal Insanity.*

68. *Smith* v. *Follette,* 445 F.2d 955, 961 (2d Cir. 1971); *Bailey* v. *United States* 386 F.2d 1 n.4 (5th Cir. 1967); *United States ex rel. Swanson* v. *Reincke,* 344 F.2d 260, 263 (1965); *People* v. *Zapata* 220 Cal. App. 2d 903, 906–907, 34 Cal. Rptr. 171, 174 (1965), *appeal dismissed for lack of juris.,* 377 U.S. 409 (1964). If addictive conduct is in truth involuntary, there seems to be no logical basis for the criminal law to deny the addict a blank check to do whatever is necessary to get the drug. Any limitations on that license would simply be arbitrary. The implications for the criminal law are "revolutionary" and disturbing. 392 U.S. at 544 (Black, J., concurring); *Powell* v. *Texas,* 397 U.S. 514, 534 (1968). But see 392 U.S. at 559 n.2 (Fortas, J., dissenting). Judge Bazelon makes this point eloquently in arguing that a poor and unskilled addict may have no "meaningful choice" but to commit a crime. *United States* v. *Carter,* 436 F.2d 200, 210 (1970).

69. See, e.g., Jaffe, "Narcotic Analgesics," in *Pharmacological Basis of Therapeutics*, p. 249.

70. *Principles,* p. 474 (there is "no valid evidence" that legitimate medical administration of opiates might "create" addicts); DeLong, "The Drugs and Their Effects," p. 79; Lasagna, "Addicting Drugs and Medical Practice," in *Narcotics* 55 (D. Wilner and G. Kassebaum, eds. 1965).

71. Villareal, "Recent Advances in the Pharmacology of Morphine-Like Drugs, in *Drug Dependence,* p. 84; J. Ball, L. Brill, R. Glasscote, J. Jaffe, and J. Susse, *The Treatment of Drug Abuse* (1972), p. 19 [hereinafter cited as Ball and Brill] report that "Iatrogenic addiction [medically induced physical dependence] appears to be an inconsequential component of the drug abuse problems."

72. One important study summarized:

[I]n the population as a whole, very few of those who could obtain morphine or heroin illegally, if they wished, become addicts. It is noteworthy that although D-amphetamine has been used very widely to counteract fatigue and sleeplessness, only an occasional person who used it became habituated to it. And despite the nearly universal exposure of the population to the "legal" psychotropic drugs (alcohol, caffeine, and nicotine), some become habituated and some do not.

Principles, p. 474. See generally Hill, "Chairman's Introduction" to *Basis of Dependence,* p. 288. With regard to opiates specifically, see Geber, "Non-Dependent Drug Use: Some Psychological Aspects," in *Basis of Dependence,* pp. 375–87; D. Louria, *Overcoming Drugs* (New York: McGraw Hill, 1971), p. 84; Wald and Hutt, "The Drug Abuse Survey Project: Summary of Findings, Conclusions and Recommendations, in *Dealing,* p. 5. Weil discusses the inadequacy of the "addict" stereotype and the individuality of patterns of use. Weil, "Altered States of Consciousness," in *Dealing,* p. 333.

73. *Principles,* p. 474.

74. With respect to government and government-related programs created for this purpose, see note 75, below. Experience in private and purely voluntary residential programs such as Synanon demonstrates that "many former compulsive drug users are able to remain drug free and to function productively so long as they remain in residence." Jaffe, "Development of a Successful Treatment Program for Narcotic Addicts in Illinois," in *Drug Abuse, Data and Debate,* ed. P. Blachly (Springfield, Ill.: Thomas, 1970), pp. 62–63. Unknown numbers simply quit drug use of their own volition. DeLong reports that "there is some evidence that a substantial number of addicts—perhaps as many as one-third—'mature out' of addiction when they reach their thirties and forties." *Dealing,* p. 214.

75. Ball and Brill; A. Lindesmith, *Addiction and Opiates* (Chicago: Aldine Pub. Co., 1968), pp. 52–54. Fraser and Grider, "Treatment of Drug Addiction," *American Journal of Medicine* 14 (1953): 571; Gearing, "Methadone Maintenance: Six Years Later," *Contemporary Drug Problems* 1 (1972): 191; Jaffe, "Development of a Successful Treatment Program," pp. 48–63. Maddux, "Hospital Management of the Narcotic Addict," in *Narcotics,* pp. 159–76. O'Donnell, "A Follow-Up of Narcotic Addicts," *American Journal of Orthopsychiatry* 34 (1964): 948; Vaillant, "A Twelve-Year Follow-Up of New York Addicts," *American Journal of Psychiatry* 122 (1966): 727 (pt. 1); *New England Journal of Medicine* 275 (1966): 1282 (pt. 2); *Archives of General Psychiatry* 15 (1966): 599 (pt. 3); Wood, "18,000 Addicts Later: A Look at California's Civil Addict Program," *Federal Probation* 37 (1973): 26. See generally Chapple, Somekh and Taylor, "A Five-Year Follow-Up of 108 Cases of Opiate Addiction," *British Journal of Addiction* 67 (1972): 33; May, "Narcotic Addiction and Control in Great Britain," in *Dealing,* pp. 545–94. For discussion of alcoholism and rehabilitation programs, see note 94, below. In the large corporate anti-alcoholism programs, which tend to identify and deal with the most advanced, chronic cases, recovery rates range from 50 percent to 77 percent, averaging 66 percent nationally. Von Wiegand, "Alcoholism in Industry (USA)," *British Journal of Addiction* 67 (1972): 181.

In reviewing eleven followup studies of narcotic addiction treatment programs in 1965, O'Donnell noted that high percentages of relapse were valid "only for a highly restricted definition of relapse" such as a single occasion of use. The studies did not indicate that "most addicts, after a period of treatment or enforced abstinence, relapse to drugs and continue to use drugs, or that addicts spend most of their time outside of institutions using drugs." O'Donnell, "The Relapse Rate in Narcotic Addiction: A Critique of Follow-Up Studies," in *Narcotics,* pp. 242–43. One study suggests that there is a reduction in criminal behavior of patients in treatment. *Drug America,* p. 177. Such a benefit is obscured by the "all or nothing" approach to assessing results.

76. L. Robins, *A Follow-Up of Vietnam Drug Users* (Interim Final Rep., Special Actions Office for Drug Abuse Prevention, Executive Office of the President, 1973).

77. Ibid., p. 22.

78. Ibid.

79. Ibid.

80. Ibid. Zinberg essentially confirms this finding on the basis of his surveys and interviews. Zinberg, "Rehabilitation of Heroin Users in Vietnam," *Contemporary Drug Problems* 1 (1972): 263, 284.

81. L. Robins, *A Follow-Up on Vietnam Drug Users,* pp. 22–23.

82. See, e.g., A. Lindesmith, *Addiction and Opiates,* p. 48; Alarcon, Rathod, and Thomson, "Observations on Heroin Abuse by Young People in Crawley New Town," in *Basis of Dependence,* p. 338.

83. Louria, Hensle, and Rosa, "Major Medical Complications of Heroin Addiction," *Annals of Internal Medicine* 67 (1967): 1–2. The reports of heroin "overdose" as the leading cause of teenage death in New York City are probably a mark of impurities or special sensitivity, since recent studies show that "overdose deaths" are not usually associated other with high concentrations of the drug or with the usual symptoms of narcotic overdose. See Cherubin, "The Medical Sequelae of Narcotic Addiction," *Annals of Internal Medicine* 67 (1967): 23; Chein, "Psychological Functions of Drug Use," in *Basis of Dependence,* pp. 14–15; Wesson, Gay, and Smith, "Treatment Techniques for Narcotic Withdrawal," in *Don't Try It,* p. 165 speak of the "monumentally poor quality" of the heroin available on the West Coast. A summary of recent studies of "street" drugs shows that less than 50 percent of samples surveyed contained the alleged ingredients, and doses varied widely. Schnoll, "Drugs and Therapy—How To Interpret What You Read and Hear," *Contemporary Drug Problems* 1 (1971–72): 15. At one point the quality of street heroin sold on the Eastern seaboard rose from about 5 percent to a 10 percent concentration; somewhat more intense withdrawal symptoms for addicts resulted. Cohen, "Patterns of Drug Abuse—1970," in *Drug Abuse* (C. Zarafonetis ed. 1972), p. 336. Plainly local fluctuations are common. This variation suggests that the persistence in the life-patterns is not a direct consequence of the physiological action of a certain dose of the drug, but is highly influenced by other (social, psychological, and cultural) factors.

84. "Because of [the highly adulterated doses generally sold] it is now easy to withdraw the majority of heavy heroin users from their drug. Even those using six to eight bags a day (a $30- to $40-a day habit) often can be rapidly withdrawn without a substitute narcotic, by using mild tranquilizer during withdrawal." D. Louria, *Overcoming Drugs,* pp. 83–84. "Discussion Remarks," in *Basis of Dependence,* p. 89 (remarks of I. Chein). Physiological dependence may also be moderate among members of the "needle cult," addicts who seem to be addicted more to using the needle on themselves (whether or not there is anything in it) than to the drug itself. See May, "Narcotic Addiction and Control in Great Britain," p. 570; notes 99, 100, 105, 107, below.

Undoubtedly there are narcotic drug users in this country who are strongly dependent physiologically as well as psychologically. One cannot say how many. No doubt significant groups within this class are the health professionals who are addicts, and the "street dealers." See, e.g., Preble and Casey, "Taking Care of Business," in *Don't Try It,* p. 106; "Discussion

Remarks," p. 89 (Chein). Both groups have ready access to reasonably potent concentrations of drugs, but far larger groups do not.

85. *Drug America*, pp. 171–72; Vaillant, "The Natural History of Urban Narcotic Drug Addiction—Some Determinants," in *Basis of Dependence*, p. 347; Wald and Hutt, "The Drug Abuse Survey Project," p. 6. This is a common finding in many studies, but of course it is related to the nature of the populations among which addictive drug use is currently prevalent. In other epochs, other results would be obtained. See Preble and Casey, "Taking Care of Business," in *Don't Try It*, pp. 100–104 (historical review); Well, "Altered States of Consciousness," in *Dealing*, p. 340 (cross-cultural review). Similar contemporary statistics are reported from England. May, "Narcotic Addiction and Control in Great Britain," p. 381.

86. R. Ashley, *Heroin—The Myths and the Facts* (New York: St. Martin's Press, 1972), p. 73; Preble and Casey, "Taking Care of Business," in *Don't Try It*, p. 116. See generally E. Brecher, *Licit and Illicit Drugs* (Boston: Little, Brown, 1972), ch. 6. Chein, "Psychological Functions of Drug Use," in *Basis of Dependence*; Vaillant, "The Natural History of Urban Narcotic Drug Addiction," in *Basis of Dependence*, p. 351.

87. See I. Chein, D. Gerard, R. Lee, and E. Rosenfeld, *The Road to H* (1964), pp. 360–61.

88. J. Douglas, *Youth in Turmoil* (New York: Time-Life Books, 1970), p. 52; Feldman, "Ideological Supports to Becoming and Remaining a Heroin Addict, *Drug Dependence* (March 1970): 10; Chein, "Psychological Functions of Drug Use," in *Basis of Dependence*, p. 23. See note 116, below.

89. Isbell, "Pharmacological Factors in Drug Dependence," in *Nonmedical Use*, pp. 36–37.

90. A. Lindesmith, *Addiction and Opiates*, p. 49.

91. R. Ashley, *Heroin—The Myths and the Facts*, p. 64, reports: "Most of what we learn about the heroin user comes from the reports of the police, physicians, psychiatrists, and social workers. As a group they are essentially middle- and upper-middle class, operating under a value system quite different from that held in the urban ghetto. . . ."

92. Vaillant, "The Natural History of Urban Narcotic Drug Addiction," in *Basis of Dependence*, p. 335, finds that addicts with a history of stable work patterns and stable early family matrices were the ones who eventually became abstinent. Von Wiegand, "Alcoholism in Industry (U.S.A.)," p. 185, reports a two-thirds average national recovery rate in the large United States corporation programs dealing mainly with advanced, chronic alcoholism in career corporate employees.

93. These policies are employed in the California Civil Commitment Program and the federal programs at the United States Public Health Service Hospital at Lexington, Kentucky. See Wood, "18,000 Addicts Later"; Vaillant, "The Natural History of Urban Narcotic Drug Addiction," in *Basis of Dependence*; Carrick, The Government's Role in Affecting Change in the Treatment of Narcotic Addiction," in *Drug Abuse: Data and Debate* (P. Blachly ed. 1970), pp. 136–52. Valliant's 12-year follow-up of New York narcotics addicts committed to the Lexington hospital reports, "Effective treatment appears to depend on the compulsory alteration of the addict's behavior for substantial periods of time. . . . [A] long prison term [nine months or more] *coupled with a year of parole* was vastly more effective than short or long prison terms alone, or hospital treatment alone. *Basis of Dependence*, pp. 355–56. A. Lindesmith, *Addiction and Opiates*, pp. 52–58, reports various studies showing that sanctions, parole, threats of job-loss or license-loss (for physician-addicts) have produced significant results in producing abstinence.

94. For many of the narcotics rehabilitation programs, variable rules of internal discipline allow increased personal freedom as the addict abstains from narcotics and pursues work assignments. See Maddux, "Hospital Management of the Narcotic Addict," in *Narcotics*, p. 75, Ball and Brill, pp. 63–241. Far more alcoholics in the United States have well developed family and career roots than do narcotics addicts. Not surprisingly, the use of carefully worked out family-job sanctions has been showing dramatic success in recent years in dealing with alcoholics. Pfeffer,

Feldman, Feibel, Frank, Cohen, Fleetwood, and Greenberger, "A Treatment Program for the Alcoholic in Industry," *Journal of the American Medical Association* 161 (1956): 827. See Mello, Mendelson, McNamee, and O'Brien, "An Experimental Approach to the Drinking Patterns of Alcoholics," in *Basis of Dependence,* pp. 259–69; Saslow, "Where Do We Go From Here?" in *Drug Abuse: Data and Debate,* pp. 247–48; Von Wiegand, "Alcoholism in Industry (U.S.A.)."

95. Lindesmith notes that introducing values that the addict accepts can positively affect the successful implementation of sanctions. A Lindesmith, *Addiction and Opiates,* p. 53.

96. See p. 308 and note 43, above. For an elaboration of the various types of hypotheses that have been proposed to account for drug dependence, see WHO Expert Committee on Drug Dependence, *Report No. 18* (Tech. Rep. Ser. No. 460, 1970). The generality and range of disciplines covered by these hypotheses reveals the utter lack of specific, or definitive causal understanding. They are cast in terms of psychiatric categories, delinquency theories, miscellaneous personal motives (e.g., pleasure, distress and crises, social ambitions, social rebellion), "metabolic lesions," conditioned responses and learning, sociocultural "pressures," and various combinations of these factors. Indeed, a later report states that "these hypotheses are nonspecific with respect to drug use." WHO Study Group, *Youth and Drugs* 20 (Tech. Rep. Ser. No. 516, 1973). In short, these theories are all very general speculations about social malaises.

The analysis which follows in the text does not critically discuss the sociologically oriented hypotheses. The assumption is that the existence of generalized social influences does not amount to the conditions for involuntary behavior in the context of criminal responsibility. It is true that there has been recent argument that for some members of alienated subcultures the social influences may reach the point of establishing irrationality and involuntariness of a kind justifying a finding of absence of criminal responsibility. This novel and highly controversial view admittedly faces formidable obstacles to acceptance in law. In any event no analysis of the bearing of such a doctrine specifically on narcotic addiction has yet been provided. See Floud, "Sociology and the Theory of Responsibility: 'Social Background' as an Excuse for Crime," in *The Science of Society and the Unity of Mankind* (R. Fletcher ed. 1974), pp. 204–21. There is good reason to suppose that social factors are very important in understanding much addictive conduct, but to say this is very different from saying or even meaning to suggest that the conduct is therefore "involuntary."

97. See, e.g., Dole and Nyswander, "Methadone Maintenance and Its Implications for Theories of Narcotic Addiction," in *The Addictive States* (A. Wikler ed. 1968), p. 359.

98. DeLong, "The Drugs and Their Effects, in *Dealing,* p. 212, summarizes the questions concerning the physiological components of addiction and concludes that there are no clear answers and that most scientists are at least skeptical about validating their effects. *Principles,* p. 474, raises the possibility that a genetic factor might explain the addictive response in the relative few who become addicts, but acknowledges a "paucity of evidence" for such a view. Specific comments such as those above are also confirmed by the more general acknowledgments that medical science today lacks *any* accepted fundamental understanding of the causes of addiction.

99. Addictive patterns of conduct are associated with the dependence-producing drugs which WHO lists as *not* producing physical dependence, e.g., cocaine. The addictive pattern of conduct can also exist when no narcotic has been used, such as in the not uncommon cases of addicts who have been unwittingly buying pure milk sugar from their dealers over substantial periods of time. Vaillant, "The Natural History of Urban Narcotic Drug Addiction," in *Basis of Dependence,* p. 352.

100. H. Beecher, *Measurement of Subjective Responses* (1959), pp. 161–66, reports that during World War II two-thirds of the wounded at Anzio did not wish pain-relieving medication, whereas four-fifths of a group of civilians with far less tissue trauma did. The gravely wounded who did not wish medication for wound-pain complained vigorously, however, at inept injections. "*Great wounds with great significance . . . are made painless by small doses of morphine, whereas fleeting experimental[ly induced] pains with no serious significance are*

not blocked by morphine." Ibid., p. 165. Beecher's experimental reports show that, generally speaking, half the pain-relieving effect of morphine is due to "placebo" reaction, a reaction to the idea that a pain reliever has been given rather than to the chemical action; the placebo effect is greater as the stress is greater. Ibid. See also A. Grollman and E. Grollman, *Pharmacology and Therapeutics,* 7th ed. (Philadelphia: Lea and Febiger, 1970), p. 99.

101. "[T]hough drugs may have specific physiological effects, their effects upon behavior and experience are largely nonspecific." A. Bernstein, L. Epstein, H. Lennard, and D. Ransom, *Mystification and Drug Misuse* (1971), p. 57.

102. *WHO Expert Commentary on Addiction-Producing Drugs,* p. 13, uses the phrase "overpowering desire."

103. See, e.g., McMorris, "Can We Punish for the Acts of Addiction?" p. 1084.

104. Glaser and Ball, who studied the literature written since 1875, found no documented case in which opiate withdrawal was "the sufficient cause of death." Glaser and Ball, "Death Due to Withdrawal of Narcotics," in *The Epidemiology of Opiate Addiction in the United States* (I. Ball and C. Chambers eds. 1970), p. 287. See, e.g., Maddux, "Hospital Management of the Narcotic Addict," in *Narcotics,* p. 168.

105. Ball and Brill, p. 10. See p. 315, notes 84–85, above.

106. Wesson, "Treatment Techniques for Narcotic Withdrawal," in *Don't Try It,* p. 165; Jaffe, "Drug Addiction and Drug Abuse," in *Pharmacological Basis of Therapeutics,* ed. L. Goodman and A. Gilman, 4th ed. (New York: Macmillan, 1970), p. 302. See Zinberg, "Rehabilitation of Heroin Users in Vietnam," p. 285.

107. Preble and Casey, "Taking Care of Business," in *Don't Try It,* p. 110.

108. See Deneau, "Psychogenic Dependence in Monkeys," in *Basis of Dependence,* pp. 199–207; Isbell, "Pharmacological Factors in Drug Dependence," in *Nonmedical Use,* pp. 36–38; Villareal, "Contributions of Laboratory Work to the Analysis and Control of Drug Dependence," in *Drug Use: Data and Debate,* p. 97. On the other hand, it should be noted that physiological dependence and consequent withdrawal stress can occur without psychological dependence, without the self-conscious cravings to use the drug and therefore without the addictive life pattern. See Eddy, et al., "Drug Dependence."

109. Blachly, "Management of the Opiate Abstinence Syndrome," *American Journal of Psychiatry* 122 (1966): 742; Fraser and Grider, "Treatment of Drug Addiction," *American Journal of Medicine* 14 (1953): 571; Maddux, "Hospital Management of the Narcotic Addict," in *Narcotics,* p. 168 (withdrawal technique in U.S. Public Health Service hospitals).

110. A. Lindesmith, *Addiction and Opiates,* pp. 34–39, takes it as "conclusively established" that under controlled conditions addicts can be deceived into thinking they have received opiates when they have been given placebos. See generally Bernstein et al., *Mystification and Drug Misuse,* pp. 57–62; Ball and Brill, p. 34; notes 99, 101, above.

111. Chein and associates report that the distress level in withdrawal depends on the setting "Alone, it can be an almost unbearable experience. In a hospital ward, remarkably little medication often stills the distress associated with quite severe physiological disturbance, e.g., painful cramps and diarrhea. Conversely, patients with minor overt symptoms may be very demanding of medication." Chein et al., *The Road to H,* pp. 247–48. See R. Phillipson, *Modern Trends in Drug Dependence and Alcoholism* (New York: Appleton, Century, Crofts; London: Butterworths, 1970), p. 1; Lennard, Epstein, and Katzung, "Psychoactive Drug Action and Group Interaction Process," *Journal of Nervous and Mental Disease* 145 (1967): 69.

112. See, e.g., Jaffe, "Development of a Successful Treatment Program," p. 48. See generally Ball and Brill.

113. *Castle v. United States,* 347 F.2d 492, 494 (D.C. Cir. 1965), *cert. denied,* 388 U.S. 915 (1967): *United States v. Henry,* 417 F.2d 267, 269 (2d Cir. 1969). See *Watson v. United States* 439 F.2d 442 (D.C. Cir. 1970) ("pharmacological duress," p. 447) ("physiological duress," p. 461) (Bazelon, C.J., concurring and dissenting).

114. *D'Aquino* v. *United States,* 192 F.2d 338 (9th Cir. 1951); *Gillars* v. *United States,* 182 F.2d 962, 974 (D.C. Cir. 1950).

115. See Freedman, "Non-Pharmacological Factors in Drug Dependence," in *Nonmedical Use,* p. 30.

116. Chein et al., *The Road to H,* p. 248: "[A]mong adolescent addicts . . . the self-identification as addicts—i.e., as persons who require opiates for comfortable functioning—is an important phenomenon in their developing addiction. . . . There is another aspect to the withdrawal syndrome; it is not merely the bane of addiction to opiates, but also its badge . . ."—a subject of much boastful humor and exaggerated story telling.

117. See, e.g., Feldman, "Ideological Supports to Becoming and Remaining a Heroin Addict"; Preble and Casey, "Taking Care of Business," in *Don't Try It*; Chein, "Psychological Functions of Drug Use," in *Basis of Dependence,* pp. 23–24, R. Ashley, *Heroin—The Myths and the Facts,* p. 73.

118. See Ball and Brill, p. 21; A. Lindesmith, *Addiction and Opiates,* p. 34; Maddux, "Hospital Management of the Narcotic Addict," in *Narcotics.*

119. Holahan reports: "[T]he habit size of a long time heavy user is often not as the level of euphoria but only at a level sufficient to suppress withdrawal or to keep the withdrawal mild." Holahan, "The Economics of Heroin," in *Dealing,* p. 290. Other commentators confirm this point. Ball and Brill, p. 11; A. Lindesmith, *Addiction and Opiates,* pp. 23–45.

120. In the addict's routine daily injections a relief and calm is achieved. Each new injection abates the tensions and discomforts that emerge as the effect of the preceding dose begins to wear off. During standard withdrawal procedures, with decreased dosages leading to abstinence, this tranquil "euphoria" is normally lost. Jaffe, "Drug Addiction and Drug Abuse," pp. 302–303.

121. For a classic discussion of these concepts, see B. F. Skinner, *The Behavior of Organisms: An Experimental Analysis* (New York: Appleton-Century, 1938); *Dealing,* pp. 133–34. Bernstein et al., *Mystification and Drug Abuse,* p. 83, point out that the capacity of the many who reside in such groups as Phoenix House to abstain refutes the hypothesis that addiction is an automatic, internally triggered pattern. See Thompson and Pickens, "Drug Self-Administration and Conditioning," in *Basis of Dependence,* pp. 177–98.

122. See Jaffe, "Development of a Successful Treatment Program." See generally Ball and Brill.

123. See, e.g., B. F. Skinner, *Beyond Freedom and Dignity* (New York: Knopf, 1971). Wald and Hutt conclude that it is a high priority "question" whether there is any inborn physiological predilection, drug-induced vulnerability, learned response to external stimuli, or none of these, that bear on addiction. See Wald and Hutt, *The Drug Abuse Survey Project,* p. 45.

124. See pp. 311–12, above. The general concept of "mental illness" has no more weight than its more specific forms taken jointly. That is, if "compulsion," "inadequate personality," "character defect," and other psychiatric diagnoses provide no independent proof of involuntariness, the generic concept, which refers vaguely to some or all of these, can do no more.

125. Bowman, "Narcotic Addiction and Criminal Responsibility under Durham," *Geo. Law Journal* 53 (1965): 1017, 1031.

126. Ibid., p. 1033 (citing an AMA Report on Narcotics Addiction). The labeling process can often simply obscure the legal issues. In *Washington* v. *United States,* 390 F.2d 444 (D.C. Cir. 1967), the court was confronted with such a situation. It commented:

> These labels and definitions were not merely uninformative. Their persistent use
> served to distract the jury's attention from the few underlying facts which were mentioned. For example, the fact that Washington's difficulties "in relating adequately to
> other people are more severe or more extreme than the avenge [person's]" was
> immersed in a dispute about whether to classify these difficulties as a "personality

defect," a "personality problem," a "personality disorder," a "disease," an "illness," or simply a "type of personality."

Ibid., p. 449.

127. Redlich and Freedman find that this characteristic may be singularly descriptive of addicts:

> It is questionable, then, whether one can speak meaningfully of an addictive person- ality beyond the tautological statement that such a person, for one or another reason, has the compulsion to take drugs. At present we are inclined to believe that addicts are a heterogeneous lot.

R. Redlich and D. Freedman, *Theory and Practice of Psychiatry* (New York: Basic Books, 1966), p. 728.

128. For discussion of the legal concepts of compulsion, coercion, and necessity, see J. Hall, *General Principles of Criminal Law* (2d ed. 1960). Of course a defendant could try to prove that the psychiatric concept of "compulsion" implied a mental disease or defect within the meaning of the insanity defense. Such proof would have to be made independently of a showing of the mere fact of addiction. See note 56, above.

129. The doctrine is set out in some of Freud's classic works, and is summarized in Redlich and Freedman, *Theory and Practice of Psychiatry*, p. 551. See generally C. Brenner, *An Elementary Textbook of Psychoanalysis* (2d ed. 1975), p. 191.

130. The remarks in text above do not imply that these general psychiatric doctrines have no use at all. They have uses *within* psychiatry: they can be helpful in gaining an overview of the human psyche, in organizing the specific insights of the clinic, and in guiding research and therapy. Moreover, the psychiatrist can make important contributions in certain aspects of the criminal trial. He or she may have insights into the mind and character of the individual on trial, or at least into a well-understood psychological type to which the defendant demonstrably belongs. However, *specific knowledge* about addicts as a "type" is lacking, although vague, speculative, and often conflicting statements abound in the psychiatric and other literatures. See Redlich and Freedman, *Theory and Practice of Psychiatry*, p. 127.

131. American Psychiatric Association, *A Psychiatric Glossary* (2d ed. 1964). This defi- nition would not necessarily preclude a finding of criminal liability. As Justice Black noted:

> When we say that appellant's [offending conduct] is caused not by "his own" voli- tion but rather by some other force, we are clearly thinking of a force that is never- theless "his" except in some special sense. The accused undoubtedly commits the proscribed act and the only question is whether the act can be attributed to a part of "his" personality that should not be regarded as criminally responsible. Almost all of the traditional purposes of the criminal law can be significantly served by punishing the person who in fact committed the proscribed act without regard to whether his action was "compelled" by some elusive "irresponsible" aspect of his personality.

Powell v. Texas, 392 U.S. 514, 560 (1968) (Black, J., concurring).

132. C. Brenner, *An Elementary Textbook of Psychoanalysis*, p. 191. See notes 86–94, 116–17, above.

133. H. English and A. English, *A Comprehensive Dictionary of Psychological and Psy- choanalytical Terms* (1958).

134. The universal characteristic common to all types of drug dependence is *psychic* dependence, a psychological compulsion to take a drug. . . . Psychic dependence is difficult to define and measure but is recognized clinically by alterations in behavior such as undergoing great risks to obtain the drug, obsession with maintaining a supply, use of the drug as the chief means of adapting to life and a strong tendency to relapse after treatment.

Isbell, "Drug Addiction and Drug Abuse," p. 361.

135 See p. 320, above The National Commission on Marijuana and Drug Abuse urges discarding of the "unidimensional concept of individual loss of self-control which has long dominated scientific and lay concepts of 'addiction' " on the grounds that it is simply inaccurate. *Drug America*, p. 139.

136. See notes 74–75, above.

137. The eminent psychiatrists Alexander and Staub acknowledge the incongruity of outlook in the two fields.

> We may for practical purposes hold the individual responsible for his acts; we assume an attitude as if the conscious Ego actually possessed the power to do what it wishes. Such an attitude *has no theoretical foundation,* but it has a practical, or still better, a tactical justification.

F. Alexander and H. Staub, *The Criminal, the Judge and the Public* (1931), pp. 72–73 (emphasis added). See, e.g., Louisell and Diamond, "Law and Psychiatry: Detente, Entente, or Concomitance?" *Cornell Law Quarterly* 50 (1965): 217, 220. Brenner, *An Elementary Textbook of Psychoanalysis,* p. 183, acknowledges that the distinction between the normal expression of character and the abnormal symptom is "necessarily an arbitrary decision" from the purely psychiatric standpoint. R. Redlich and D. Freedman, *Theory and Practice of Psychiatry,* p. 350, say the distinction is "very difficult or impossible" to make. See Fingarette, *The Meaning of Criminal Insanity,* p. 39.

138. This imputation of motive rests upon inferences that seem repeatedly apparent as one reads the court records, and psychiatrists' statements about the irrelevance and inappropriateness of the criminal law in the areas of mental disease and addiction. See Fingarette, *The Meaning of Criminal Insanity,* pp. 57–52.

139. *United States* v. *Moore,* 486 F.2d 1139, 1159 (D.C. Cir.) (Wilkey, J.), *cert. denied,* 414 U.S. 390 (1973).

140. *Marshall* v. *United States,* 414 U.S. 417, 427–29 (1974) (Burger, C.J.).

141. A recent polar formulation reflects a common doctrinaire approach: "Medicine views the drug misuser as a patient who needs treatment: law enforcement views him as a criminal who must be punished." Group for the Advancement of Psychiatry, *Drug Misuse* (New York: Scribner, 1971), p. 12. Too often such a formulation merely sidesteps a set of complex personal, social, legal, and spiritual problems:

> Oftentimes . . . the desire to avoid the implications of criminality while maintaining formal control has resulted in compulsory treatment of an "illness" which has never been adequately defined. The Commission warns against the tendency to assume that when its motives are benevolent, society need not attend to the philosophical and constitutional issues raised by its actions.

Drug America, p. 257, Goldstein and Katz, "Abolish the Insanity Defense—Why Not?"

142. See notes 93–95 above.

143. See H. L. A. Hart, *Punishment and Responsibility* (New York: Oxford University Press, 1968), p. 23:

> Criminal punishment as an attempt to secure desired behavior differs from the manipulative techniques of the Brave New World (conditioning, propaganda, etc.) or the simple incapacitation of those with antisocial tendencies, by taking a risk. It defers action till harm has been done: its primary operation consists simply in announcing certain standards of behavior and attaching penalties for deviation, making it less eligible, and then leaving individuals to choose. This is a method of social control which maximizes individual freedom within the coercive framework of law. . . .

Part Eight

State-Supported and Court-Ordered Treatment for Addiction Is Unconstitutional (and Counterproductive)

28

The First Amendment and Drug Alcohol Treatment Programs: To What Extent May Coerced Treatment Programs Attempt to Alter Beliefs Relating to Ultimate Concerns and Self-Concept?

Ellen Luff

Many courts are ordering persons convicted of DWI [driving while intoxicated] and other alcohol- and drug-related offenses to attend Alcoholics Anonymous [AA] or another Twelve-Step Program.[1] These programs meet the legal definition of a religion[2] because, among other things, they counsel "turning our will and our lives over to the care of God, as we understood Him" (Third Step); and "working" the steps culminates in a "spiritual awakening" (twelfth step).[3] Therefore, state-coerced attendance constitutes an establishment of a religion and violates the Establishment Clause of the First Amendment.[4] In addition, forcing an atheist to attend a theistic program constitutes a violation of the Free Exercise Clause of the First Amendment.[5]

The issue of forced AA attendance violating First Amendment rights has been raised by numerous individuals in the past, but has typically resulted in no definitive judicial decision and a settlement of limited application.[6] In 1987, John Norfolk, an atheist from the Eastern Shore of Maryland convicted of driving while intoxicated, objected to being forced to attend AA and refused to follow the court order compelling his attendance at the meetings. He contacted the ACLU who represented him at the hearing on his violation of probation. The case received extensive press coverage. Mr. Norfolk lost in the Queen Anne's County District Court.[7] But on appeal, Circuit Court Judge John Sause ruled for Mr. Norfolk, stating that the state should not be forcing people to attend programs such as AA. Judge Sause then enunciated a new policy to be henceforth followed in his court: After a defendant is found guilty of a crime involving drugs or alcohol, if probation is to be granted, the

Originally published in *Drug Policy 1989–90: A Reformer's Catalogue* (Washington, D.C.: Drug Policy Foundation). Reprinted by permission of the Drug Policy Foundation.

defendant will be given several weeks to devise his or her probation program. After the program is reviewed by the probation department, the court will then sentence the defendant to comply with the terms of probation the defendant has designed. If the defendant does not comply with the agreed-upon terms, then he or she will be incarcerated.[8]

Judge Sause's decision was the best conceivable outcome. It not only cured Mr. Norfolk's objection, but it anticipated First Amendment objections which could have been made to court[s] ordering only "secular therapies."

As has been observed by various writers,[9] secular psychotherapy has many of the characteristics of a religion. It is likely that forcing someone into a therapy which contains basic underlying assumptions contrary to those of the probationer would be considered a First Amendment violation even if the therapy was not as obviously religious as AA. The bottom line is—although the state has an interest in preventing certain behavior and may use various methods, including probation with therapy and support groups, to achieve that end—it may not attempt to alter people's beliefs concerning metaphysical issues, "ultimate concerns," or self-concept. Professor Lawrence Tribe in describing the essence of the First Amendment has stated:

> Not surprisingly the [Supreme] Court has insisted that activities actually going on within the head are absolutely beyond the power of government to control. . . . In a society whose whole constitutional heritage rebels at the thought of giving the government the power to control men's minds, the governing institutions, and especially the courts, must not only reject direct attempts to exercise forbidden domination over mental processes; they must strictly examine as well oblique intrusions likely to produce, or designed to produce, the same result.[10]

Those making drug policy must be wary of trampling on the First Amendment in their zeal to help or cure drug and alcohol abusers. First Amendment infringements are common in this area since many eminent psychologists believe a conversion or spiritual experience is necessary for remission from alcoholism or drug addiction. William James stated "the only cure for dipsomania is religiomania.' Carl Jung, in his correspondence with Bill Wilson, the co-founder of AA, stated that alcoholism resulted from an unrecognized spiritual need and could be counteracted by religious insight.[11] But if the state becomes a party to attempting to precipitate a conversion experience, the First Amendment has been violated.[12]

In addition, a state-promoted treatment program may be subject to attack on First Amendment grounds if it attempts to persuade clients to change basic beliefs and presents a comprehensive explanation of the world or what constitutes and produces happiness. It would also be subject to attack if it seeks to persuade the client to adopt a different identity or self-concept as, for instance, an "alcoholic" or "addict."[13] The fact that the program claims it is "secular" and disavows that it is a religion,[14] is not controlling. The courts have held that Transcendental Meditation is a religion for First Amendment purposes, despite TM's vigorous objection to being so characterized.[15]

First Amendment cases involving the Free Exercise Clause may permit some curtailment of the exercise of the right if another recognized state interest is being advanced, but only if the method used is the least intrusive means possible.[16] Applying this analysis to drug alcohol treatment programs which seek to cause people to change their beliefs, the least possible intrusion into the person's belief system or mind should be attempted in order to further the legitimate state interest in preventing people from driving while intoxicated. It is permissible for the state to require all probationers convicted of DWI-related offenses to attend educational classes designed to persuade them to cease driving while under the influence of drugs or alcohol. It is not permissible to intrude further into the probationer's mind by forcing sustained attendance in programs designed to alter other more remotely related beliefs, such as their belief in God or their self-identity.

In addition to First Amendment problems, reasoning similar to that set forth above could be applied to Employee Assistance Programs (EAPs). Title VII of the Civil Rights Act prohibits discrimination based on religion. Courts have held that coercing attendance at staff meetings which begin with prayers is employment discrimination.[17] If employers insist employees attend programs which would be objectionable on First Amendment grounds if coerced by the state, then employers could be subject to a Title VII suit. A Georgia U.S. District Court suit brought by an ACLU attorney against an employer for requiring employees to attend an EST type training program (no drug alcohol issue was involved) was recently settled in the employees' favor.[18]

SUMMARY

State agencies and employers can avoid violating people's right to freedom of thought and belief by restricting the mandatory component of their program to alcohol education and permitting the person to select a therapy or support group in which he or she wishes to participate.

NOTES

1. The problem addressed by this chapter would be unaffected by legalization or decriminalization of drugs, since there would still be criminal sanctions against operating automobiles, airplanes, and boats while intoxicated or impaired by drugs. Employers dissatisfied with job performance would still be demanding that drug abusers receive treatment. First Amendment problems inherent in coerced treatment are identical for alcohol- and drug-treatment programs.

2. In *United States v. Seeger*, 380 U.S. 163, 13 Led 2d 733, 85 S.Ct. 850 (1965) stated

the test to be applied was: "whether the Church occupies a place in the lives of its members parallel to that filled by the orthodox belief in God in religions more widely accepted in the United States." And in *United States* v. *Kuch,* 288 F. Supp. 439, 444 (DC 1968), in holding that the Neo American Church was not a religion, the court noted that one claiming that a group is a religion should be able to demonstrate: "belief in a supreme being, a religious discipline, a ritual, and tenets to guide one's daily existence." In *Theriault* v. *Silber,* 547 F.2d 1279, 1281 (5th 1977), the court stated: 'To the extent that *Kuch* includes within its test criteria the require-ment that one possess a belief in a Supreme being and such criterion excludes, for example agnosticism and conscientious atheism, for the Free Exercise and Establishment shields, that requirement is too narrow."

In Note, "Toward a Constitutional Definition of Religion," *Harvard Law Review* 91 (1978): 1056, the author proposes a definition of religion based on Paul Tillich's characteriza-tion of religion as that which deals with "ultimate concerns." See also Choper, "Defining 'Reli-gion' in the First Amendment," *University of Illinois Law Review* (1982): 579, where extratem-poral consequences is proposed as the hallmark of a religion.

3. Chapter 5, "How It Works," pages 58 through 61 of *Alcoholics Anonymous* (AA World Services 1986) which sets forth the Twelve Steps. Chapter 4, "We Agnostics," pages 55 through 57, describes how someone who came into AA an atheist was later converted to theism. Simi-larly, *Came to Believe,* (AA World Services 1977) in "The Belief Will Come" pages 46 to 48 and "An Atheist's Journey," pages 79 through 81, atheists are converted to theism. A conver-sion experience or a "spiritual awakening" is actually deemed necessary since it is an AA doc-trine that alcoholism is a spiritual, as well as emotional and physical disease, *Alcoholics Anon-ymous,* p. 64, and that only faith in a Higher Power will result in continued sobriety, ibid. p. 70. c.f. *Not God,* note 15 below.

For an excellent anthropological study of AA, see Antze, "Symbolic Action in Alcoholics Anonymous," in Ed. Douglas, *Constructive Drinking, Perspectives on Drinking from Anthro-pology* (Cambridge: Cambridge University Press, 1987) where AA is compared with several other non-Western religions. See also Roberts and Smithwick, "Finding God at the Bottom of a Bottle—Thousands of Baltimore Alcoholics turn Addiction to Salvation," *Baltimore Maga-zine,* April 1989; Elpenor, "A Drunkard's Progress—AA and the Sobering Strength of Myth," *Harper's Magazine,* October 1986.

4. "Congress shall make no law respecting an establishment of religion, or prohibiting the free exercise thereof. . . ."

Although AA gets no money from the state for its services, it is established in that state employees are "monitoring" AA attendance, and probation officers and rehab workers even assist DWI defendants to "work the steps." Read, "The Alcoholic, the Probation Officer, and AA: A Viable Team Approach to Supervision," *Federal Probation,* March 1987, pp. 11, 15.

In *Engel* v. *Vitale,* 370 U.S. 421, 431 (1962), a case invalidating a school prayer statute, the Supreme Court stated:

> [The Establishment Clause]'s first and most immediate purpose rested on the belief that a union of government and religion tends to destroy government and degrade religion. The history of governmentally established religion, both in England and in this country, showed that whenever government had allied itself with one particular form of religion, the inevitable result had been that it had incurred the hatred, disre-spect and even contempt of those who held contrary beliefs. The same history showed that many people had lost their respect for any religion that had relied upon the support of government to spread its faith. The Establishment Clause thus stands as an expression of principle on the part of the Founders of our Constitution that reli-gion is too personal, too sacred, too holy, to permit its "unhallowed perversion" by a civil magistrate.

5. The First Amendment protects the right to nonbelief as well as belief, *Torcaso* v. *Watkins*, 367 U.S. 488. 6. Led 2d 982, 81 S.Ct.1680 (1961), and even protects the practice of "a myriad of seldom heard of, off-brand, off-beat religious concepts." *McMillan* v. *State*, 258 Md. 147. 265 A.2d 453 (1970).

6. See *Alcoholism, the National Magazine*, February 1985, concerning settlement of a case against the Veterans Administration. Cases where issue was raised but decided adverse to parole violator on other grounds: *Youle* v. *Edgar*, No 4-88-0005 The Appellate Court of Illinois Fourth District, unreported opinion; *Farmer* v. *Coughlin*, 1987 WL 27664 (S.D.N.Y.) (Not reported in F. Supp.); *Jaco* v. *Shields*, 507 F. Supp 67 (1981). Cases are presently pending or anticipated in Alaska, North Carolina, and Washington. Both ACLU and American Jewish Congress are interested in participating in litigation to prohibit state-compelled AA.

7. Queen Anne County District court, Cit. No. D713675. The judge based his decision largely on his supposition that "AA seems to be the only thing that has proven successful in the treatment of the alcoholic" (p. 8). This supposition is not supported by any studies, and research using control groups suggests that there may be a negative correlation between AA attendance and continued sobriety. Miller and Hester, "The Effectiveness of Alcoholism Treatment—What Research Reveals," from Miller and Heather (eds.), *Treating Addictive Behaviors* (New York: Plenum, 1986), pp. 121, 135.

8. Queen Anne's County Criminal Case No. 3588, decided March 16, 1989. Besides stating that the "subjective nature of alcohol and drug problems made it inappropriate to coerce participation, Judge Sause further stated that the state had no right to add to the "burden" of AA members by sending to their meetings unwilling people who might be disruptive and breach anonymity. He stated that just because AA members were "good natured" and did not turn people away, did not give the state the right to make this "valid" and "worthwhile" organization a state agency. The issue of AA being imposed upon was not specifically raised by the defendant or state, and AA, in accordance with its tradition of avoiding public controversy, took no position in the case. The judge's knowledge of the negative public reaction to the inundation of AA meetings with court-ordered people apparently came from the reading local newspapers. In Maryland, because many AA groups refused to sign court slips, the probation departments in many areas attempted to verify attendance by requiring court-ordered people to take notes on the name of the person who was the main speaker at a meeting as well as on what transpired in the meetings. In other areas state employees were paid to attend meetings for the purpose of checking attendance.

9. James Hillman, *The Myth of Analysis* (Evanston: Northwestern University Press, 1972); Thomas Szasz, *The Myth of Psychotherapy* (Syracuse, N.Y.: Syracuse University Press, 1988).

10. Tribe, *Constitutional Law* (2d ed. 1988) p. 1315.

11. "Spiritus contra Spiritum: The Bill Wilson/C. G. Jung Letters—The Roots of the Society of Alcoholics Anonymous," *Parabola*, Summer 1987.

12. Although the Supreme Court has approved of farming out some state functions to religious groups, such as teenage chastity counseling, *Bowen* v. *Kendrick*, 56 LW 4818 (decided June 29, 1988), it specifically noted that the programs, although run by religious groups, were not attempting to inculcate religious beliefs.

13. The Supreme Court has recognized that individuals need to be protected from state interference with the "ability independently to define one's identity that is central to any concept of liberty." *Roberts* v. *U.S. Jaycees*, 468 U.S. 609, 619, 104 S.Ct. 3244, 3250 (1984). c.f. Discussion of "self-identification" in Karst, "The Freedom of Intimate Association," (1980) *Yale Law Journal* 89 (1980): 624, 635.

14. AA literature states it is "spiritual" and not "religious," maintaining that it is not a religious society since it "requires no definite religious belief as a condition of membership." *44 Questions* (Pamphlet, AA World Services), p. 15. For a discussion of why AA developed this characterization of itself see Paul Kurtz, "The Context of the History of Religious Ideas," chap.

8 of *Not God—A History of Alcoholics Anonymous* (Minneapolis: Hazelton, 1979). Although many varieties of Christianity stress doctrinal conformity, many religions have no requirement that their members hold definite beliefs concerning ultimate concerns.

15. *Malnik* v. *Yogi,* 529 F.2d 197 (3rd. Cir. 1979), affirming 440 F. Supp. 1284 (D.C. NJ 1977).

16. *Robinson* v. *Price,* 614 F.2d 1097 (5th Cir. 1980).

17. *Young* v. *Southwestern,* 509 F.2d 140 (5th Cir. Tex.) (Unitarian atheist, employer held staff meetings which began with a short religious talk followed by a prayer); EEOC Decision No. 73-0528, CCH EEOC Dec Sec 6316 (employees merely "urged to attend"); EEOC Dec No. 72-1114, CCH EEOC Dec Sec 6347; *Towley Mfgr Co.* (9th Cir., Judge Snead, 1988).

18. *Civil Liberties,* Winter 1989, p. 10.

29

Thinking about Drinking:
The Power of Self-Fulfilling Prophecies*

Jeffrey A. Schaler

The beliefs people have about addiction—what they think about drinking, for instance—have a powerful effect on their behavior. This relationship between belief and behavior is known as a self-fulfilling prophecy. The more people believe in their ability to moderate their consumption of drugs and alcohol, the more likely they will moderate. The inverse is true, too: The more people believe in their inability to moderate their consumption of drugs and alcohol, the more likely they will not moderate.

The beliefs of addiction-treatment providers are important as well. What we believe about drugs, addiction, disease, authority, and personal and "higher" powers largely dictates our behavior toward clients. Knowing more about the beliefs that treatment providers hold dear can thus help us to build better treatment policies. In my research on the beliefs addiction-treatment providers have about addiction, I have observed a conflict about what addiction is and isn't, which is known as the "disease-model controversy." Regardless of whether treatment providers' beliefs about addiction are true or false, rational or irrational, those beliefs largely shape their actions.

One example is the influence of adults' beliefs on the nature of drug-use prevention programs for children. Our children are taught false information about drugs and addiction. They are the targets of scare tactics by antidrug fundamentalists. We know that many children discount anything adults tell

Originally published in the *International Journal of Drug Policy* 7, no. 3 (1996). Reprinted by permission.

*I thank Mr. Wayne Sowan and Ms. Doris Greyeyes of Treaty 6 First Nations of Alberta for inviting me to speak at their "ground-breaking" conference, "Alternative Approaches to Addictions and Destructive Habits," at Edmonton, November 7, 1995, and Joel E. Schaler, M.D. for introducing me to the Navajo concept of *hozho*.

them about the dangers of drug use. That's because children know that much of what they're taught is false. They see their friends and others using drugs with consequences different from the ones they're taught to expect. As a result of that misinformation, adults' credibility with children is diminished, with dangerous results. In other words, by teaching certain myths about drugs in often coercive ways, e.g., that drugs are universally addicting substances and that drug users are sick, antidrug propagandists succeed in teaching children something completely different from what they originally intended to teach them, i.e., that people cannot hurt themselves with drugs. Moreover, they fail to understand that children learn more from the way adults think and behave than from what they say.

Something similar has happened in our attempts to help drug users in what is called addiction "treatment." Because treatment is based on certain beliefs people assert as truth about addiction, treatment is a disaster—it's a problem masquerading as a solution. In other words, our inaccurate and essentially religious-based beliefs about addiction become self-fulfilling prophecies (Schaler, 1996). Yet the prophecies created are the exact opposite of those treatment providers allegedly intended to create. We are moving in reverse in the name of moving forward.

It is important to clarify two terms: addiction and self-efficacy. The literal definition of addiction simply means someone likes to do something, moves toward something, someone, etc. It means we choose to say yes to something, to some experience or activity (Schaler, 1991). As Alexander and Schweighofer (1988) pointed out several years ago, addiction can be positive or negative, drug- or nondrug-related, and characterized by tolerance and withdrawal or no tolerance and withdrawal. A positive addiction enhances the values we hold dear. Through a positive addiction we pull our life together, creating meaning and purpose. Obviously, that sense of meaning and purpose varies from person to person. A negative addiction pulls our life apart. By engaging in a negative addiction we live in conflict with ourselves, which again bears on the sense of meaning and purpose in our lives.

One of the most powerful addictions we almost all experience at one time or another is, of course, love. Peele and Brodksy (1975) have written extensively about this. Love is a non-drug experience, and it is certainly characterized by physical symptoms of tolerance and withdrawal. As in a relationship characterized by love, many people use allegedly addictive drugs for long periods of time, choose to give up those drugs, and experience virtually no symptoms of withdrawal and tolerance, let alone irresistible cravings causing them to continue to use drugs at any expense.

Another important concept in contemporary psychology is self-efficacy. Technically, self-efficacy is people's confidence in their ability to achieve a specific goal in a specific situation. It refers to the capability people believe they possess to effect a specific behavior or to accomplish a certain level of performance. Self-efficacy is not the skills one has but rather one's judgment of what one can do with those skills (Bandura, 1977, 1986).

As Bob Dylan sang: "You don't need a weatherman to know which way the wind blows." You don't need psychologists to know that having confidence in your ability to achieve something for yourself has much to do with whether you will actually make the effort to succeed at something you set your mind to do. While self-efficacy is a scientific concept, tested by psychologists in various settings, it is also common sense. When you believe you can do something, you are more likely to be successful at it. When you believe you cannot do something, you are more likely to be unsuccessful at it.

That sounds simple enough. We tend to do what we believe we can do. We tend not to do what we believe we cannot do. This thinking can be applied to the consumption of drugs and alcohol.

Doesn't it make sense to say that the more people believe in their ability to moderate their consumption of drugs and alcohol, the more likely they will be to moderate? The inverse is true, too: The more people believe in their inability to moderate their consumption of drugs and alcohol, the more likely they will be not to moderate. Most treatment programs for drug addiction teach people to believe they lack the ability to moderate their consumption of drugs. The more treatment programs convince clients this is true, the more likely the clients are to prove them "correct." That's because consuming drugs irresponsibly (like consuming drugs moderately) involves the intention to do so. There is no force alien to oneself that is responsible for one's behavior. Believing a disease makes people drink is illogical; it ignores empirical findings on self-efficacy. It goes against common sense. It also individualizes and depoliticizes the cultural context within which drug consumption occurs.

While treatment providers routinely "diagnose" drug users as being in denial, they deny the fact that treatment generally doesn't work. At best, treatment tends to be as effective as no treatment at all (Edwards et al., 1977). This failure likely has much to do with the beliefs of treatment providers and their attempts to brainwash clients. It might be useful to look at the development of their beliefs historically (Levine, 1978).

In colonial America there was no such thing as alcoholism. People drank a great deal and drinking was encouraged by ministers and physicians alike. Alcohol was called "the good creature of God." Problems with excessive consumption were attributed to social interaction, i.e., whom the drinker was drinking with and where they drank, e.g., a particular tavern.

Gradually, religious leaders started calling excessive drinking a sin, an indication the drinker was indulging in "lust" and "passions." In 1785, Benjamin Rush, a signer of the U.S. Declaration of Independence and the "father of American psychiatry," invented (not discovered) the idea that alcoholism is a disease. This was part of a trend of Dr. Rush's to medicalize socially deviant behavior. Religious leaders pushing the "sin" model of alcoholism welcomed his authority. Then the members of what came to be known as the "temperance movement" integrated those sin and medical models of alcoholism, claiming Rush as their founder. This new view of alcoholism culminated in Prohibition. During that time alcohol was considered universally addictive. Anybody who drank would become an alcoholic. Drinking problems were attributed to the alcohol itself. Drinking was a sin that caused a disease. The "good creature of God" had become "demon rum," "that engine of the devil." As alcohol was universally addicting, prohibition was the only "cure."

Prohibition failed for many reasons. One seldom mentioned is the myth that alcohol was universally addictive. People realized that most people drank responsibly. People did not believe the temperance movement's propaganda about alcohol and drunkenness.

Next, alcoholism was decriminalized through remedicalization. Immediately after the repeal of Prohibition in 1933, Alcoholics Anonymous (AA) was founded as a self-help, spiritual fellowship for heavy drinkers. AA advanced "new" beliefs about alcoholism that actually weren't new at all: They were recycled beliefs from the temperance movement masquerading as medical discoveries. AA did invent the idea that 10 percent of the population had something wrong with their bodies, which was called the disease of alcoholism. It allegedly kept people from being able to control their consumption of alcohol. For them, prohibition was still needed, only this time it was politically incorrect to call such a recommendation "prohibition." So AA and others called it "abstinence."

Ever since, AA members and supporters have been seeking scientific validation for the idea that alcoholism is a disease. The cornerstone of the disease concept of alcoholism (and now addiction generally) is that the person afflicted with this mythical disease can never learn to control his or her consumption of alcohol and other universally addicting drugs. That part of the disease concept is the loss-of-control theory. While it remains a potent idea in most addiction-treatment practice and policy today, it has been repeatedly disproved scientifically since the early 1960s.

AA and other twelve-step recovery programs are the foundation of most addiction-treatment programs in the United States and Canada today. Many people consider these treatment programs to have more in common with religious indoctrination than with objective medicine. And U.S. courts are increasingly viewing state involvement with twelve-step programs as violating the U.S. Constitution's First Amendment—the free exercise and establishment clauses guaranteeing separation of church and state (Luff, 1989; Murray, 1996).

Here is the "holy trinity" of the disease concept of addiction: To get better you must turn over your life to a "higher power." This "higher power" can be anything as long as it is not you. (Ironically, self-empowerment is a sin according to the disease concept.) You must "admit" that you are powerless and that you have a disease. And you must never consume drugs again (prohibition or abstinence).

Today, the main beliefs of disease-model thinking are (Schaler, 1997):

1. Most addicts don't know they have a problem and must be forced to recognize they are addicts.
2. Addicts cannot control themselves when they drink or take drugs.
3. The only solution to drug addiction and/or alcoholism is treatment.
4. Addiction is an all-or-nothing disease: A person cannot be a temporary drug addict with a mild drinking or drug problem.
5. The most important step in overcoming an addiction is to acknowledge that you are powerless and can't control it.
6. Abstinence is the only way to control alcoholism/drug addiction.
7. Physiology, not psychology, determines whether one drinker will become addicted to alcohol and another will not.
8. The fact that alcoholism runs in families means that it is a genetic disease.
9. People who are drug addicted can never outgrow addiction and are always in danger of relapsing.

It's important to understand that none of these beliefs has been proved scientifically. Not one of them. In fact, they are consistently proved false. Yet these beliefs dominate addiction-treatment programs throughout the world. Now consider each of these beliefs within the commonsense context of self-efficacy principles.

Believing in the above myths is likely to cause treatment failure. In other words, teaching people in treatment for addiction problems that they "don't know they have a problem" creates a problem for them. Teaching them that they cannot control themselves convinces them that they cannot control themselves. Teaching them to believe that treatment is the only solution to their problem convinces them that they cannot solve problems on their own. It reinforces dependency. Teaching them that addiction is all or nothing brainwashes them into believing they can never be anything other than sick.

Teaching them that they are powerless enables them to act powerless. Teaching them that abstinence is the only way to control their addiction convinces them that whenever they are not abstinent, they are out of control. Then, when they drink, they do go out of control. There is no middle ground. Teaching them that they are physically different from "normal" people gives them permission to act irresponsibly when they consume too many drugs or too much alcohol, as does teaching them that alcoholism runs in families. Teaching them that they can never mature out of their addiction and are always in danger of relapsing makes them feel hopeless and helpless. Their behavior is determined by their beliefs. There is nothing they can do about it!

In fact, there is nothing they can ever do to change their behavior except abstain and pray.

The commonsense concept of self-efficacy is consistent with the Navajo concept of "*hozho,* the most important concept in traditional Navajo culture, which combines the concepts of beauty, goodness, order, harmony, and everything that is positive or ideal" (Carrese and Rhodes, 1995).

> Navajos say, "think and speak in a positive way." This theme is encompassed by the Navajo phrases *hoshooji nitsihakees* and *hoshooji saad.* The literal translations are, "think in the Beauty Way" and "talk in the Beauty Way." The prominence of these themes reflects the Navajo view that thought and language have the power to shape reality and control events . . . [they reflect] the Navajo view that health is maintained and restored through positive ritual language. Providers should "avoid thinking or speaking in a negative way." This theme is approximated by the Navajo phrase, *Doo djiniidah.* The literal translation is "Don't talk that way!" (Carrese and Rhodes, 1995)

Reconsider the nine beliefs integral to disease-model thinking, and reconsider treatment failure—and even consider irresponsible drug use. From the self-efficacy, scientific, and Navajo points of view, not only are disease-model beliefs inaccurate, they are destructive. The disease model creates more of the very problems it allegedly solves. In other words, its nine beliefs become self-fulfilling prophecies.

What can we replace those beliefs with? How about the truth about addiction and recovery? How about ideas consistent with the self-efficacy, scientific, and Navajo points of view? The following beliefs based on the free-will model of addiction meet those criteria:

1. The best way to overcome addiction is to rely on your own will power.
2. People can stop relying on drugs or alcohol as they develop other ways to deal with life.
3. Addiction has more to do with the environments people live in than with the drugs they are addicted to.
4. People often outgrow drug and alcohol addiction.
5. Alcoholics and drug addicts can learn to moderate their drinking or cut down on their drug use.
6. People become addicted to drugs/alcohol when life is going badly for them.
7. Drug addicts and alcoholics can find their own ways out of addiction, without outside help, given the opportunity.
8. Drug addiction is a way of life people rely on to cope with the world.

The prevailing treatment policy should not only be changed on the basis of identifying negative beliefs that lead to self-fulfilling prophecies, but also replaced by beliefs proved to be scientifically valid and culturally consistent with Navajo principles of positive thinking. Those self-fulfilling prophecies we can live with.

Those prophecies encourage people to recognize the will power they have to control their life. As people come to believe they can develop other ways to deal with life instead of relying on drugs or alcohol, they gain confidence in their ability to determine their own destiny. As they come to believe addiction has more to do with the environments they live in than with the drugs they use, they may further realize they have the power to change those environments in order to help themselves. They may recognize they are the "higher power." And that, of course, is the most sacrilegious idea to disease modelists.

When people realize how many people outgrow drug and alcohol addiction, they realize their own addiction problems are solvable. When heavy drinkers and drug users learn they have the ability to moderate their drinking or drug use, they are naturally more likely to fulfill that belief in their ability. When they recognize drug and alcohol addiction is a behavior they choose to engage in when life is going badly, they are more likely to do something to improve their life. When people believe they can rely on themselves to overcome an addiction, they are more likely to mobilize the necessary inner strength to change their behavior. When drug addicts and alcoholics believe they can find their own ways out of addiction, without outside help, given the opportunity, they are more likely to wake from their drug-induced despair and build a life they value more than a life of drugs alone. Most importantly when people believe drug addiction is mainly a way of life, a behavior people engage in as a way to cope with the world—and not something they are hopelessly imprisoned in—they may be more inclined to make the necessary changes not only in their own world but in the world they live in. People can learn what's necessary to live a meaningful life and put that knowledge to positive effect.

Each of these beliefs results in a more positive and commonsense outlook consistent with scientific principles established through self-efficacy research and consistent with the Navajo concept of *hozho*. We all create self-fulfilling prophecies for ourselves based on our beliefs. What people believe to be true about themselves dictates how they behave in the world.

Our task is not to indoctrinate people with religious pseudoscientific myths about addiction as a disease. It is to recognize the commonsense truths supported by scientific research over the past thirty-five years and to encourage heavy drinkers and drug users to recognize those truths. Changing their behavior is then up to them. But recognizing those truths, the likelihood will increase that they will create new self-fulfilling prophecies based on accurate recognition of their own personal power (not some alien "higher power," or the power of some fanciful disease said to govern their behavior, or the power of a drug). That's the Navajo way.

REFERENCES

Alexander, B. K., and A. R. F. Schweighofer. (1988). "Defining 'Addiction.' " *Canadian Psychology* 29: 151–62.

Bandura, A. (1977). "Self-Efficacy: Towards a Unifying Theory of Behavioral Change." *Psychological Review* 84: 191–215.

———. (1986). *Social Foundations of Thought and Action: A Social Cognitive Theory.* Englewood Cliffs, N.J.: Prentice-Hall.

Carrese J. A., and L. A. Rhodes. (1995). "Western Bioethics on the Navajo Reservation. Benefit or Harm." *Journal of the American Medical Association* 274: 826–29.

Edwards, G., J. Orford, S. Egert, S. Guthrie, A. Hawker, C. Hensman, M. Mitcheson, E. Oppenheimer, and C. Taylor (1977). "Alcoholism: A Controlled Trial of Treatment and 'Advice.' " *Journal of Studies on Alcohol* 38: 1004–31.

Levine, H. G. (1978). "The Discovery of Addiction: Changing Conceptions of Habitual Drunkenness in America." *Journal of Studies on Alcohol* 39: 43–74.

Luff, E. (1989). "The First Amendment and Drug Alcohol Treatment Programs: To What Extent May Coerced Treatment Programs Attempt to Alter Beliefs Relating to Ultimate Concerns and Self-Concept?" In A. S. Trebach and K. B. Zeese, eds. *Drug Policy 1989–1990: A Reformer's Catalogue.* Washington, D.C.: Drug Policy Foundation. pp. 260–6.

Murray F. J. (1996). "Courts Hit Sentencing DWIs to AA, Fault Religious Basis." *The Washington Times* 4 November: A10 (news item).

Peele, S., and A. Brodsky. (1975). *Love and Addiction.* New York: Taplinger.

Schaler, J. A. (1991). "Drugs and Free Will." *Society* 28: 42–9.

———. (1995). "The Addiction Belief Scale. *International Journal of the Addictions* 30: 117–34.

———. (1996). "Spiritual Thinking in Addiction-Treatment Providers: The Spiritual Belief Scale." *Alcoholism Treatment Quarterly* 14: 7–33.

———. (1997). "Addiction Beliefs of Treatment Providers: Factors Explaining Variance." *Addiction Research* 4: 367–84.

List of Contributors

Bruce K. Alexander, Ph.D., professor of psychology at Simon Frazer University in British Columbia, is the author of *Peaceful Measures: Canada's Way Out of the "War on Drugs"* (University of Toronto Press).

George J. Annas, J.D., M.P.H., is professor of health law at Boston University Schools of Medicine and Public Health.

Randy E. Barnett, J.D., is Austin B. Fletcher Professor at Boston University School of Law. He was an assistant state's attorney asigned to the Felony Trial Division of the Cook County State's Attorney's Office in Chicago, Illinois, from 1977 to 1981.

William J. Bennett, Ph.D., former Secretary of Education and director of the Office of National Drug Control Strategy, is John M. Olin Distinguished Fellow in Cultural Policy Studies at the Heritage Foundation in Washington, D.C.

Joseph R. Biden Jr. is a Democratic U.S. Senator from Delaware.

Robert B. Coambs, Ph.D., is an associate of the University of Toronto's Centre for Health Promotion.

David T. Courtwright, Ph.D., is a professor of history at the University of North Florida. He is the author of *Dark Paradise: Opiate Addiction in America before 1940* (1982), *Addicts Who Survived* (1989), and *Violent Land: Single Men and Social Disorder from the Frontier to the Inner City* (1996).

Robert J. DuPont, M.D., a psychiatrist, is a former director of the National Institute on Drug Abuse.

Patricia Erickson, Ph.D., a senior scientist at the Addiction Research Foundation in Toronto, is an adjunct professor in the department of sociology at the University of Toronto.

Herbert Fingarette, Ph.D., is emeritus professor of philosophy at the University of California, Santa Barbara, and most recently author of *Death: Philosophical Soundings* (Open Court Publishers).

Milton Friedman is Senior Research Fellow at the Hoover Institution at Stanford University and Nobel Laureate in Economics.

Daryl F. Gates is the former Chief of Police for Los Angeles and creator of Drug Awareness Resistance Education (D.A.R.E.).

Ronald L. Goldfarb, a Washington, D.C., attorney, is a literary agent, author, and former Justice Department prosecutor.

Patricia Hadaway, Ph.D. (deceased), was a psychologist who conducted primary research on the anti-tobacco war with Dr. Barry Beyerstein at Simon Fraser University.

Dwight B. Heath, Ph.D., is professor of anthropology and director of the Center for Latin American Studies at Brown University.

John E. Helzer, Ph.D., is professor of psychiatry at the University of Vermont College of Medicine.

Michi N. Hesselbrock, Ph.D., is professor of research at the University of Connecticut School of Social Work.

John Kaplan (deceased) was a professor at the School of Law, Stanford University, and author of *The Hardest Drug: Heroin and Public Policy* (University of Chicago Press).

Jerome P. Kassirer, M.D., is editor-in-chief of *The New England Journal of Medicine.*

Dr. Rushworth M. Kidder is founder and president of the Institute for Global Ethics in Camden, Maine.

Morton M. Kondracke is a nationally syndicated columnist and executive editor of *Roll Call* in Washington, D.C.

Charles Krauthammer, M.D., formerly a psychiatrist, is a nationally syndicated columnist.

Ellen M. Luff (deceased), an ACLU-Md. panel attorney who specialized in the First Amendment, is credited for writing and implementing passage of Maryland's Equal Rights Amendment in 1972.

David F. Musto, M.D., is professor of psychiatry (Child Study Center) and of the history of medicine at the Yale School of Medicine.

Charles B. Rangel (D-NY) is the former chairman of the House Select Committee on Narcotics Abuse and Control.

Lee N. Robbins, Ph.D., is professor of psychiatry at Washington University School of Medicine in St. Louis.

Jeffrey A. Schaler, Ph.D., a psychologist, is Adjunct Professor of Justice, Law, and Society at American University's School of Public Affairs in Washington, D.C. He is currently writing a book on addiction for Open Court Publishers.

Anton R. F. Schweighofer, a practicing psychologist, is a doctoral candidate in clinical psychology at Simon Fraser University. His thesis is on temperance mentality among Canadian psychologists.

Thomas S. Szasz, M.D., emeritus professor of psychiatry at the SUNY Health Sciences Center in Syracuse, New York, is author of *The Meaning of Mind: Language, Morality, and Neuroscience* (Praeger).

Timothy R. Weber is a research associate with the Social and Evaluation Research Department of the Addiction Research Foundation in Toronto.

James Q. Wilson, Ph.D., is Professor of Organization and Strategy, and holds the James A. Collins Chair in Management at the University of California, Los Angeles.

Eric D. Wish, Ph.D., is director of the Center for Substance Abuse Research (CESAR) at the University of Maryland, College Park.